Stroke: Clinical Neurology

Stroke: Clinical Neurology

Edited by Lenny Cowan

AMERICAN
MEDICAL PUBLISHERS
www.americanmedicalpublishers.com

American Medical Publishers,
41 Flatbush Avenue,
1st Floor, New York,
NY 11217, USA

Visit us on the World Wide Web at:
www.americanmedicalpublishers.com

ISBN: 978-1-63927-330-0

Cataloging-in-Publication Data

Stroke : clinical neurology / edited by Lenny Cowan.
p. cm.
Includes bibliographical references and index.
ISBN 978-1-63927-330-0
1. Cerebrovascular disease. 2. Cerebrovascular disease--Treatment. 3. Brain--Diseases.
4. Neglect (Neurology). I. Cowan, Lenny.
RC388.5 .S77 2022
616.81--dc23

Table of Contents

Preface

The branch of medicine which deals with the disorders of the nervous system is known as neurology. Some of the diseases which are studied under neurology are stroke, dementia and meningitis. When a biological cell ceases to carry out its functions properly, it results in poor blood flow to the brain giving rise to stroke. There are two main categories of stroke - ischemic and hemorrhagic. The ischemic stroke occurs due to interruption of the blood supply to brain. Hemorrhagic strokes arise from the rupture of a blood vessel or an abnormal vascular structure. The reasons of ischemic stroke include blood clotting, embolism, decrease in blood supply, and cerebral venous sinus thrombosis. A hemorrhagic stroke is caused by bleeding directly into the brain or into the space between its membranes. High blood pressure is the primary risk factor for stroke. Medical imaging techniques like MRI scan and CT scan are used for its diagnosis. This book traces the progress of this field and highlights some of its key concepts and applications. It will serve as a valuable source of reference for graduate and post-graduate students. This book explores all the important aspects of stroke in the present day scenario.

Significant researches are present in this book. Intensive efforts have been employed by authors to make this book an outstanding discourse. This book contains the enlightening chapters which have been written on the basis of significant researches done by the experts.

Finally, I would also like to thank all the members involved in this book for being a team and meeting all the deadlines for the submission of their respective works. I would also like to thank my friends and family for being supportive in my efforts.

Editor

1

Lower serum uric acid level strongly predict short-term poor functional outcome in acute stroke with normoglycaemia

Shuolin Wu[1,2], Yuesong Pan[2,3,4,5], Ning Zhang[1,2], Wang Yong Jun[2,3,4,5], Chunxue Wang[1,2,3,4,5*] On Behalf of the Investigators for the Survey on Abnormal Glucose Regulation in Patients With Acute Stroke Across China (ACROSS-China)

Abstract

Background: Conflicting results on the correlation between hyperuricemia and the prognosis of stroke had been reported and the close association between serum uric acid (SUA) and abnormal glycomatabolism might further complicate the assessment of the correlation. We aimed to investigate SUA in predicting the prognosis of acute stroke in different glycometabolism status.

Methods: A total of 2907 patients aged from 18 to 85 (1220 diabetes mellitus (DM), 777 prediabetes and 910 normoglycemia) were selected from the Abnormal Glucose Regulation in Patients with Acute Stroke across China (ACROSS-China) study. The patients were divided into groups according to the SUA quartile as well as decile. The correlations between SUA and the poor outcome (mRS > 2) at discharge were assessed stratified by glucose metabolism status. Multivariate logistic regression was used to analyze the potential risk factors of poor in-hospital outcome of stroke and the risk-adjustment of the correlation between SUA and the prognosis of stroke. $P < 0.05$ was considered statistically significant.

Results: SUA were divided first as Quartile1 to 4 (Quartile1 < 221 μmol L^{-1}; Quartile2 (221–286) μmol L^{-1}; Quartile3 (286–352) μmol L^{-1} and Quartile4 > 352 μmol L^{-1}), then as decile1 to 10. In normoglycaemia, SUA quartiles, deciles and continuous SUA concentration were independently significantly associated with poor outcome. Q1 was independently associated with the higher possibility of poor functional outcome (compared to Q4, odds ratios (ORs) with 95% confidential interval (CI) was 3.79 (1.23–8.67) in Q1); Lower level of SUA in DM was also associated with poor functional outcome at discharge compared to the highest level of SUA(Q4)(OR with 95% CI, 2.07 (1.05–4.08)), however, lower SUA level was also related to severer stroke at admission in DM as well as in prediabetes ($P < 0.001$ in DM and 0.023 in prediabetes) and severer stroke resulted in worse functional outcome at discharge (OR with 95% CI, 12.15 (8.08–18.21) in DM and 11.58 (7.50–23.25) in prediabetes). But in normoglycamic stroke, SUA levels did not differ in stroke severity at admission ($P = 0.066$).

Conclusions: Low SUA level (<221 μmol L^{-1}) independently and strongly predicts the short-term poor functional outcome in acute stroke with normoglycaemia other than diabetes or prediabetes.

Keywords: Uric acid, Diabetes mellitus, Stroke, Risk factors

* Correspondence: wangchunxuefate@126.com
[1]Department of Neuropsychiatry and Behavioral Neurology and Clinical Psychology, Beijing Tiantan Hospital, Capital Medical University, Beijing, China
[2]China National Clinical Research Center for Neurological Diseases, Beijing, China
Full list of author information is available at the end of the article

Background

The association between hyperuricemia and cardiovascular disease has been well documented for a very long time. However, conflicting results on the correlation between hyperuricemia and the incidence and prognosis of stroke had been reported. In a meta-analysis study, Kim, et al. reported that hyperuricemia increased the risk of both the ischemic stroke and the hemorrhagic stroke as well as the risk of post-stroke mortality [1]. Several other groups also found that the post-stroke hyperuricemia could significantly exacerbate the outcome of stroke [2–4]. Other study suggested that the effect of pre-stroke hyperuricemia on poor post-stroke outcome, especially in diabetic patients, was still questionable [5]. Holme and his group also suggested that hyperuricemia might be rather a complementary indicator than an independent risk factor of AS [6]. Kramer et al. found that the importance of the pre- cardiovascular disease hyperuricemia in predicting cardiovascular disease mortality was only significant in the pre-diabetic and type 2 diabetic patients but not in the normoglycemic patients [7]. Some investigators even found that post-stroke hyperuricemia might have played a protective role in the prognosis of stroke [8–12]. Miedema et al. found no evidence to support the association between the SUA level and the outcome of stroke in their study [13].

Hyperuricemia, hyperglycaemia and cardiovascular disease are found to be co-morbid disease [14]. Hyperuricaemia is also positively associated with prediabetes diagnosed according to impaired fasting glucose criteria other than subjects with normal fasting glucose [15]. A meta-analysis also ascertain that hyperglycaemia is contributed to the development of diabetes and impaired fasting glucose [16]. Even in normal range of SUA, uric acid is related to diabetes onset in healthy lean women [17]. Since the close and complicated association between SUA and prediabetes as stated above and diabetes was a well-known risk factor of stroke [18], it is in very need to assess and compare the effect of SUA on stroke prognosis stratified by different glycometabolism status. Newman et al. reported that a combination of the post-stroke hyperuricemia and diabetes could significantly increase the risk of adverse events, including recurrent stroke, cardiovascular events even death, in post-stroke patients [3]. In another study, Zhang et al. found that the post-stroke hyperuricemia was associated with better short-term outcome of stroke in non-diabetes patients [12]. However they failed to distinguish between the pre-diabetes and the normoglycemia patients in their study. In our study, the association between SUA and the outcome of acute primary stroke would be assessed in both diabetes and normoglycemia patients. The pre-diabetes patients were excluded in our study.

Methods

Patient selection

ACROSS-CHINA" was a large prospective cohort study conducted in China from 2008 to 2009 that investigated on abnormal glucose regulation in acute first-ever stroke (within 14 days), in which a total of 3450 patients with ischemic stroke, intracerebral hemorrhage (ICH) or subarachnoid hemorrhage (SAH) were successively recruited from 34 hospitals across China [19, 20]. Acute stroke was diagnosed according to World Health Organization combined with CT or MRI confirmation [21].

All the patients without previous DM were required to perform a standard oral glucose tolerance test (OGTT) at the day 14 ± 3 after stroke onset or before discharge according to the World Health Organization criteria [22]. Patients were categorized as diabetes, pre-diabetes or normoglycemia according to their OGTT results. One hundred and forty-four patients without SUA values and 399 patients with missing OGTT results were excluded respectively. In the remaining 2,907 patients, there were 1220 diabetics, 777 prediabetics and 910 normoglycaemic patients (Fig. 1).

Data collection

Demographic, education degree, tobacco use and alcohol consumption, physical exam and a National Institute of Health Stroke Scale (NIHSS) score were obtained at admission. A detailed history of previous diseases, such as hypertension, coronary artery disease and atrial fibrillation, were also recorded. Body mass index (BMI) was

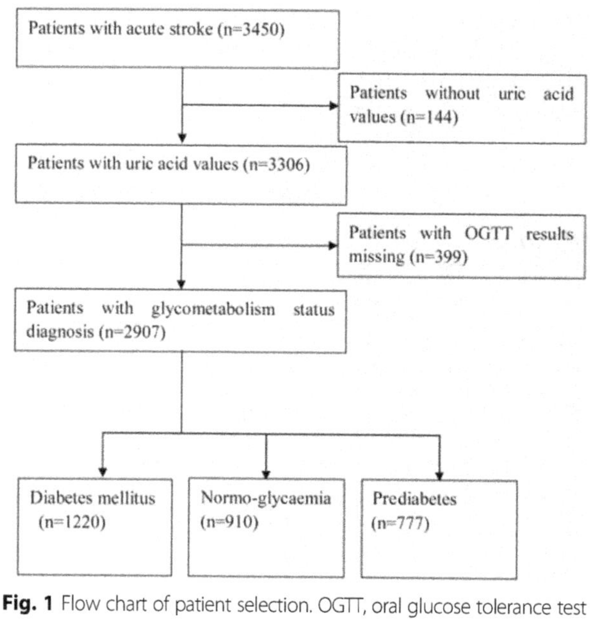

Fig. 1 Flow chart of patient selection. OGTT, oral glucose tolerance test

defined as body weight (kg)/the square of height (m). Participants without a history of diabetes were required to take an OGTT test within 24 h after the hospital admission. The lab tests included blood routine test, high density lipoprotein, low density lipoprotein, creatinine, SUA, homocysteine, glucose and insulin level, et al. All the lab tests were performed within 24 h after admission at fasting condition by the certified central laboratory. SUA was measured by the urine enzyme endpoint method. The index of insulin resistance was calculated with the Homeostasis Model Assessment 2- Insulin Resistance (HOMA2-IR) method [23]. A Modified Rankin Scale (mRS) was calculated in every participant at discharge to evaluate the in-hospital outcome of stroke.

The criteria of diagnosing abnormal glycometabolism

The OGTT result and the blood glucose level were used to divide patients into three categorise based on the 1999 World Health Organization (WHO) criteria. The details were as follow: (1) Diabetes mellitus (DM) was defined as fasting plasma glucose (FPG) ≥ 7.0 m mol L^{-1} and/or 2-h value (2-h-value) ≥ 11.1 m mol L^{-1}; (2) Prediabetes consisted of both impaired glucose tolerance (IGT) and impaired fasting glucose (IFG). IGT was defined as FPG < 7.0 m mol L^{-1} and a 2-h-value between 7.8 mmol/L and 11.1 m mol L^{-1}. IFG was defined as fasting glucose value between 6.1 m mol L^{-1} and 7.0 m mol L^{-1} with a normal 2-h-value; (3) normoglycemia was defined as FPG < 6.1 m mol L^{-1} and a 2-h-value < 7.8 m mol L^{-1}. Patients who had a history of DM or had ever received hyperglycemic agents for at least 6 months were also assigned to the DM group. All the prediabetics were newly-diagnosed.

Other variables definition

Tobacco use was categorized as 'current', 'previous' or 'never' smoking. 'Current smoking' was defined as that the individual was an active smoker at the time of the stroke. 'Previous smoking' was defined as that the individual had quit smoking 1 year prior to the stroke. 'Never smoking' was defined as that the individual had never smoked prior to the stroke. Alcohol consumption was categorized as 'never drinking', 'mild drinking', moderate to severe drinking'. 'Moderate or severe drinking' was defined as that the individual consistently consumed ≥2 standard size alcoholic beverages per day. 'Mild drinking' was defined as that the individual consumed <2 standard size alcoholic beverages per day. 'Never drinking' was defined as that the individual had never consumed any alcoholic beverages. Stroke severity was categorized by the NIHSS score as mild stroke (NIHSS < 9) or severe stroke (NIHSS ≥ 9) [4].

Outcome assessment

The primary endpoint comprised death and dependency with mRS >2 [24, 25]. Death (mRS = 6) was recorded within 14 ± 3 days after admission to the hospital. Dependency (mRS = 3 to 5) was assessed at 14 ± 3 days after the index date of hospital admission or at hospital discharge. Death indicated all-cause death according to the International Classification of Diseases, 10th Revision. Neurological improvement and deterioration were used as supplemental indicators to describe the association between SUA and stroke outcome. Neurological improvement was defined as 4 point decrease in NIHSS during hospitalization or a 0 point status on NIHSS at discharge. Neurological deterioration was defined as 1 point increase in NIHSS during hospitalization [24, 26, 27].

Statistical analysis

Baseline clinical features were compared stratified by different diabetes diagnosis and functional outcome. All continuous variables were presented as mean ± standard deviation for normal distribution and median (Quartile 1 to 3) for skewed distribution. Kolmogorov-Smirnov test was used for normal distribution test. Categorical variables were presented as frequencies and/or prevalence/incidence rate. For the continuous variables, when the group numbers were more than two, if the variable was normal distribution, one-way ANOVA test was used to perform the comparison (LSD-test for variables with homogeneity of variance and Games-Howell test for variables with heterogeneity of variance), otherwise Kruskal-Wallis H test was performed instead; when the group numbers were just two, if the variable was normal distribution, *T*-test was used to perform the comparison, otherwise Mann–Whitney *U* test was used instead. For categorical variables, the comparisons were used Chi-square test and Fisher exact test. The adjustment of the correlation between different variables was done by multivariate logistic regression. Variables with a *P* value < 0.1 in univariate analysis were included in the multivariate regression test. Variables, which had shown potential association to the outcome of stroke during the literature search, were also included in the multivariate regression test. The independent factors included in the multivariate analysis were age, gender, education degree, tobacco use, alcohol consumption, BMI, high density lipoprotein, low density lipoprotein, creatinine, systolic and diastolic blood pressure, HOMA2-IR, homocysteine, a history of coronary heart disease, a history of hypertension, a history of atrial fibrillation, stroke types and stroke severity at admission. The use of Aspirin, Diuretics and Coumadin [28], which could influence SUA concentration, were also analyzed. SUA was compared between "use" and "non-use" of them respectively and stratified by different glycometabolism first, then it will be recognized as a confounding factor if $P < 0.05$ and entered into the according multivariate analysis. The fitness of the models was evaluated by using the Hosmer and Lemeshow goodness-of-fit test and a P value > 0.2 was considered as a good fit. All the statistical analyses were done with SPSS ver. 19.0 software (SPSS Inc., Chicago, IL). A $P < 0.05$ was considered statistically significant.

Results

Comparison of the characteristics of patients in different glucose metabolism groups

Patients with normoglycemia accounted for 31.3% of the study population. The differences in the characteristics of patients among different groups were shown in Table 1. The normoglycemia group had highest percentage of males (67.7% vs. 64.5%vs. 58.3%, $P < 0.001$) and higher prevalence of current smoking ($P = 0.036$). The mean level of age in this group was significantly younger than that of the DM or prediabetes group ($P < 0.001$). In the physical exam and the lab test, the patients in the normoglycemia group had significantly lower blood pressure, BMI, NIHSS score, low density lipoprotein level and HOMA2-IR than that in the DM or prediabetes group (all $P < 0.05$). The high density lipoprotein, homocysteine in the normoglycemia group were significantly higher than that in the DM or prediabetes group (all $P < 0.05$). Previous histories of coronary heart disease, hypertension or atrial fibrillation in thenormoglycaemia group were significantly less common than that in the DM group (all $P < 0.05$). Ischemic stroke was the most common type of stroke in all groups, followed by intracerebral hemorrhage and SAH. The percentages of stroke types

Table 1 Baseline Clinic features according to glycometabolism diagnosis by OGTT

Clinic features	Diabetes mellitus ($n = 1220$)	Prediabetes ($n = 777$)	Normoglycemia ($n = 910$)	P
Age, y (median, Q_{1-3})	64 (55, 73)	61 (52,72)	58 (49, 69))	<0.001
Male, n (%)	711(58.3)	501 (64.5%)	616 (67.7)	<0.001
Tobacco use, n (%)				0.036
Never	712 (58.4)	428 (55.1)	480 (52.7)	
Quit	110 (9.0)	74 (9.5)	79 (8.7)	
Current	351 (28.8)	246 (31.7)	320 (35.2)	
Alcohol consumption, n (%)				0.164
Mild	213 (17.5)	132 (17.0)	171 (18.8)	
Moderate to severe	165 (13.5)	131 (16.9)	152 (16.7)	
Never	817 (67.0)	494 (63.6)	564 (62.0)	
BMI, kg/m^2 (median, Q_{1-3})	25.0 (22.9,27.3)	24.5 (22.5,26.8)	24.2 (22.0,26.2)	<0.001
NIHSS (median,Q_1-Q_3)	5 (2–9)	5 (2,9)	4 (2–8)	0.002
Creatinine,m mol L^{-1} (median, Q_{1-3})	71.2 (58.0, 87.0)	72.0 (60.0, 87.0)	71.8 (59.9, 86.7)	0.425
LDL, m mol L^{-1} (median, Q_{1-3})	3.0 (2.4, 3.6)	2.9 (2.3, 3.5)	2.8 (2.3, 3.4)	0.001
HDL,m mol L^{-1}(median, Q_{1-3})	1.1(1.0, 1.3)	1.2 (1.0, 1.4)	1.2 (1.1, 1.4)	<0.001
Systolic blood pressure, mmHg (median, Q_{1-3})	150 (138, 160)	143 (130, 160)	146 (130, 160)	<0.001
Homocysteine, μ mol L^{-1}, (median, Q_{1-3})	14.4 (11.5, 18.7)	15.5 (12.0, 21.9)	15.7 (12.3, 22.8)	<0.001
HOMA2-IR (median, Q_{1-3})	2.5 (1.6, 4.0)	1.9 (1.1, 3.0)	1.6 (0.9, 2.5)	<0.001
Past medical history, yes, n (%)				
Coronary artery disease	172 (14.1)	87 (11.2)	90 (9.9)	0.009
Hypertension	795 (65.2)	470 (60.5)	514 (56.5)	<0.001
Atrial fibrillation	66 (5.4)	54 (6.9)	31 (3.4)	0.006
Stroke types, n (%)				<0.001
IS	1015 (83.2)	541 (69.6)	675 (74.2)	
ICH	174 (14.3)	185 (23.8)	198 (21.8)	
SAH	31 (2.5)	51 (6.6)	37 (4.1)	

OGTT the oral glucose tolerance test, *BMI* body mass index, *LDL* low density lipoprotein, *HDL* high density lipoprotein, *NIHSS* the National Institutes of Health Stroke Scale, *HOMA2-IR* the correctly solved computer model for homeostasis model assessment of insulin resistance, *IS* ischemic stroke, *ICH* intra-cerebral hemorrhage, *SAH* subarachnoid hemorrhage were significantly different in patients with different glycometabolism status ($P<0.001$).

Comparison of the characteristics of patients with different functional outcomes of the stroke

There were no significant differences between the favorable outcome group and the poor outcome group in the mean level of age, BMI, HOMA2-IR, low density lipoprotein level, high density lipoprotein level, the prevalence of the histories of coronary heart disease or hypertension. Compared to the favorable outcome group, the mean level of creatinine was significantly lower in the poor outcome group, whereas the blood pressure and homocysteine level were significantly higher in the poor outcome group. The percentage of moderate to severe alcohol consumption as well as the percentage of severe stroke and atrial fibrillation in the poor outcome group was significantly higher than that in favorable outcome group. The percentage of mild drinking was significantly higher in favorable outcome group than that in the poor outcome group. Ischemic stroke was the most common type of stroke in both groups. Cardioembolic ischemic stroke was only accounted for 5.7% ($n=91$) of the total patients with poor functional outcome. The intracerebral hemorrhage was more commonly seen in the poor outcome group than that in the favorable outcome group while ischemic stroke and SAH were more prevalent in the favorable outcome group. DM was more prevalent in the poor outcome while normoglycemia were more commonly seen in the favorable outcome group (Table 2).

Analysis on medication use and SUA concentration

There are 1542 patients with data on aspirin, 20 patients on Coumadin and 124 patients on Diuretics. SUA levels were compared between "use" and "non-use" of them respectively and stratified by different glycometabolism. After that a significant association was found between Aspirin use and SUA level among normal glycemic stroke patients (Additional file 1: Table S3, Additional file 2: Table S4 and Additional file 3: Table S5). Aspirin use was then entered into the multivariate analysis on SUA and the outcome among normoglycaemic stroke patients.

Correlation between SUA and poor functional outcome at discharge

Univariate analysis of SUA quartiles on poor outcome

The patients were divided into quartile groups (Q1 to Q4) based on their SUA level. The concentrations of SUA in these groups were as follow: Q1 < 221 μmol L^{-1}, Q2 221-286 μmol L^{-1}, Q3 286-352 μmol L^{-1} and Q4 > 352 μmol L^{-1} (DM group, N_{Q1}=307, $N_{Q2}=306$, $N_{Q3}=310$, $N_{Q4}=291$; Prediabetes group, N_{Q1}=184, $N_{Q2}=198$, $N_{Q3}=190$, $N_{Q4}=198$; Normoglycaemia group, N_{Q1}=229, $N_{Q2}=218$, $N_{Q3}=211$, $N_{Q4}=248$). In both diabetic and normoglycemic strokes, the occurrence of stroke poor outcome decreased across the increasing SUA levels from Q1 to Q4($P=0.019$ in DM, 0.016 in normoglycemia), however, it didn't differ in SUA quartiles in prediabeteic strokes ($P=0.110$ in prediabetes) (Fig. 2).

Multivariate analysis of SUA quartiles on poor functional outcome at discharge

To further evaluate the correlation between the SUA level and the poor post-stroke outcome, the SUA level along with other potential risk factors of poor post-stroke outcome were introduced into a regression model as independent variables and the multivariate logistic regression was used to assess the adjusted correlation between the SUA level and the outcome of stoke. The NIHSS score was entered into the regression model as an ordinal variable with the cut-off point of 9 first and then as a continuous one.

The final results of the regression showed that there was a negative correlation between the SUA level and the occurrence rate of poor outcome of stroke in normoglycemic group. In the normoglycemic group, the occurrence rate of poor outcome in Q1 group was also significantly higher than that in the Q4 group (OR = 3.79, 95% CI 1.23–8.67, $P=0.020$) (Fig. 3); In DM group, the possibility of poor outcome in lowest SUA group (Q1) was significantly higher than that in Q4 (OR = 2.07, 95% CI 1.05–4.08). The possibility of poor outcome in Q2 and Q3 groups were not significantly higher than that in Q4 (Q2: OR = 1.33, 95% CI 0.71–2.47; Q3: OR = 1.79, 95% CI 0.99–3.26). In prediabetes, the possibility of poor outcome did not differ in SUA quartiles (all $P>0.05$). The Hosmer and Lemeshow goodness-of-fit test results (χ^2, P) were (8.839, 0.356), (110.982, 0.215) and (4.558, 0.755) in the DM, prediabetes and the normoglycemia group, respectively (Fig. 3).

In normoglycaemic stroke patients, NIHSS was then entered as a continuous variable into multivariate analysis instead of NIHSS as a binary variable. The association was still significant after the new adjustment (Additional file 4: Table S7).

In normoglycaemic stroke patients, further analysis was performed stratified by sex (Additional file 5: Table S6). There was 620 male and 290 female in normoglycaemic group. In male, after adjusted for the same variables as the above, the lowest level of SUA is still an independent risk factor for the poor functional outcome (OR with 95% CI 5.06(1.17–12.05), $P=0.031$). However it was not the case in female patients (OR with 95% CI 9.21(0.98–38.66), $P=0.158$).

Table 2 Baseline Clinic features according to poor functional outcomes evaluated by mRS > 2

Clinic features	Favorable outcomes (*n* = 1305)	Poor functional outcomes (*n* = 1602)	*P*
Age, y	60 (52, 71)	62 (53, 72)	0.003
Male, *n* (%)	954 (73.1)	1089 (68.0)	<0.001
Tobacco use, *n* (%)			0.036
Never	692 (53.0)	928 (57.9)	
Quit	126 (9.7)	137 (8.6)	
Current	436 (33.4)	481 (30.0)	
Alcohol consumption, *n* (%)			0.006
Never	811 (62.1)	1064 (66.4)	
Mild	266 (20.4)	250 (15.6)	
Moderate to severe	192 (14.7)	256 (16.0)	
BMI(kg/m^2)	24.6 (22.5,26.7)	24.5 (22.4,26.8)	0.637
NIHSS scales			<0.001
<9	1256 (96.2)	996 (62.2)	
9–18	30 (2.3)	474 (29.6)	
> 18	7 (0.5)	124 (7.7)	
Creatinine (m mol L^{-1})	72.7 (60.0, 87.5)	70.0 (57.5,85.0)	0.002
LDL(m mol L^{-1})	2.8 (2.3,3.5)	2.9 (2.3,3.5)	0.290
HDL(m mol L^{-1})	1.2 (1.0,1.4)	1.2 (1.0,1.4)	0.125
Systolic blood pressure (mmHg)	140 (130,160)	150 (134,161)	<0.001
Homocysteine (μmol L^{-1})	14.6 (11.4,19.8)	15.8 (12.3,21.4)	<0.001
HOMA2-IR	1.8 (1.1,3.0)	2.0 (1.2,3.1)	0.055
Past medical history, yes, *n* (%)			
Coronary heart disease	146 (11.2)	203 (12.7)	0.230
Hypertension	785 (60.2)	994 (62.0)	0.296
Atrial fibrillation	53 (4.1)	98 (6.1)	0.013
Stroke types, n (%)			<0.001
Ischemic stroke	1059 (81.1)	1172 (73.2)	<0.001
Cardioembolic	44 (3.4)	91 (5.7)	
Large-artery atherosclerosis	565 (43.3)	819 (51.1)	
Small-artery occlusion Lacunar	367 (28.1)	200 (12.5)	
Other demonstrated or undemonstrated	38 (2.9)	25 (1.6)	
ICH	176 (13.5)	381(23.8)	
SAH	70 (5.4)	49 (3.1)	
Glycometabolism status			**<0.001**
Diabetes mellitus	500 (38.3)	720 (44.9)	
Prediabetes	348 (26.7)	429 (26.8)	
Normoglycaemia	457 (35.0)	453 (28.3)	

mRS modified Rankin scale, *BMI* body mass index, *LDL* low density lipoprotein, *HDL* high density lipoprotein, *NIHSS* the National Institutes of Health Stroke Scale, *HOMA2-IR* the correctly solved computer model for homeostasis model assessment of insulin resistance, *IS* ischemic stroke, *ICH* intra-cerebral hemorrhage, *SAH* subarachnoid hemorrhage

Multivariate analysis of SUA deciles on poor functional outcome

SUA was re-divided into decile groups (D1 to D10) in different glucose metabolism groups. The SUA quartile groups in previous regression model were replaced with SUA deciles and a new regression model was calculated. The ORs of the incidence rate of poor outcome obtained from the regression model were used in the curve-fitting

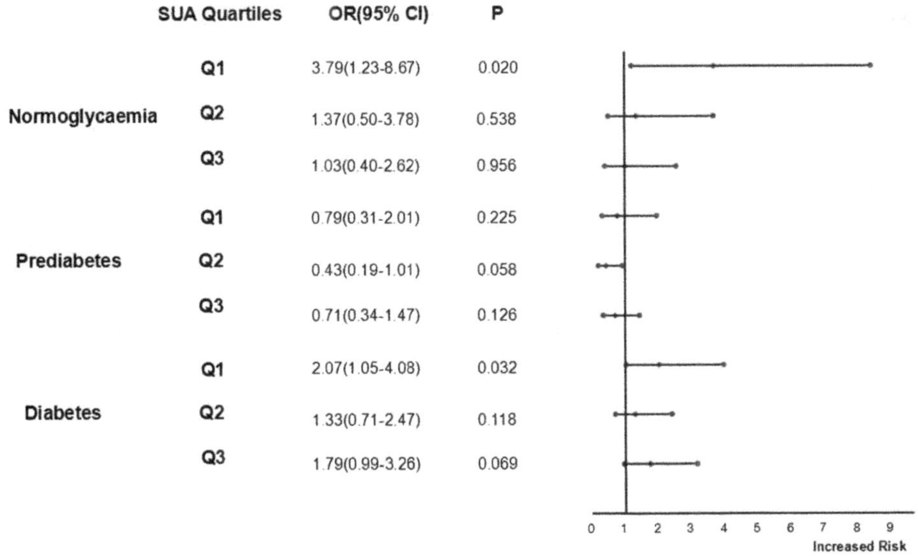

Fig. 3 Association between uric acid quartiles and poor outcomes in multivariate logistic regression analysis [a] ([a] adjusted for age, gender, stroke types, tobacco use, alcohol consumption, education level received, a history of hypertension, coronary artery disease or atrial fibrillation, NIHSS <9 VS ≥9, body mass index, homocysteine, systolic blood pressure, diastolic blood pressure, HOMA-IR, low density lipoprotein, high density lipoprotein, creatinine. In normoglycaemic subjects, Aspirin use was included as a binary variable in the analysis). NIHSS indicates the National Institutes of Health Stroke Scale; HOMA2-IR indicates the correctly solved computer model for homeostasis model assessment of insulin resistance

analysis. The curve-fitting results showed a U-shape curve and the cubic curve had the highest R^2 value in both the DM group and the normoglycemia group (Fig. 4a and c). The occurrence of poor outcome significantly decreased across SUA deciles from D1 to D9 in both normoglycemia and DM strokes (P for trend0.003 and 0.010, respectively), while it did not differ from D1-10 in prediabetes group (Fig. 4 b, P for trend, 0.568).

Multivariate analysis of continuous SUA concentration on poor functional outcome

SUA were further reintroduced into the multivariate analysis as a continuous variable. After adjusting for the same confounding factors as the above, higher SUA was still significantly independently associated with the less possibility of poor outcome in patients with normoglycaemia, while the association did not

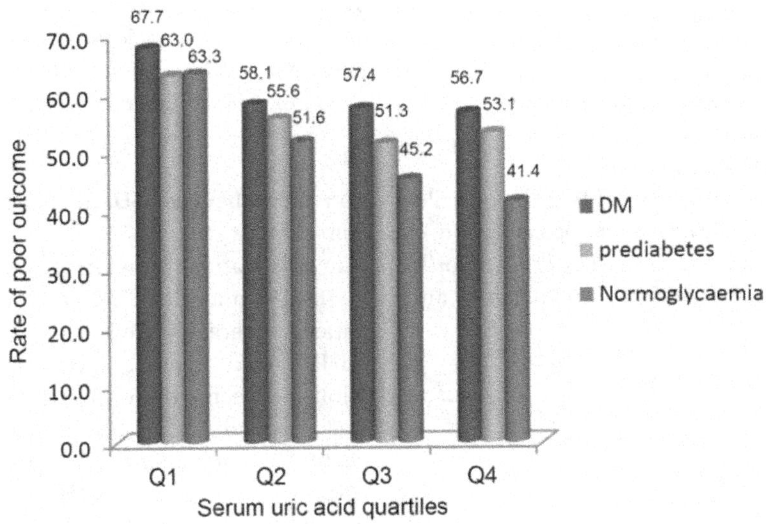

Fig. 2 Poor outcome rates depending on serum uric acid quartiles stratified by glycometabolism status. OGTT, the oral glucose tolerance test. Q1-4 indicates serum uric acid levels by quartiles. Q1 to Q4 were Q1, <221 μmol L^{-1}; Q2, (221–286) μmol L^{-1}; Q3, (286–352) μmol L^{-1} and Q4, >352 μmol L^{-1}

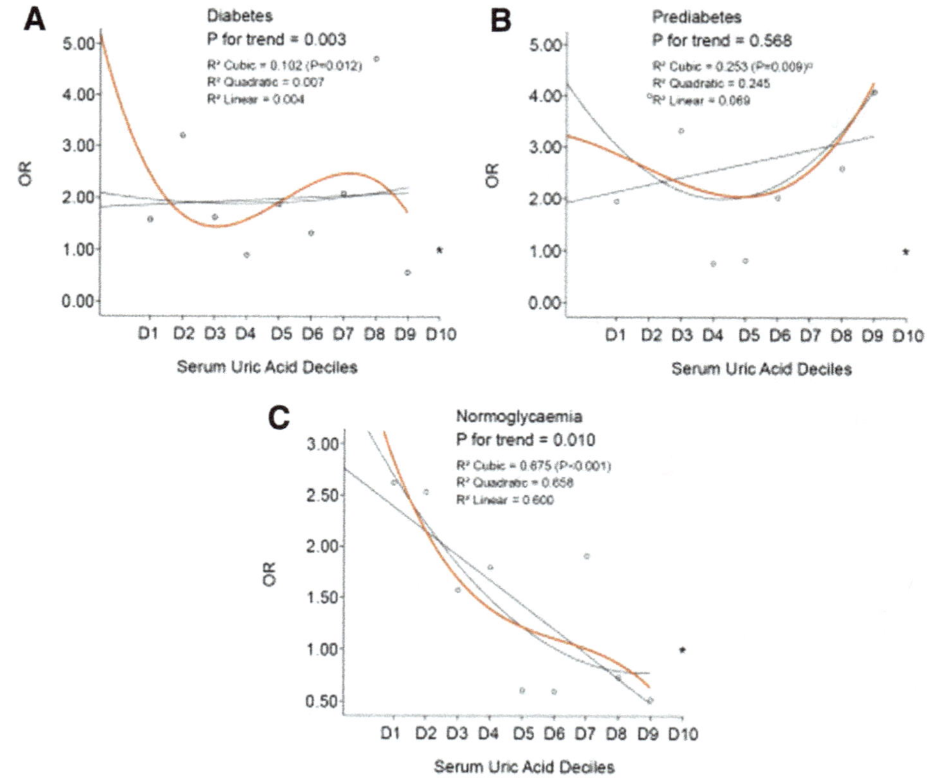

Fig. 4 Association between serum uric acid deciles and poor outcomes in multivariate logistic regression analysis[a] ([a] adjusted for the same variables as those in Fig. 3). *indicates the reference OR (the OR of D10 = 1). Reference point not included as basis for fit of regression lines. D1-10 indicates 1st decile to the 10th decile of serum uric acid. D1 to D10 (μmol L^{-1}) in 'Diabetes' were <169, 169–206, 206–235, 235–261, 261–286, 286–308, 308–334, 334–368, 368–424, >424. D1 to D10 (μmol L^{-1}) in "Prediabetes" were <155, 155–208, 208–237, 237–266, 266–287, 287–314, 314–342, 342–380, 380–438, >438. D1-10 (μmol L^{-1}) in 'Normoglycaemia' were <151, 151–201, 201–235, 235–260, 260–288, 288–316, 316–343, 343–381, 381–425, >425

exist in patients with DM or prediabetes (Table 3). The Hosmer and Lemeshow goodness-of-fit test results (χ^2, P) were (9.873, 0.274) in DM, (4.719, 0.787) in prediabetes and (5.621, 0.690) in normoglycemia group, respectively.

SUA concentration and Neurological functional change stratified by glycometabolism

SUA and Neurological improvement

In diabetic and prediabetic stroke patients, SUA quartiles were significantly associated with neurological improvement. Patients with the lowest level of SUA (<221umol/L) occupied 28.5% and 30.6% within the diabetes and prediabetes being neurological improved (both P <0.05. Additional file 6: Table S1. Additional file 7: Figure S1).

Table 3 Association between SUA as a continuous variable and poor outcome stratified by glycometabolism status[a]

Glycometabolism status	Odds ratio with 95% confidence intervals	*P*
Diabetes mellitus	0.98 (0.97–1.00)	0.135
Prediabetes	1.00 (1.00–1.01)	0.105
Normoglycaemia	0.99 (0.98–1.00)	0.022

[a]adjusted for the same variables as those in Fig. 3

SUA and Neurological deterioration

There were no significant association between SUA and neurological deterioration in all the glycometabolism statuses (Additional file 8: Table S2. Additional file 9: Figure S2).

Correlation between SUA levels and stroke severity at admission

The correlation between stroke severity (NIHSS < 9, 9–18,>18) and the SUA level was also analyzed. The patients were divided into 3 groups according to NIHSS of <9, 9–18 and >18, respectively. The correlation between stroke severity and the SUA quartile was calculated (Fig. 5). In DM and prediabetes, the percentage of patients with low SUA (Q1) in the severe stroke group (NIHSS > 18) was significantly higher than that in the mild stroke group (NIHSS < 9) (P < 0.001for DM and 0.023 for prediabetes). There were no significant differences in the SUA level across

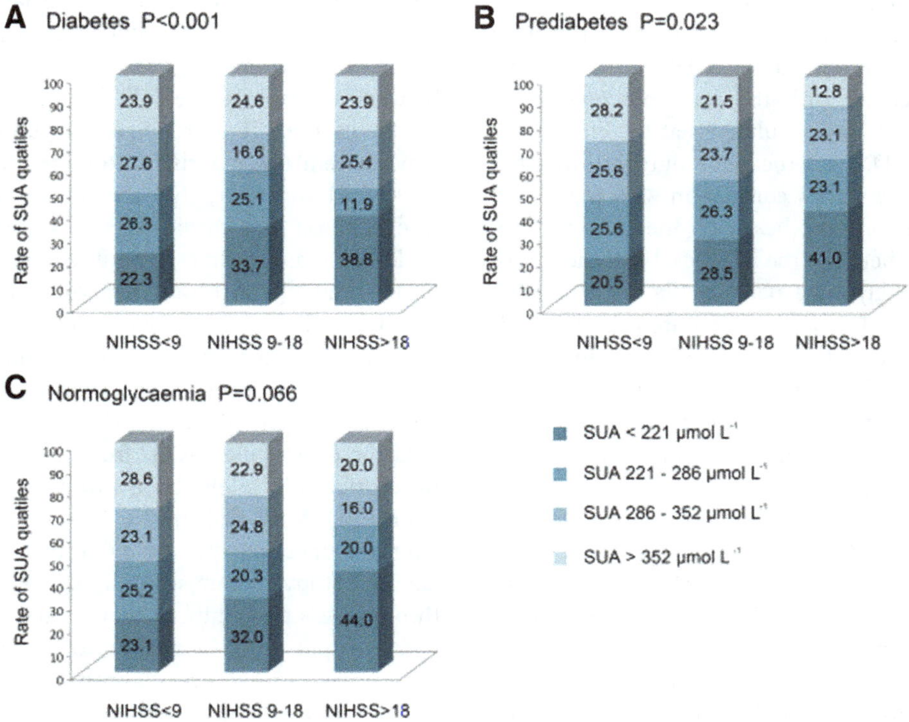

Fig. 5 Association between serum uric acid levels and stroke severity stratified by glycometabolism status. SUA indicates serum uric acid. NIHSS indicates the National Institutes of Health Stroke Scale

different stroke severity in the normoglycemia group ($P = 0.066$).

Other variables associated with the poor functional outcome of the stroke in multivariate analysis

NIHSS ≥9 was a significant risk factor of the poor outcome in all patients (In diabetes, 12.15 (8.08–18.21); In prediabetes, 11.58 (7.50–23.25); In normoglycemia, 18.40 (7.90–25.45)). In normoglycemia group, higher BMI as well as higher systolic blood pressure were also related to significantly higher risk of poor outcome (BMI 1.09 (1.02–1.18), systolic blood pressure 1.02 (1.01–1.18)).

Discussion

Most of previous studies suggested that hyperuricemia was a risk factor of stroke. In the present study, SUA values in predicting poor functional outcomes after stroke differed in 3 glycometabolism statuses. Lower SUA level (SUA < 220 μmol L^{-1}) was an independent risk predictor of the short-term prognosis of the acute first-ever stroke in patients with normoglycemia other than DM or prediabetes and such an effect might has gender difference. In the present study, the relationship is much more robust in male than in female normoglycaemic stroke patients.

Difference in the association of SUA level and post-stroke poor functional outcome among different glycometabolism status

The correlation between the SUA level and the poor post-stroke outcome in the normoglycemia patients was different from that in the DM or prediabetes patients in our study. Low SUA level was an independent predictor of the poor outcome of stroke in the normoglycemia patients but not in DM or prediabetes group. In DM group, a paradox association was found: 1) the association between the lowest SUA quartile (Q1) and the poor outcome was observed as significant (Fig. 3. $P = 0.032$) but the trend from Q1-Q4 was not (Fig. 3. P for trend = 0.109); 2) the association between SUA deciles and poor outcome was in a significant trend (Fig. 4 a. P for trend 0.003); 3) however, the significant association disappeared when assessment was performed between the continuous SUA concentration and the poor outcome (Table 3 . $P = 0.135$). In prediabetes group, possibility of poor outcome in the lower SUA levels was similar to that in the higher SUA levels either SUA was introduced into the multivariate analysis as a categorical variable or a continuous variable.

These debated results might be attributed to the negative association between SUA levels and stroke severity in DM and prediabetes (Fig. 5 a and b. $P < 0.001$ for DM and 0.023 for prediabetes). The percentage of the lower

SUA level was significantly increased across the aggravated stroke severity in diabetes and prediabetes group, and stroke severity (measured as NIHSS level) was also significantly associated with the poor outcome in the multivariate analysis, we speculated that the effect of the low SUA level in DM on the poor outcome of stroke might be carried out via its correlation with the severity of stroke. On the contrary, based on the fact that there was no correlation between the SUA level and the severity of stroke in normoglycemia patients (Fig. 5c. $P = 0.066$), the association of SUA and poor outcome was independent of stroke severity at baseline in normoglycemia patients. Therefore, SUA in normoglycaemia was an independent risk factor of poor outcome, whereas SUA in DM was only a complementary but not an independent one.

Zhang et al. reported their findings of a similar study in 2012 [12]. The correlation between the SUA level and the poor outcome of stroke in patients with normoglycemia and DM in their study was in line with us; Although the patients in their study were young and mid-age adults (18–45 years old) which was different with us (from 18 to 85 years old), the results were similar. It is a pity that they did not differentiate the prediabetes patients from the 'real' normoglycemia patients. Further than their research, we examine the association in prediabetes. Though we did not found a significant association between SUA and poor outcome in prediabetes, concerning the results that the association was much more significant and prominent in normoglycaemia patients than those with abnormal glycometabolism, it was highly implied that glucose metabolism might deeply affect the influence of SUA on post-stroke short-term outcome.

Till now, the effect of SUA on the prognosis of stroke in abnormal glucose metabolism is still debatable. Kramer et al. in their 2010 study reported that hyperuricemia was a significant risk factor for the mortality of cardiovascular disease in patients with prediabetes and typeIIdiabetes, but it did not increase the risk of mortality in patients with normoglycemia [7]. Their findings contradicted to our results. The conflicting results might be caused by the different race (Caucasian vs. Chinese) and age (mid-age to elders vs. 18 to 85) of the participants as well as the different sampling time of SUA (pre-event vs. post-event different phases).

Gender difference is attributed to SUA concentration [29, 30], thus effect of SUA on poor functional outcome differs in gender. There is no significant association found in female subgroup in the present study, which is mainly caused by the not large enough sample size (only 290 female stroke patients with normoglycaemia).

The possible mechanisms of the association between post-stroke SUA levels and the outcomes after stroke

There were conflicting results about the association between the post-stroke SUA level and the prognosis of stroke in the literature. Several studies reported that hyperuricemia was a risk factor for the poor outcomes [2–4] and suggested that the follow adverse effects of uric acid on the cardiovascular system might be the underline reasons: first, Hyperuricemia could cause insulin resistance [31]; second, hyperuricemia could increase the risk of hypertension and further aggravated atherosclerosis [32]; third, hyperuricemia could directly or indirectly impair the self-regulation of the arteriole and increased the risk of stroke [33].

At the meanwhile, results from other studies suggested hyperuricaemia might be a protective factor of stroke [8–12, 34]. Most of them [8, 10–12, 34] were published after the meta-analysis study from Kim, et al. [1]. In another study, administration of uric acid during the thrombolysis procedure in acute ischemic stroke patients had been proven to be neuro-protective [35]. It had also been proven in another study that low SUA was associated with larger infarction area and worse neurological deficit in the stroke patients [36]. The possible mechanisms of this protective effect of SUA included: (1) SUA was one of the most important serum antioxidant factors and an anti-inflammatory factor [37–40]; (2) SUA could stabilize endothelia progenitor cells (EPCs) [41]; (3) SUA could decrease the degradation of the extracellular superoxide dismutase-3(SOD_3) [42]; (4) In the chronic disease, hyperuricaemia was a reaction of the negative feedback mechanism to counterbalance the increased level of reactive oxygen species (ROS) [43]. It had been proven that Xanthine Oxidase (XO) expression increased after acute ischemic cerebral lesion and the increased XO would further lead to the uric acid level in local brain tissue to increase significantly. The rate of the change in XO and local uric acid level was positively correlated with the severity of the ischemic damage of the brain tissue [44, 45]. In 2010, Brouns, et al. reported the rate of SUA decrease in the first 7 days after stroke was positively correlated with the severity of the stroke as well as the incidence rate of poor post-stroke outcome [46]. Therefore, the concentration of peripheral SUA post stroke is most possibly in a dynamically decreasing pattern but it is still unknown exactly.

This dynamically decreasing pattern of SUA post stroke would attribute to the contradictory results on SUA and poor outcome. Of all the researches, SUA values from the different measurement timing post stroke (some were within 3 days, some were within 14 days, others were within several hours, etc.) could not stand for the SUA level in a concordant post-stroke phase. Since its dynamic changes, the association of

SUA and poor outcome was altered concerning a specific population (poor outcome or favorable outcome). For example, as for the patients with poor outcome, when the timing of SUA evaluated was just at the phase of higher SUA level, we might find an adverse effect of SUA on poor outcome, otherwise the effect might find to be protective. Therefore, the diverse investigations on SUA at different phases post stroke might come to paradox results. Further investigation needs to be carried out on figuring out the pattern of SUA concentration post stroke and its association as well the abnormal glucose metabolism on poor prognosis.

Advantages and limitations

ACROSS-CHINA is a nationwide, prospective, multiple-center study. In our study, pre-diabetic patients were excluded by OGTT test result to eliminate their possible interference to the results. There were some limitations in our study. First, only patients with SUA data were included in the study and this might cause selection bias. Second, there were no data of the dynamic change of SUA level. Third, only a few data on medications that might affect the SUA level were collected and no data on non-VKA oral anticoagulants (NOACs). Fourth, lack of data on exercise pre- and post- stroke. Exercise is also a major factor to influence SUA concentration [47].

Conclusions

The associations between post-stroke SUA and poor functional outcome at discharge differ in diverse abnormal glycometabolism populations. In acute stroke patients with normoglycemia, low SUA level (<220 μmol L-1) is an independent risk predictor of poor short-term outcome other than DM or prediabetes. The debated conclusion on the association between SUA and the poor outcome after stroke might be due to the diverse post-stroke time of blood sample for SUA in those different studies. Further research will be conducted on the association between the pattern of SUA change in stroke patients with different time of stroke onset, different glycoemtabolism status, different gender, through recording the dynamic value of SUA post stroke and the poor functional outcome and stratifying the study group by diagnosing glycometabolism status.

Additional files

Additional file 1: Table S3. Aspirin use and SUA levels stratified by glycometabolism.

Additional file 2: Table S4. Coumadin use and SUA levels stratified by glycometabolism.

Additional file 3: Table S5. Diuretics use and SUA levels stratified by glycometabolism.

Additional file 4: Table S7. SUA quartile and poor functional outcome at discharge with NIHSS adjusted as a continuous variable.

Additional file 5: Table S6. Multivariate analysis on SUA and poor functional outcome in normoglycaemic stroke stratified by gender.

Additional file 6: Table S1. Uric acid level and neurological improvement stratified by glycometabolism status.

Additional file 7: Figure S1. (TIF 740 kb)

Additional file 8: Table S2. Uric acid level and neurological deterioration stratified by glycometabolism status.

Additional file 9: Figure S2. (TIF 721 kb)

Additional file 10: Which involves 2907 patients' information across from the essential information such as age,gender,educational level, etc., to the variables including in our data analysis such as SUA levels, diagnosis of glycometabolism status, functional outcomes (poor or good) and so on. Each variable has its meaning and number 1,2,3 or more stands for the different meanings of each variable. For example, as for the variable "gender", 1 stands for "male" and 2 stands for "female".

Additional file 11: (PDF 29 kb)

Abbreviations

ACROSS-China: The abnormal glucose regulation in patients with acute stroke across China study; BMI: Body mass index; CI: Confidential interval; D1 to D10: Decile1 to Decile 10; DM: Diabetes mellitus; EPCs: Endothelia progenitor cells; FPG: Fasting plasma glucose; HOMA2-IR: The Homeostasis Model Assessment 2-Insulin Resistance; ICH: Intracerebral hemorrhage; IFG: Impaired fasting glucose; IGT: Impaired glucose tolerance; mRS: Modified Rankin Scale; NIHSS: The National Institutes of Health Stroke Scale; NOACs: Non-VKA oral anticoagulants; OGTT: Oral glucose tolerance test; ORs: Odds ratios; Q1 to Q4: Quartile 1 to quartile 4; ROS: Reactive oxygen species; SAH: Subarachnoid hemorrhage; SUA: Serum uric acid; WHO: World Health Organization; XO: Xanthine Oxidase

Acknowledgements

We thank all the participants in the study.

Funding

The study was supported by Beijing Municipal Science and Technology Commission NO.Z151100004015127 and NO.Z151100003915117. The funding didn't have a role in the design of the study, collection, analysis, interpretation of data or in writing the manuscript.

Authors' contributions

SLW drafted the manuscript; NZ helped to collect the data; SLW and YSP performed the statistically analysis; CXW participated the design of the study and explanation of the data; YJW participated the design of the study. All authors read and approved the final manuscript.

Competing interests

The authors declare that they have no competing interesets.

Author details

[1]Department of Neuropsychiatry and Behavioral Neurology and Clinical Psychology, Beijing Tiantan Hospital, Capital Medical University, Beijing,

China. [2]China National Clinical Research Center for Neurological Diseases, Beijing, China. [3]Department of Neurology, Beijing Tiantan Hospital, Capital Medical University, Beijing, China. [4]Center of Stroke, Beijing Institute for Brain Disorders, Beijing, China. [5]Beijing Key Laboratory of Translational Medicine for cerebrovascular Disease, Beijing, China.

References

1. Kim SY, Guevara JP, Kim KM, et al. Hyperuricemia and risk of stroke: a systematic review and meta-analysis. Arthritis Rheum. 2009;61:885–92.
2. Weir CJ, Muir SW, Walters MR, et al. Serum urate as an independent predictor of poor outcome and future vascular events after acute stroke. Stroke. 2003;34:1951–6.
3. Karagiannis A, Mikhailidis DP, Tziomalos K, et al. Serum uric acid as an independent predictor of early death after acute stroke. Circ J. 2007;71:1120–7.
4. Newman EJ, Rahman FS, Lees KR, et al. Elevated serum urate concentration independently predicts poor outcome following stroke in patients with diabetes. Diabetes Metab Res Rev. 2006;22:79–82.
5. Chiquete E, Ruiz-Sandoval JL, Murillo-Bonilla LM, et al. Serum uric acid and outcome after acute ischemic stroke: PREMIER study. Cerebrovasc Dis. 2013; 35:168–74.
6. Zoppini G, Targher G, Bonora E. The role of serum uric acid in cardiovascular disease in type 2 diabetic and non-diabetic subjects: a narrative review. J Endocrinol Invest. 2011;34:881–6.
7. Holme I, Aastveit AH, Hammar N, et al. Uric acid and risk of myocardial infarction, stroke and congestive heart failure in 417,734 men and women in the Apolipoprotein MOrtality RISk study (AMORIS). J Intern Med. 2009;266:558–70.
8. Kramer CK, von Mühlen D, Jassal SK, et al. A prospective study of uric acid by glucose tolerance status and survival: the Rancho Bernardo Study. J Intern Med. 2010;267:561–6.
9. Logallo N, Naess H, Idicula TT, et al. Serumuri acid: neuroprotection in thrombolysis. The Bergen NORSTROKE study. BMC Neurol. 2011;11:114.
10. Chamorro A, Obach V, Cervera A, et al. Prognostic significance of uric acid serum concentration in patients with acute ischemic stroke. Stroke. 2002;33:1048–52.
11. Zhang B, Gao C, Yang N, et al. Is elevated SUA associated with a worse outcome in young Chinese patients with acute cerebral ischemic stroke? BMC Neurol. 2010;10:82.
12. Amaro S, Urra X, Gómez-Choco M, et al. Uric acid levels are relevant in patients with stroke treated with thrombolysis. Stroke. 2011;42 Suppl 1:S28–32.
13. Zhang B, Gao C, Hou Q, et al. The potent different risk factors for cerebral infarction in young patients with and without type 2 diabetes: subanalysis of the Young Cerebral Infarction Study (YCIS). Atherosclerosis. 2012;221:215–20.
14. Miedema I, Uyttenboogaart M, Koch M, et al. Lack of association between serum uric acid levels and outcome in acute ischemic stroke. J Neurol Sci. 2012;319:51–5.
15. Winnard D, Wright C, Jackson G, et al. Gout, diabetes and cardiovascular disease in the Aotearoa New Zealand adult population: co-prevalence and implications for clinical practice. N Z Med J. 2012;126:53–64.
16. Wu J, Qiu L, Yan WH, et al. Serum gamma-glutamyltransferase and uric acid levels are associated with impaired fasting glucose in adults from Inner Mongolia, China. BMC Public Health. 2013;13:294.
17. Jia Z, Zhang X, Kang S, Wu Y. Serum uric acid levels and incidence of impaired fasting glucose and type 2 diabetes mellitus: a meta-analysis of cohort studies. Diabetes Res Clin Pract. 2013;101(1):88–96.
18. Shani M, Vinker S, Dinour D, Leiba M, Twig G, Holtzman EJ, Leiba A. High Normal Uric Acid Levels Are Associated with an Increased Risk of Diabetes in Lean, Normoglycemic Healthy Women. J Clin Endocrinol Metab. 2016; 101(10):3772–8.
19. Jia Q, Zhao X, Wang C, et al. Diabetes and poor outcomes within 6 months after acute ischemic stroke:the China National Stroke Registry. Stroke. 2011; 42:2758–62.
20. Jia Q, Zheng H, Zhao X, et al. Abnormal glucose regulation in patients with acute stroke across China: prevalence and baseline patient characteristics. Stroke. 2012;43:650–7.
21. Task WHO. Force on Stroke and other Cerebrovascular Disorders. Stroke-1989: Recommendations on stroke prevention, diagnosis, and therapy. Report of the WHO Task Force on Stroke and other Cerebrovascular Disorders. Stroke. 1989;20:1407–21.
22. American Diabetes Association. Diagnosis and classification of diabetes mellitus. Diabetes Care. 2006;29:43–8.
23. Levy JC, Matthews DR, Hermans MP. Correct homeostasis model assessment (HOMA) evaluation uses the computer program (Letter). Diabetes Care. 1998;21:2191–2.
24. Kamouchi M, Matsuki T, Hata J, et al. Prestroke glycemic control is associated with the functional outcome in acute ischemic stroke: the Fukuoka Stroke Registry. Stroke. 2011;42:2788–94.
25. Theofanidis D. Validation of international stroke scales for use by nurses in Greek settings. Top Stroke Rehabil. 2016:1–8. [Epub ahead of print] PubMed PMID: 27680397.
26. Yong M, Kaste M. Dynamic of hyperglycemia as a predictor of stroke outcome in the ECASS-II trial. Stroke. 2008;39:2749–55.
27. Weimar C, Mieck T, Buchthal J, Ehrenfeld CE, Schmid E, Diener HC. Neurologic worsening during the acute phase of ischemic stroke. Arch Neurol. 2005;62:393–7.
28. Menon RK, Mikhailidis DP, Bell JL, Kernoff PB, Dandona P. Warfarin administration increases uric acid concentrations in plasma. Clin Chem. 1986;32(8):1557–9.
29. Chou P, Lin KC, Lin HY, Tsai ST. Gender differences in the relationships of serum uric acid with fasting serum insulin and plasma glucose in patients without diabetes. J Rheumatol. 2001;28(3):571–6.
30. Antón FM, García Puig J, Ramos T, González P, Ordás J. Sex differences in uric acid metabolism in adults: evidence for a lack of influence of estradiol-17 beta (E2) on the renal handling of urate. Metabolism. 1986;35(4):343–8.
31. Klein BE, Klein R, Lee KE. Components of the metabolic syndrome and risk of cardiovascular disease and diabetes in Beaver Dam. Diabetes Care. 2002;25:1790–4.
32. Rich MW. Uric acid: is it a risk factor for cardiovascular disease? Am J Cardiol. 2000;85:1018–21.
33. Johnson RJ, Kang DH, Feig D, et al. Is there a pathogenetic role for uric acid in hypertension and cardiovascular and renal disease? Hypertension. 2003;41:1183–90.
34. Wu H, Jia Q, Liu G, et al. Decreased Uric Acid Levels Correlate with Poor Outcomes in Acute Ischemic Stroke Patients, but Not in Cerebral Hemorrhage Patients. J Stroke Cerebrovasc Dis. 2014;23(3):469–75.
35. Amaro S, Planas AM, Chamorro A. Uric acid administration in patients with acute stroke: a novel approach to neuroprotection. Expert Rev Neurother. 2008;8:259–70.
36. Leinonen JS, Ahonen JP, Lönnrot K, et al. Low plasma antioxidant activity is associated with high lesion volume and neurological impairment in stroke. Stroke. 2000;31:33–9.
37. Nieto FJ, Iribarren C, Gross MD, et al. Uric acid and serum antioxidant capacity: a reaction to atherosclerosis? Atherosclerosis. 2000;148:131–9.
38. Ames BN, Cathcart R, Schwiers E, et al. Uric acid provides an antioxidant defense in humans against oxidant- and radical-caused aging and cancer: a hypothesis. ProcNatlAcadSci U S A. 1981;78:6858–62.
39. Davies KJ, Sevanian A, Muakkassah-Kelly SF, et al. Uric acid-iron ion complexes. A new aspect of the antioxidant functions of uric acid. Biochem J. 1986;235:747–54.
40. Zare F, Magnusson M, Bergström T, et al. Uric acid, a nucleic acid degradation product, down-regulates dsRNA-triggered arthritis. J Leukoc Biol. 2006;79:482–8.
41. Patschan D, Patschan S, Gobe GG, et al. Uric acid heralds ischemic tissue injury to mobilize endothelial progenitor cells. J Am SocNephrol. 2007;18: 1516–24.
42. Hink HU, Santanam N, Dikalov S, et al. Peroxidase properties of extracellular superoxide dismutase: role of uric acid in modulating in vivo activity. ArteriosclerThrombVasc Biol. 2002;22:1402–8.
43. Doehner W, Landmesser U. Xanthine oxidase and uric acid in cardiovascular disease: clinical impact and therapeutic options. SeminNephrol. 2011;31:433–40.
44. George J, Struthers AD. Role of urate, xanthine oxidase and the effects of allopurinol in vascular oxidative stress. Vasc Health Risk Manag. 2009;5:265–72.
45. Higgins P, Ferguson LD, Walters MR. Xanthine oxidase inhibition for the treatment of stroke disease: a novel therapeutic approach. Expert Rev CardiovascTher. 2011;9:399–401.
46. Brouns R, Wauters A, Van De Vijver G, et al. Decrease in uric acid in acute ischemic stroke correlates with stroke severity, evolution and outcome. ClinChem Lab Med. 2010;48:383–90.
47. Green HJ, Fraser IG. Differential effects of exercise intensity on serum uric acid concentration. Med Sci Sports Exerc. 1988;20(1):55–9.

2

Cilostazol improves endothelial function in acute cerebral ischemia patients: a double-blind placebo controlled trial with flow-mediated dilation technique

Seong-Joon Lee[1], Jin Soo Lee[1], Mun Hee Choi[1], Sung Eun Lee[1], Dong Hoon Shin[2] and Ji Man Hong[1,3*]

Abstract

Background: In order to evaluate the impact of cilostazol on endothelial function, we compared the changes of flow-mediated dilation (FMD) between aspirin and cilostazol groups in patients with acute cerebral ischemia.

Methods: Patients presenting with acute cerebral ischemic events were randomly assigned into aspirin ($n = 40$) or cilostazol ($n = 40$) group in a double-blinded manner. FMD was measured at baseline (T0) and 90 days (T1). We measured L-arginine at baseline (a precursor of biologically active nitric oxides). Serious and non-serious adverse events were described.

Results: Despite no difference in the baseline FMD values ($p = 0.363$), there was a significant increase of FMD values in cilostazol group (7.9 ± 2.4 to 8.9 ± 2.3%, $p = 0.001$) and not in aspirin group (8.5 ± 2.6 to 9.3 ± 2.8%, $p = 0.108$). In the multiple regression analysis performed in cilostazol group, serum L–arginine levels were inversely correlated with FMD at T1 (ß = −0.050, SE: 0.012, $p < 0.001$) with age, total cholesterol levels, and C-reactive protein as confounders. While T0 FMD values in both aspirin and cilostazol groups did not show any correlation with serum L-arginine levels, the correlation is restored in the cilostazol group at T1 ($r = 0.467$, $p = 0.007$), while such is not shown in the aspirin group. There was no difference of serious adverse events between the two groups ($p = 0.235$). Adverse events were more common in the cilostazol group (35/40 vs. 25/40, $p = 0.010$), due to frequent headaches (14/40 vs. 3/30, $p = 0.003$) which was well tolerated.

Conclusion: Cilostazol improved endothelial function in acute cerebral ischemia patients. It also restored an inverse correlation between 3-month FMD and baseline L-arginine levels.

Keywords: Endothelium, Cilostazol, Cerebral infarction, Transient ischemic attack, Arginine

Background

Cilostazol is a selective phosphodiesterase (PDE) 3 inhibitor with therapeutic focus on cyclic adenosine monophosphate (cAMP) [1]. It inhibits platelet aggregation and plays a role as a direct arterial vasodilator [2, 3]. It prevents the occurrence of restenosis after coronary angioplasty and stenting and reduced growth of carotid intima-media thickness in diabetic patients [4, 5]. In cerebrovascular disease, the progression rate of symptomatic intracranial artery stenosis was significantly lower in the cilostazol aspirin combination group than in the aspirin monotherapy group [6]. These findings suggest antiatherogenic effects of cilostazol, previously known to be through actions on PDE3 in vascular smooth muscle cells [7], lipoprotein metabolism [8], and prevention of endothelial apoptosis [9].

In the development of atherosclerosis, endothelial dysfunction is a key step in its development and can be used as a prognostic marker in predicting future stroke

* Correspondence: dacda@hanmail.net
[1]Department of Neurology, Ajou University School of Medicine, Suwon, Republic of Korea
[3]Department of Neurology, Ajou University School of Medicine, 164, World cup-ro, Yeongtong-gu, Suwon-si, Gyeonggi-do 16499, South Korea
Full list of author information is available at the end of the article

and heart attacks [10, 11]. Endothelial function can be noninvasively assessed by the ultrasound measurement of brachial artery flow-mediated dilation (FMD), which represents the endothelium-dependent relaxation of an artery in response to reactive hyperemia [12]. FMD is comprised of two cellular mechanisms, endothelial nitric oxide (NO) synthesis from its precursor L-arginine, by mechanical shear-stress of vessel wall [13], and concurrent vascular smooth muscle cell relaxation through actions of NO. Accordingly, improvement of FMD can be a biomarker for protection against atherogenesis.

Therefore, we hypothesized that in acute cerebral ischemia patients, antiatherogenic effects of cilostazol can be represented by improvements in flow-mediated vasodilation, representing its positive effects in endothelial function. To achieve this goal, in acute stroke patients randomized to aspirin control group versus cilostazol group in a double-blinded manner, the value of FMD at admission, 3 months, and its improvement was compared, along with its association with baseline L-arginine levels as well as other known vascular risk factors.

Methods

Study design and participants

This investigator-initiated, randomized, double–blind trial was prospectively conducted with two-arm parallel treatment groups and a single dose scheme: 100 mg aspirin daily and cilostazol placebo twice daily versus aspirin placebo daily and 100 mg cilostazol twice daily. The dosage of each drug was planned according to previous prospective studies [1, 6, 14]. Randomization was performed by a computer generation block card randomization procedure. This study was conducted from March 2012 to October 2014. The institutional review board of Ajou University Hospital approved the protocol and all participants provided written informed consent.

Eligible patients were over 30 years of age and had an (1) acute ischemic stroke confirmed by diffusion weighted imaging, or a (2) transient ischemic attack (TIA) within 7 days. Patients were excluded if (1) there is intracranial hemorrhage on imaging study, (2) patients is previously taking antiplatelets, vitamin K antagonists, factor Xa antagonists, or chronic treatment with systemic steroidal and non-steroidal anti-inflammatory drugs, (3) patients who received fibrinolytics within the previous 48 h, (4) cognitive impairment interfering with the possibility of obtaining informed consent, (5) pregnancy, (6) participation in another pharmacological study, (7) peptic ulcer disease or hematological abnormality, (8) initial modified Barthel index <30 points, and (9) liver function tests exceeding a 2-fold upper range value. A total of 80 eligible patients were prospectively recruited. All included patients underwent diagnostic studies including routine blood tests and cardiologic work-ups. The primary outcome was differences in endothelial function in the two groups measured by means of FMD on admission and at 3 months. According to previous studies, the adverse effects in two groups were investigated. A flowchart for the study population is shown in Additional file 1: Figure S1.

Flow-mediated dilation (FMD) protocol

Endothelial function was evaluated by measurement of FMD of the brachial artery in response to hyperemia according to methods previously described [15]. The subjects were instructed to fast after dinner on the day before assessment and to refrain from smoking, alcohol, or caffeine 6 h before the start of evaluation. They were fully rested before the FMD measurements. Briefly, a blood pressure cuff is placed on the forearm. Occlusion is created by inflating the cuff to at least 50 mmHg above the subject's systolic pressure for 5 min. The pressure is then released quickly to induce hand and forearm hyperemia and subsequent brachial artery reactive vasodilation. FMD is defined as the maximal percent change in brachial artery diameter after reactive hyperemia compared with baseline. The FMD values of 60 individuals without vascular disease consisting of normal volunteers, primary headache patients, or essential tremor patients were used as reference (FMD value: 8.8 ± 2.7%, age: 57.7 ± 14.9). FMD was examined at baseline (T0) before administration of antiplatelet agents, and after 3 months of randomized antiplatelet treatment (T1).

Specimen collection and measurement of serum l-arginine

Venous blood samples were initially collected in 3.2% sodium citrate (Becton Dickinson, USA). The serum L-arginine levels were measured by Arginine ELISA Assay Kit (Eagle Biosciences). The concentrations of analytes into the samples were estimated from the standard curve and expressed as micromole per liter.

Statistical analysis

The statistical power of the study was set at 85%, given a mean difference of 2 and a standard deviation of 2.7 (based on our hospital laboratory results), with a type I error of 0.05 for FMD. A sample of 34 patients per group was calculated based on Dunnett's procedure of comparing several treatments with a control (PASS 2008, USA). To allow for a 15% drop-out rate, 40 patients were randomly assigned per each group. Categorical variables were analyzed using a χ^2 test or Fisher's exact test. Numeric were analyzed using a Student's *t*-test between two groups. First, comparison between the aspirin group and cilostazol group was performed to verify occurrences of adverse events and their baseline characteristics. The change of FMD values at the initial and follow-up period were compared using a paired t-test between the control and cilostazol groups. To validate the factors associated with T1 FMD values, multiple linear regression analysis was performed, including potentially significant variables in the correlation analysis ($p < 0.200$). To evaluate the effects of baseline serum L-arginine levels on FMD outcomes, correlation analysis between FMD and L-arginine levels at T0 and at T1 in both groups were compared. Statistical analyses were performed using commercially available software (SPSS, version 22.0, USA). *P*-values <0.05 were considered significant.

Results

Baseline clinical characteristics and adverse events

A total of 40 patients were enrolled to each group. In the aspirin group, 3 patients were excluded due to serious adverse events (SAE) (intracerebral hemorrhage, thrombocytopenia, and femur fracture), 2 patients were lost on follow up, and 1 withdrew consent. A total of 34 patients were enrolled for the final analysis. In the cilostazol group, 2 patients were excluded due to SAE (acute cholecystitis, and ischemic stroke), 1 were excluded due to adverse event (hypoglycemia), and 5 patients were lost on follow up. A total of 32 patients were included in the final analysis.

Baseline clinical factors such as age, sex, diagnosis of hypertension (HTN), diagnosis of diabetes mellitus (DM), and history of smoking did not differ between the two groups. Baseline laboratory data such as hemoglobin, glucose, lipid profiles, and serum L-arginine levels did not differ between the two groups (Table 1). When initial FMD values and mean age of aspirin and cilostazol groups were compared to reference group, there was no statistical difference (FMD values: 8.5 ± 2.6 vs. 7.9 ± 2.4 vs. 8.8 ± 2.7%, $p = 0.257$, age: 79.5 ± 11.7 vs. 57.4 ± 12.7 vs. 57.7 ± 14.9, $p = 0.787$).

5 patients experienced SAE (intracerebral hemorrhage, thrombocytopenia, femur fracture, bell's palsy, and infectious enterocolitis) in the aspirin group, while 2 patients experienced SAE (acute cholecystitis and ischemic stroke) in the cilostazol group ($p = 0.235$). Compared to aspirin group, the number of patients who experienced adverse events was significantly higher in the cilostazol group (62.5% vs. 87.5%, $p = 0.01$) due to higher frequency of headaches (7.5% vs. 35.0%, $p = 0.003$). The number of other adverse events did not differ (Table 2).

Table 1 Baseline clinical and laboratory factors of the aspirin group and cilostazol group

	Aspirin (*n* = 34)	Cilostazol (*n* = 32)	*P*
Age	59.5 ± 11.7	57.4 ± 12.7	0.494
Male sex	20 (58.8%)	23 (71.9%)	0.266
TOAST classification			0.233
Atherosclerosis	1 (2.9%)	3 (9.4%)	
Small artery disease	28 (82.4%)	28 (87.5%)	
Unknown	3 (8.8%)	0 (0.0%)	
Transient ischemic attack	2 (5.9%)	1 (3.1%)	
HTN	28 (82.4%)	22 (68.8%)	0.197
DM	10 (29.4%)	5 (15.6%)	0.182
Cardiac problems	3 (8.8%)	2 (6.3%)	0.693
Hyperlipidemia	13 (38.2%)	14 (43.8%)	0.649
Metabolic syndrome	20 (58.8%)	14 (43.8%)	0.324
BMI	24.9 ± 3.1	24.6 ± 3.0	0.994
Smoking	16 (47.1%)	13 (40.6%)	0.599
Previous statin use	1 (2.9%)	2 (6.3%)	0.519
Laboratory data			
Hemoglobin (mg/dL)	14.0 ± 2.0	14.2 ± 1.4	0.638
Glucose (mg/dL)	147.9 ± 62.9	130.2 ± 37.8	0.173
CRP (mg/dL)	0.2 ± 0.3	0.2 ± 0.3	0.692
Fibrinogen (mg/dL)	319.4 ± 70.4	327.1 ± 78.7	0.678
Homocysteine (mg/dL)	12.0 ± 4.5	12.3 ± 6.4	0.84
L-arginine (mmol/L)	98.3 ± 42.6	95.0 ± 25.1	0.706
Lipid			
Total cholesterol (mg/dL)	192.6 ± 35.6	193.6 ± 38.6	0.913
Triglyceride (mg/dL)	157.7 ± 102.4	135.0 ± 67.4	0.296
HDL (mg/dL)	45.0 ± 12.8	44.7 ± 9.7	0.921
LDL (mg/dL)	118.5 ± 29.7	121.8 ± 33.1	0.669

HTN hypertension; *DM* diabetes mellitus; *BMI* body mass index; *CRP* C reactive protein; *HDL* high density lipoprotein; *LDL* low density lipoprotein

Patient management and FMD changes

Apart from randomized use of antiplatelets, other stroke managements such as blood pressure control, statins or glucose management was performed according to previously published guidelines [16]. In terms of medication, the choice of antihypertensive use did not significantly differ. While statin use was more common in the cilostazol group, all patients received lipid lowering agents. Vitamin supplementation or choice in oral hypoglycemic agents did not differ (Table 3).

Despite no difference in the baseline FMD between the groups ($p = 0.363$), there was a significant increase of FMD values in the cilostazol group (7.9 ± 2.4 to 8.9 ± 2.3%, $p = 0.001$) while not in the aspirin group (8.5 ± 2.6 to 9.3 ± 2.8%, $p = 0.108$). Increase in maximal brachial artery diameter was also seen in the cilostazol group (5.2 ± 0.7 to 5.4 ± 0.7, $p = 0.041$) (Fig. 1).

Factors associated with FMD at T1 in cilostazol group

In the multiple linear regression analysis for evaluation of factors associated with increase in FMD values at T1, factors that were potentially associated with FMD levels in the correlation analysis ($p < 0.200$) were included (Table 4). In the multivariate analysis, baseline L–arginine

Table 2 Comparison of adverse events between the two groups

	Aspirin (n = 40)	Cilostazol (n = 40)	P
Serious adverse events	5	2	0.235
Acute cholecystitis	0	1	NC
Ischemic stroke recurrence	0	1	NC
Bell's palsy	1	0	NC
Intracerebral hemorrhage	1	0	NC
Thrombocytopenia	1	0	NC
Femur fracture	1	0	NC
Infectious enterocolitis	1	0	NC
Adverse events	25	35	0.010
Headache	3	14	0.003
Anxiety/Palpitation	3	9	NC
Dizziness	2	4	NC
Heartburn /Dyspepsia	4	1	NC
Diarrhea	1	1	NC
Hand tremor	2	1	NC
Itching/skin rash	3	2	NC
Dysuria	1	0	NC
Depression	1	0	NC
Acute rhinitis	1	1	NC
Food allergy	1	0	NC
Hyperglycemia/Hypoglycemia	0	2	NC
Muscle pain	1	0	NC
Liver enzyme elevation	1	0	NC
Tinnitus	1	0	NC

levels were inversely correlated with FMD at T1 (ß = −0.050, SE: 0.012, p < 0.001), as also seen in baseline C-reactive protein levels (ß = −3.267, SE = 0.984, p = 0.001) (Table 4).

Serum L-arginine levels and FMD

Figure 2 shows the correlation analysis between serum L-arginine levels and FMD at initial and 3 month. At T0, both cilostazol (r = 0.231, p = 0.204) and aspirin (r = 0.26, p = 0.883) groups do not show correlation between serum L-arginine levels and FMD. At T1, cilostazol group shows restored correlation between serum L-arginine levels and FMD (r = 0.467, p = 0.007), while such is not shown in the aspirin group (r = 0.174, p = 0.324).

Discussion

To the best of our knowledge, this is the first study to investigate the effect of cilostazol on endothelial function by FMD in patients with acute cerebral ischemia. Our study results show that administration of cilostazol had

Table 3 Treatment factors according to aspirin and cilostazol treatment groups

	Aspirin (n = 34)	Cilostazol (n = 32)	P
Admission MBP (mmHg)	107.6 ± 11.8	106.6 ± 15.0	0.770
3 month MBP (mmHg)	98.1 ± 11.9	95.6 ± 10.2	0.370
MBP reduction (mmHg)	9.5 ± 16.9	11.3 ± 14.5	0.659
Antihypertensives	27 (79.4%)	22 (68.8%)	0.322
ARB	27 (79.4%)	21 (65.6%)	0.209
CCB	11 (32.4%)	8 (25.0%)	0.510
BB	2 (5.9%)	0 (0.0%)	0.164
Lipid lowering agents			0.024
Statins	29 (85.3%)	32 (100.0%)	
Fibrates	5 (14.7%)	0 (0.0%)	
Vitamin Supplementation	4 (11.8%)	4 (12.5%)	0.927
Oral Hypoglycemic agents			
Metformin	8 (23.5%)	3 (9.4%)	0.123
Glimepiride	2 (5.9%)	3 (9.4%)	0.592
DPP-4 inhibitors	3 (8.8%)	1 (3.1%)	0.332

MBP mean blood pressure; *ARB* angiotensin receptor blockers; *CCB* calcium channel blockers; *BB* beta blockers; *DPP* dipeptidyl peptidase

a beneficial effect on endothelial function in acute cerebral ischemia patients. Furthermore, cilostazol treated patients showed significant relationship between baseline serum L-arginine levels and FMD, while such findings are not seen in the aspirin group. Our study results emphasize the use of cilostazol in acute ischemic stroke [17], for cilostazol induced improvements in endothelial function may be an underlying surrogate marker for its

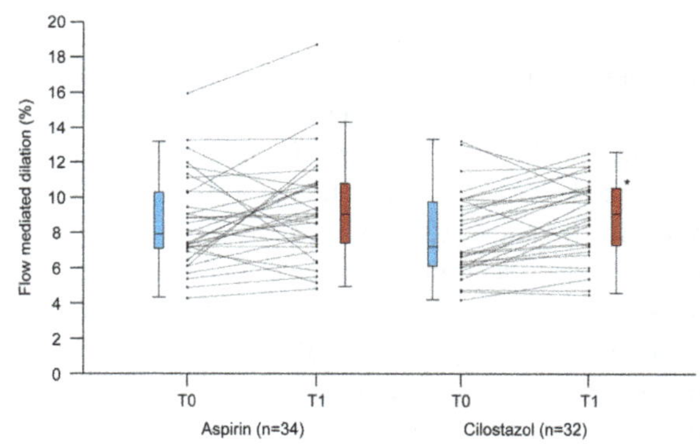

	Aspirin Baseline	Aspirin 3 months	p	Cilostazol Baseline	Cilostazol 3 months	p
FMD (%)	8.5±2.6	9.3±2.8	0.108	7.9±2.4	8.9±2.3	0.001
Baseline diameter (mm)	4.8±0.7	4.7±0.7	0.244	4.9±0.7	5.1±0.7	0.173
Maximal diameter (mm)	5.1±0.8	4.9±0.7	0.023	5.2±0.7	5.4±0.7	0.041

Fig. 1 The FMD parameters on enrollment and at 3 months. A significant increase of FMD values in the cilostazol group is seen, while not in the aspirin group

Table 4 Factors that are correlated with 3 month FMD values of the cilostazol group in multiple linear regression analysis

	Univariate analysis		Multivariate analysis (r^2 = 0.695)			
Factors	r	p	ß	SE	95% CI	p
Age	−.286	0.113	−0.036	0.024	(−0.086, 0.013)	0.145
Initial mean BP	.003	0.988				
3 month mean BP	−.007	0.968				
Hemoglobin	.003	0.988				
Glucose	.122	0.507				
Total cholesterol	.249	0.170	0.009	0.008	(−0.008, 0.025)	0.290
Triglyceride	.162	0.376				
HDL	.017	0.927				
LDL	.219	0.228				
ESR	−.004	0.982				
CRP	−.352	0.048	−3.267	0.984	(−5.285, −1.248)	0.003
L-arginine	−.508	0.003	−0.050	0.012	(−0.075, −0.024)	<0.001

FMD flow mediated dilation; *BP* blood pressure; *HDL* high density lipoprotein; *LDL* low density lipoprotein; *ESR* erythrocyte sedimentation rate; *CRP* c-reactive protein

role in prevention of atherogenesis [6] and blocking small-vessel pathology [18].

Previous studies on FMD and cilostazol have shown conflicting results. Results of studies involving smokers have shown improvement in endothelial function, and younger smokers are more likely to respond to treatment [19–21]. Preclinical studies supporting such findings have shown that cilostazol increases NO synthesis in interleukin-1 beta-stimulated smooth muscle cells, at least partially through a cAMP-dependent pathway [22, 21]. Furthermore, cilostazol increased production of NO and concentration dependent vasodilation in porcine thoracic aorta. This finding was more obvious with intact epithelium compared to denuded aorta, suggesting that cilostazol-induced vasodilation was dependent on endothelial release of NO [23].

However, an FMD study involving Raynaud syndrome patients [24] and a recent study involving coronary artery disease patients [25] both showed no improvement of FMD with oral cilostazol use for 6 weeks and 6–9 months respectively, while significant improvement in brachial artery diameter was seen in both studies. The negative results of the two recent disease oriented studies represent the multifactorial causes of endothelial dysfunction

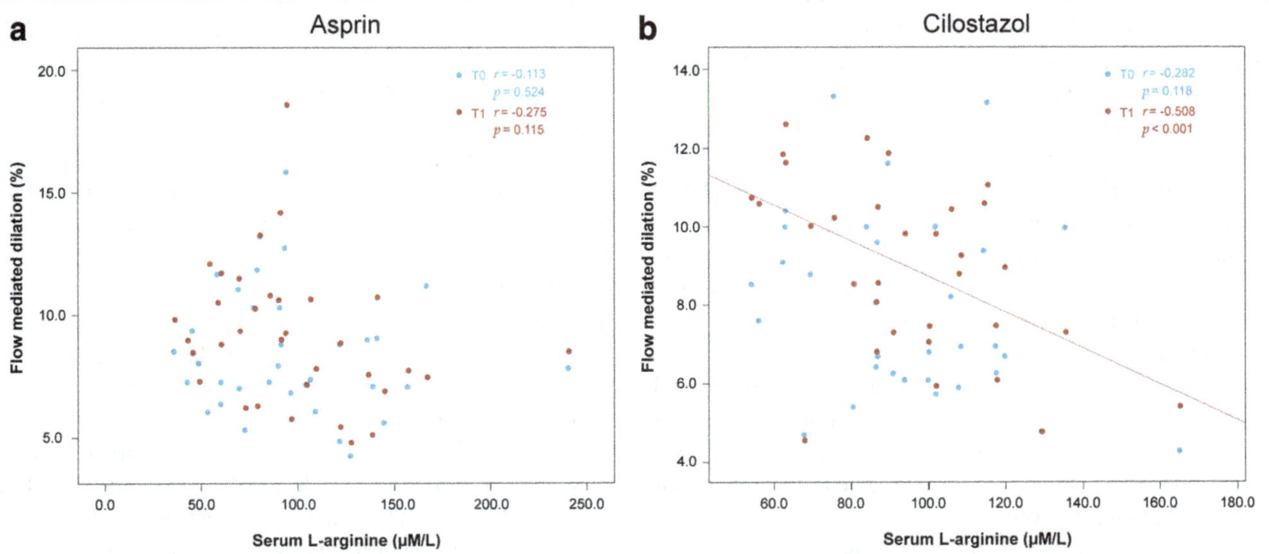

Fig. 2 Correlation between initial serum L-arginine levels and FMD at enrollment and at 3 months. Blue dots denote FMD at enrollment (T0), and red dots denote FMD at 3 months (T1). **a** In the aspirin group FMD values and L-arginine levels do not show correlation at T0 and at T1. **b** In the cilostazol group, T0 FMD values and L-arginine levels do not show correlation, but an inverse correlation between the two values is revealed at T1

encountered in clinical settings. Patients with overt coronary artery disease or peripheral arterial obstructive disease have multiple vascular risk factors such as dyslipidemia [26], hypertension [27], or diabetes [28] that lead to impaired NO bioavailability by multiple mechanisms such as endothelial nitric oxide synthase (eNOS) uncoupling, increased NO breakdown by reactive oxygen species, or increase in asymmetric dimethylarginine (ADMA) [29]. A single agent such as cilostazol may not be sufficient for improvements in endothelial function in such complex situations, and furthermore, the effect of cilostazol may have been masked by other medications known to have effect on endothelial function. In this regard, the positive results seen in our study may have been due to the somewhat homogenous inclusion criteria of patients that had not used antithrombotic agents previously.

A subsequent result of our study is the inverse correlation seen between serum L-arginine levels and FMD in the cilostazol group after 3 months. One might presume that higher levels of L-arginine, a substrate for NO, may be associated with higher FMD values. However, endothelial function is known to be more dependent on ADMA levels, a competitive inhibitor of NO synthase; namely the L-arginine paradox. Furthermore, because L-arginine-dependent metabolic pathways are critical determinants of several pathophysiological conditions, its levels are generally tightly regulated [30]. In hypertensive patients [31] and end-stage renal disease patients [32], endothelium dependent vasodilation showed inverse relations with plasma L-arginine levels along with ADMA levels [31]. In the case of hypercholesterolemia, serum L-arginine levels did not differ much in contrast to ADMA levels showing inverse correlation with endothelial function [33]. Overall, plasma L-arginine levels seem to show inverse relation with endothelial function. Such inverse relation was seen only in the 3 month cilostazol group, while this relation was altered in the acute stroke phase of both population, and 3 month aspirin group. Thus, only the 3 month FMD values of cilostazol group are in line with the L-arginine paradox. While our study results itself lack further explanation, we presume that accumulation of multiple risk factors and acute ischemia systemically affects endothelial function, resulting in alteration of normal endothelial physiology. Cilostazol seems to induces improvements in suppressed eNOS bioactivity by phosphorylation of activation sites [34], restoring the physiologic relation between plasma L-arginine levels and FMD, while such finding is not seen in the aspirin group.

Our study enlightens another clinically important issue of pharmacotherapy. The use of cilostazol and L-arginine co-supplementation. Although physiological range of L-arginine are in a range that enables full activity of its enzyme [30], there is still evidence that oral supplementation doses improve endothelial function in certain patient groups [35, 36]. By combined use of L-arginine supplementation and cilostazol, further improvements in endothelial function may be achieved, for L-arginine acts as a substrate for NO synthesis, while cilostazol activates eNOS via phosphorylation of its activation sites. Further clinical studies may be needed to address this issue.

The current study has some limitations. First, plasma L-arginine levels were measured only on admission due to limitations in study design. Accordingly, the serial changes in its values and its association with FMD values could not be evaluated. Also, serum ADMA levels were not measured in our study. However, previous studies have revealed that plasma L-arginine levels are known to correlate with plasma ADMA levels [31], and previous reports that L-arginine supplementation successfully improved the FMD in special populations [33] support our study results. We hope to address these limitations in future studies using cilostazol and L-arginine co-supplementation. Another limitation is the small number of patients included, that led to intergroup difference. While insignificant, the percentage of patients with comorbidity of DM and HTN tends to be higher in the aspirin group, which may have biased the results in favor of cilostazol group. In terms of lipid lowering therapy, statin use was higher in the cilostazol group, while all patients received lipid lowering agents. This may have influenced our results, for statin therapy can be associated with improvements in endothelial function [37]. In interpretation of the FMD values, while insignificant, the initial FMD values tended to be higher in the aspirin group, and this baseline difference may have affected the FMD changes. Considering the reference FMD values of our lab, there may be chance that elevations in FMD values of both groups reach a plateau at some point, and the lower baseline FMD values in cilostazol group may have biased the results. However, to our knowledge, no previous study addressing improvements of FMD have considered the issue of FMD reaching plateau levels, and such issues need to be clarified in future studies.

Conclusions

In acute cerebral ischemia patients, we compared the changes of FMD after 3 month double blinded randomized treatment with aspirin and cilostazol. Cilostazol improved endothelial function in acute cerebral ischemia patients, but aspirin did not. It also restored an inverse correlation between 3-month FMD and baseline L-arginine levels. The action of cilostazol in its roll of improving endothelial function seems to be due to activation of eNOS, as previous studies have shown. Our study emphasizes the role of cilostazol in the acute phase of cerebral ischemia, as it holds its roll in stabilization of dysfunctional endothelium, and remodeling of vessel wall structure. L-arginine and cilostazol co-administration may be considered for further improvement in endothelial function.

Abbreviations
ADMA: asymmetric dimethylarginine; cAMP: cyclic adenosine monophosphate; DM: diabetes mellitus; eNOS: endothelial nitric oxide synthase; FMD: flow mediated dilation; HTN: hypertension; NO: nitric oxide; PDE: phosphodiesterase; SAE: serious adverse events; TIA: transient ischemic attack

Acknowledgements
The authors have nothing to declare.

Funding
This study was funded by Otsuka Pharmaceutical Company, South Korea. The study sponsor provided drugs containing cilostazol and aspirin placebo, or aspirin and cilostazol placebo in the tablet form of same size, shape and color. They had no role in the study design; in the collection, analysis, and interpretation of data; in the writing of the report; and in the decision to submit the article for publication.

Authors' contributions
SJL contributed to patient data acquisition, and preparation and review of the manuscript. JSL, MHC and SEL contributed to patient data acquisition and review of the manuscript. DHS contributed to study design and patient data acquisition. JMH contributed to study design, patient data acquisition, and preparation and review of the manuscript. All authors read and approved the final manuscript.

Competing interests
The authors declare that they have no competing interests.

Author details
[1]Department of Neurology, Ajou University School of Medicine, Suwon, Republic of Korea. [2]Department of Neurology, Gachon University Gil Hospital, Incheon, Republic of Korea. [3]Department of Neurology, Ajou University School of Medicine, 164, World cup-ro, Yeongtong-gu, Suwon-si, Gyeonggi-do 16499, South Korea.

References
1. Huang Y, Cheng Y, Wu J, Li Y, Xu E, Hong Z, Li Z, Zhang W, Ding M, Gao X, et al. Cilostazol as an alternative to aspirin after ischaemic stroke: a randomised, double-blind, pilot study. The Lancet Neurology. 2008;7(6):494–9.
2. Ikeda Y, Kikuchi M, Murakami H, Satoh K, Murata M, Watanabe K, Ando Y. Comparison of the inhibitory effects of cilostazol, acetylsalicylic acid and ticlopidine on platelet functions ex vivo. Randomized, double-blind cross-over study. Arzneimittelforschung. 1987;37(5):563–6.
3. Tanaka T, Ishikawa T, Hagiwara M, Onoda K, Itoh H, Hidaka H. Effects of cilostazol, a selective cAMP phosphodiesterase inhibitor on the contraction of vascular smooth muscle. Pharmacology. 1988;36(5):313–20.
4. Ahn CW, Lee HC, Park SW, Song YD, Huh KB, Oh SJ, Kim YS, Choi YK, Kim JM, Lee TH. Decrease in carotid intima media thickness after 1 year of cilostazol treatment in patients with type 2 diabetes mellitus. Diabetes Res Clin Pract. 2001;52(1):45–53.
5. Park SW, Lee CW, Kim HS, Lee NH, Nah DY, Hong MK, Kim JJ, Park SJ. Effects of cilostazol on angiographic restenosis after coronary stent placement. Am J Cardiol. 2000;86(5):499–503.
6. Kwon SU, Cho YJ, Koo JS, Bae HJ, Lee YS, Hong KS, Lee JH, Kim JS. Cilostazol prevents the progression of the symptomatic intracranial arterial stenosis: the multicenter double-blind placebo-controlled trial of cilostazol in symptomatic intracranial arterial stenosis. Stroke. 2005;36(4):782–6.
7. Takahashi S, Oida K, Fujiwara R, Maeda H, Hayashi S, Takai H, Tamai T, Nakai T, Miyabo S. Effect of cilostazol, a cyclic AMP phosphodiesterase inhibitor, on the proliferation of rat aortic smooth muscle cells in culture. J Cardiovasc Pharmacol. 1992;20(6):900–6.
8. Wang T, Elam MB, Forbes WP, Zhong J, Nakajima K. Reduction of remnant lipoprotein cholesterol concentrations by cilostazol in patients with intermittent claudication. Atherosclerosis. 2003;171(2):337–42.
9. Shin HK, Kim YK, Kim KY, Lee JH, Hong KW. Remnant lipoprotein particles induce apoptosis in endothelial cells by NAD(P)H oxidase-mediated production of superoxide and cytokines via lectin-like oxidized low-density lipoprotein receptor-1 activation: prevention by cilostazol. Circulation. 2004;109(8):1022–8.
10. Celermajer DS, Sorensen KE, Gooch VM, Spiegelhalter DJ, Miller OI, Sullivan ID, Lloyd JK, Deanfield JE. Non-invasive detection of endothelial dysfunction in children and adults at risk of atherosclerosis. Lancet. 1992;340(8828):1111–5.
11. Ross R. The pathogenesis of atherosclerosis: a perspective for the 1990s. Nature. 1993;362(6423):801–9.
12. Deanfield JE, Halcox JP, Rabelink TJ. Endothelial function and dysfunction: testing and clinical relevance. Circulation. 2007;115(10):1285–95.
13. Durante W. Role of arginase in vessel wall remodeling. Front Immunol. 2013;4:111.
14. Katakami N, Kim YS, Kawamori R, Yamasaki Y. The phosphodiesterase inhibitor cilostazol induces regression of carotid atherosclerosis in subjects with type 2 diabetes mellitus: principal results of the diabetic atherosclerosis prevention by Cilostazol (DAPC) study: a randomized trial. Circulation. 2010;121(23):2584–91.
15. Shin DH, Lee JS, Hong JM, Kim SY. Cross-section imaging with M-mode as an alternative method for the measurement of brachial artery flow-mediated vasodilation. Journal of clinical ultrasound : JCU. 2013;41(3):158–63.
16. Jauch EC, Saver JL, Adams HP Jr, Bruno A, Connors JJ, Demaerschalk BM, Khatri P, McMullan PW Jr, Qureshi AI, Rosenfield K, et al. Guidelines for the early management of patients with acute ischemic stroke: a guideline for healthcare professionals from the American Heart Association/American Stroke Association. Stroke. 2013;44(3):870–947.
17. Lee YS, Bae HJ, Kang DW, Lee SH, Yu K, Park JM, Cho YJ, Hong KS, Kim DE, Kwon SU, et al. Cilostazol in acute ischemic stroke treatment (CAIST trial): a randomized double-blind non-inferiority trial. Cerebrovasc Dis. 2011;32(1):65–71.
18. Fujita Y, Lin JX, Takahashi R, Tomimoto H. Cilostazol alleviates cerebral small-vessel pathology and white-matter lesions in stroke-prone spontaneously hypertensive rats. Brain Res. 2008;1203:170–6.
19. Oida K, Ebata K, Kanehara H, Suzuki J, Miyamori I. Effect of cilostazol on impaired vasodilatory response of the brachial artery to ischemia in smokers. J Atheroscler Thromb. 2003;10(2):93–8.
20. Kim KS, Park HS, Jung IS, Park JH, Ahn KT, Jin SA, Park YK, Kim JH, Lee JH, Choi SW, et al. Endothelial dysfunction in the smokers can be improved with oral cilostazol treatment. Journal of cardiovascular ultrasound. 2011;19(1):21–5.
21. Jeong IS, Park JH, Jin SA, Kim JH, Lee JH, Choi SW, Jeong JO, Seong IW. Oral sarpogrelate can improve endothelial dysfunction as effectively as oral cilostazol, with fewer headaches, in active young male smokers. Heart Vessel. 2013;28(5):578–82.
22. Ikeda U, Ikeda M, Kano S, Kanbe T, Shimada K. Effect of cilostazol, a cAMP phosphodiesterase inhibitor, on nitric oxide production by vascular smooth muscle cells. Eur J Pharmacol. 1996;314(1–2):197–202.
23. Nakamura T, Houchi H, Minami A, Sakamoto S, Tsuchiya K, Niwa Y, Minakuchi K, Nakaya Y. Endothelium-dependent relaxation by cilostazol, a phosphodiesteras III inhibitor, on rat thoracic aorta. Life Sci. 2001;69(15):1709–15.
24. Rajagopalan S, Pfenninger D, Somers E, Kehrer C, Chakrabarti A, Mukherjee D, Brook R, Kaplan MJ. Effects of cilostazol in patients with Raynaud's syndrome. Am J Cardiol. 2003;92(11):1310–5.
25. Mori H, Maeda A, Wakabayashi K, Sato T, Sasai M, Tashiro K, Iso Y, Ebato M, Suzuki H. The effect of Cilostazol on endothelial function as assessed by flow-mediated dilation in patients with coronary artery disease. J Atheroscler Thromb. 2016;23(10):1168–77.
26. Creager MA, Cooke JP, Mendelsohn ME, Gallagher SJ, Coleman SM, Loscalzo J,

Dzau VJ. Impaired vasodilation of forearm resistance vessels in hypercholesterolemic humans. J Clin Invest. 1990;86(1):228–34.
27. Bragulat E, de la Sierra A, Antonio MT, Coca A. Endothelial dysfunction in salt-sensitive essential hypertension. Hypertension. 2001;37(2 Pt 2):444–8.
28. Watts GF, Playford DA. Dyslipoproteinaemia and hyperoxidative stress in the pathogenesis of endothelial dysfunction in non-insulin dependent diabetes mellitus: an hypothesis. Atherosclerosis. 1998;141(1):17–30.
29. Landmesser U, Hornig B, Drexler H. Endothelial function: a critical determinant in atherosclerosis? Circulation. 2004;109(21 Suppl 1):II27–33.
30. Boger RH. The pharmacodynamics of L-arginine. J Nutr. 2007;137(6 Suppl 2):1650S–5S.
31. Perticone F, Sciacqua A, Maio R, Perticone M, Maas R, Boger RH, Tripepi G, Sesti G, Zoccali C. Asymmetric dimethylarginine, L-arginine, and endothelial dysfunction in essential hypertension. J Am Coll Cardiol. 2005;46(3):518–23.
32. Zoccali C, Bode-Boger S, Mallamaci F, Benedetto F, Tripepi G, Malatino L, Cataliotti A, Bellanuova I, Fermo I, Frolich J, et al. Plasma concentration of asymmetrical dimethylarginine and mortality in patients with end-stage renal disease: a prospective study. Lancet. 2001;358(9299):2113–7.
33. Boger RH, Bode-Boger SM, Szuba A, Tsao PS, Chan JR, Tangphao O, Blaschke TF, Cooke JP. Asymmetric dimethylarginine (ADMA): a novel risk factor for endothelial dysfunction: its role in hypercholesterolemia. Circulation. 1998;98(18):1842–7.
34. Hashimoto A, Miyakoda G, Hirose Y, Mori T. Activation of endothelial nitric oxide synthase by cilostazol via a cAMP/protein kinase A- and phosphatidylinositol 3-kinase/Akt-dependent mechanism. Atherosclerosis. 2006;189(2):350–7.
35. Bode-Boger SM, Muke J, Surdacki A, Brabant G, Boger RH, Frolich JC. Oral L-arginine improves endothelial function in healthy individuals older than 70 years. Vasc Med. 2003;8(2):77–81.
36. Bode-Boger SM, Scalera F, Ignarro LJ. The L-arginine paradox: importance of the L-arginine/asymmetrical dimethylarginine ratio. Pharmacol Ther. 2007;114(3):295–306.
37. Frick M, Alber HF, Hugel H, Schwarzacher SP, Pachinger O, Weidinger F. Short- and long-term changes of flow-mediated vasodilation in patients under statin therapy. Clin Cardiol. 2002;25(6):291–4.

3

Current smoking is associated with extracranial carotid atherosclerotic stenosis but not with intracranial large artery disease

Ruijun Ji[1,2,3,4,5], Yuesong Pan[2,3], Hongyi Yan[2,3], Runhua Zhang[2,3], Gaifen Liu[1,2,3,4], Penglian Wang[1,2,3,4], Yilong Wang[1,2,3,4], Hao Li[2,3], Xingquan Zhao[1,2,3,4], Yongjun Wang[1,2,3,4,6*] On behalf of The Chinese Intracranial Atherosclerosis (CICAS) Study investigators

Abstract

Background: Accumulating evidence has shown that cigarette smoking is an important risk factor for ischemic stroke. However, it is not clear about the potential mechanisms through which cigarette smoking affects stroke risk. In the study, we aimed to investigate the relationship between cigarette smoking and the occurrence of extracranial (ECAS) and intracranial atherosclerotic stenosis (ICAS).

Methods: We analyzed patients enrolled in the Chinese intracranial atherosclerosis (CICAS), which was a prospective, multicenter, hospital-based cohort study. Smoking status was classified into never, former and current smoking. For those patients with current smoking, data on time duration (year) and extent (the number of cigarette smoked per day) was recorded and pack year of smoking was calculated. ICAS was evaluated with 3-dimentional time-of-flight MRA and ECAS was evaluated with cervical ultrasonography or contrast-enhanced MRA. Multivariable Logistic regression was performed to identify the association between smoking status and the occurrence of ECAS and ICAS.

Results: A total of 2656 patients (92.7%) of acute ischemic stroke and 208 (7.3%) of transient ischemic attack were analyzed. The mean age was 61.9 ± 11.2 and 67.8% were male. There were 141 (4.9%) patients had only ECAS, 1074 (37.5%) had only ICAS, and 261 (9.1%) had both ECAS and ICAS. Current smoking was significantly associated with the occurrence of ECAS (adjusted OR = 1.47, 95% CI = 1.09–1.99, $P < 0.01$). In addition, with 1 year of smoking increment, the risk of ECAS increased by 1.1% (adjusted OR = 1.011; 95% CI = 1.003–1.019; $P = 0.005$); with one cigarette smoked per day increment, the risk of ECAS increased by 1.0% (adjusted OR = 1.010; 95% CI = 1.001–1.020; $P = 0.03$); and with one pack year of smoking increment, the risk of ECAS increased by 0.7% (adjusted OR = 1.007; 95% CI = 1.002–1.012; $P < 0.01$). However, no significant association was found between smoking status and the occurrence of ICAS.

Conclusion: A dose–response relationship was identified between cigarette smoking and the occurrence of ECAS, but not ICAS. Further studies on molecular mechanisms were warranted.

Keywords: Stroke, Smoking, Extracranial atherosclerotic stenosis, Intracranial atherosclerotic stenosis, Association

* Correspondence: yongjunwang1962@gmail.com
[1]Department of Neurology, Tiantan Comprehensive Stroke Center, Tiantan Hospital, Capital Medical University, Beijing, China
[2]China National Clinical Research Center for Neurological Diseases, Beijing, China
Full list of author information is available at the end of the article

Background

Cigarette smoking is responsible for approximately five million deaths every year and there are still an estimated 1.1 billion smokers worldwide [1–3]. Accumulating evidence has shown that cigarette smoking is an important risk factor for first ischemic stroke [4]. In contrast to extensive data on association between cigarette smoking and risk for first stroke, data on its association with recurrent stroke are sparse [5]. In the Cardiovascular Health Study, cigarette smoking was associated with a 2-fold increased risk for stroke recurrence in the elderly [6].

The mechanisms through which cigarette smoking affects stroke risk have been a topic of interest over the last several years. Although it is not fully understood, cigarette smoking likely contributes to increased stroke risk through both short-term effect on thrombus generation in atherosclerotic arteries and long-term effect related to the development of atherosclerotic stenosis [7]. Clinically, atherosclerotic stenosis of cervicocephalic arteries could be classified into extracranial (ECAS) and intracranial atherosclerotic stenosis (ICAS). ECAS is the most common vascular lesion found in stroke patients of White. In contrast, ICAS is found more common among stroke patients of Asian, Black, and Hispanic ancestry [8]. Thus far, limited is known about the potential role of cigarette smoking in the development of ECAS and ICAS.

In the present study, we aimed to clarify the relationship between time duration, the number of cigarette smoked per day and pack years of smoking and the occurrence of ECAS and ICAS.

Methods

Study population

This study was based on the Chinese intracranial atherosclerosis (CICAS) study [9], which was a prospective, multicenter, hospital-based cohort study aimed at clarifying the prevalence and risk of recurrent stroke in patients with intracranial large artery occlusive disease. Briefly, 22 general hospitals covering a wide geographic area in China participated in the CICAS. The inclusion criteria of CICAS study were: (1) age between 18 and 80 years; (2) hospitalized with a primary diagnosis of acute ischemic stroke (AIS) or transient ischemic attack (TIA) according to the World Health Organization criteria; (3) stroke confirmed by head computerized tomography (CT) and/or brain magnetic resonance imaging (MRI); (4) time from symptom onset to hospitalization < 7 days. The CICAS study excluded those patients who were: (1) with known source for cardioembolism; (2) disabled before admission (modified Rankin Scale [mRS] score > 2); (3) physically or subjectively unable to comply with MRI examination; (4) clinically unstable or required close monitoring or were moribund. The CICAS study had been approved by the institutional review board (IRB) at each participating hospital. All participants provided written informed consent.

Study variables

Clinical characteristics

In the CICAS network, a standardized case report form (CRF) was used for data collection. For the present study, the following candidate variables were analyzed: (1) demographics (age and gender); (2) stroke risk factors: hypertension (defined by a history of hypertension, or being treated with an antihypertensive agent before admission, or diagnosed at discharge), diabetes mellitus (defined by a history of diabetes mellitus, or being treated for diabetes mellitus or glycosylated hemoglobin ≥ 7%, or diagnosis at discharge), dyslipidemia (defined as a self-reported history, current use of lipid-lowering medications, total cholesterol level ≥ 5.7 mmol/L, or triglyceride level ≥ 1.7 mmol/L on admission), family history of stroke, history of cerebral ischemia (including a history of ischemic stroke and TIA), history of hemorrhagic stroke (including intracerebral hemorrhage and subarachnoid hemorrhage), heart disease (defined as a history of myocardial infarction, angina pectoris, and congestive heart failure), smoking status, and heavy drinking (drinking >2 units per day on average for men or >1 unit per day on average for women); (3) comorbidities: chronic obstructive pulmonary disease (COPD), hepatic cirrhosis, peptic ulcer or previous gastrointestinal bleeding (GIB), arthritis, Alzheimer's disease/dementia, cancer and peripheral angiopathy; (4) Admission systolic (SBP) and diastolic blood pressure (DBP) (mmHg); (5) Admission National Institutes of Health Stroke Scale (NIHSS) score; (6) admission blood tests: fasting blood glucose (mmol/L), triglyceride (TG) (mmol/L), cholesterol (TC) (mmol/L), high density lipoprotein (HDL) (mmol/L) and low density lipoprotein (LDL) (mmol/L).

Smoking status

In the CICAS study, smoking status was classified into never, former and current smoking. Current smoking was defined as a patient who had smoked continuously for 6 months with at least one cigarette per day. Former smoking was defined as a patient who was used to smoke but not satisfied the criteria of current smoking. For those patients with current smoking, data on time duration (year) and extent (the number of cigarette smoked per day) was recorded and pack year of smoking was calculated. The pack year is a unit for measuring the amount a person has smoked over a long period of time. It is calculated by multiplying the number of packs of cigarettes smoked per day by the number of years the person has smoked.

Vascular imaging of ECAS and ICAS

In the CICAS study, all patients underwent conventional MRI on a 3.0-T or 1.5-T MR scanner, including sequences of 3-D time-of-flight MRA, T_2/T_1-weighted imaging, fluid-attenuated inversion recovery sequences (FLAIR), and diffusion-weighted imaging (DWI). All MRI and MRA images were read centrally by two readers who were blinded to patients' clinical information. Disagreement involving more than 10% degree of stenosis was resolved by an appointed senior reader who decided the final classification. The following arterial segments were assessed: 1) bilateral extracranial and intracranial internal carotid artery (ICA), anterior cerebral artery (ACA) A1/A2, middle cerebral artery (MCA) M1/M2, posterior cerebral artery (PCA) P1/P2 and basilar artery (BA). The degree of intracranial stenosis on MRA was calculated using the method of the WASID study [10] and was classified into four groups: <50% or no stenosis, 50% to 69%, 70% to 99%, and occlusion. The extracranial internal carotid artery was evaluated with ultrasonography according to the published diagnostic criteria [11] or by contrast-enhanced MRA. In the present study, significant stenosis was defined as a more than 50% atherosclerotic stenosis or occlusion of the large intracranial and/or extracranial arteries. Based on the presence and location of cerebral atherosclerotic stenosis, patients were classified into four groups: 1) without ECAS or ICAS; 2) with only ECAS; 3) with only ICAS; and 4) with both ECAS and ICAS.

Statistical analysis

Continuous variables were summarized with mean and standard deviation (SD) or median and interquartile range (IQR); categorical variables were summarized as proportions. In univariate analysis, Chi-square or Fisher exact test was used to compare categorical variables and one way analysis of variance or Kruskal-Wallis test was employed to compare continuous variables. In multivariable analysis, Logistic regression was performed to assess association between smoking status (never, former and current smoking) and the occurrence of ECAS, ICAS and specific location of ICAS (intracranial ICA, MCA, ACA, PCA and BA). Logistic regression adjusted for demographics (age and gender), stroke risk factors, comorbidities, admission NIHSS score, admission SBP and DBP, and admission blood tests. All tests were 2-tailed and statistical significance was determined at α level of 0.05. Statistical analysis was performed using SAS 9.1 (SAS Institute, Cary, NC) and SPSS 17.0 (SPSS Inc., Chicago, IL).

Results

Patient characteristics

Patient characteristics are shown in Table 1. A total of 2864 patients (2656 [92.7%] of AIS and 208 [7.3%] of TIA) were enrolled in the CICAS network. The mean age was 61.9 ± 11.2 and 67.8% were male. There were 1568 (54.8%) patients who never smoked, 247 (8.6%) with former smoking and 1049 (36.6%) with current smoking. A total number of 1476 (51.5%) patients had either ECAS or ICAS. Compared with patients without ECAS or ICAS, those developed ECAS or ICAS were more common for older age, male gender, presence of diabetes mellitus, hypertension, dyslipidemia and cerebral ischemia, family history of stroke, current or former smoking, higher NIHSS score, higher blood glucose, and lower blood HDL (Table 1).

Proportion of ECAS and ICAS

The proportions of ECAS and ICAS in the CICAS study are shown in Additional file 1: Table S1. A total number of 141 (4.9%) patients had only ECAS, 1074 (37.5%) had only ICAS, and 261 (9.1%) had both ECAS and ICAS. For those patients developing ICAS, the most frequent location was MCA stenosis (29.6%), then followed by PCA stenosis (18.6%), ACA stenosis (7.7%), BA stenosis (6.3%), and intracranial ICA (2.3%) (Additional file 1: Table S1).

Association between smoking status and ECAS or ICAS

Association between smoking status and the occurrence of ECAS or ICAS is shown in Table 2. Compared with patients never smoked, those with current smoking were significantly associated with the occurrence of ECAS (adjusted OR = 1.47, 95% CI = 1.09–1.99, $P < 0.01$). Although there is a trend that former smoking was associated with ECAS (adjusted for age, gender, and stroke risk factors), it did not reach statistical significance after adjusting all potential confounders (adjusted OR = 1.42, 95% CI = 0.92–2.18, $P = 0.11$). When combining former and current smoking together, ever smoking was significantly associated with the occurrence of ECAS (adjusted OR = 1.46, 95% CI = 1.09–1.94, $P < 0.01$). However, no similar association was found between cigarette smoking and the occurrence of ICAS or specific location of ICAS (intracranial ICA, MCA, ACA, PCA and BA) (Table 2).

Association between time duration of smoking and ECAS or ICAS

Association between time duration of smoking and the occurrence of ECAS or ICAS was investigated in the subgroup of patients who were with never and current smoking ($n = 2617$). The risk of ECAS increased steadily with longer time duration of smoking (Fig. 1a). After adjusting for all potential confounders, significant association was found between time duration of smoking and the occurrence of ECAS. With 1 year of smoking increment, the risk of developing ECAS increased by 1.1% (adjusted OR = 1.011; 95% CI = 1.003–1.019; $P = 0.005$).

Table 1 Baseline characteristics

Variables	Overall (*n* = 2864)	No ECAS or ICAS (*n* = 1388)	Only ECAS (*n* = 141)	Only ICAS (*n* = 1074)	ECAS + ICAS (*n* = 261)	*P* value
Age (Mean ± SD)	61.9 ± 11.2	61.2 ± 11.2	64.7 ± 10.4	62.1 ± 11.5	63.6 ± 10.1	<0.001
Gender (male)	1944(67.8)	938(67.6)	110(78.0)	696(64.8)	200(76.6)	<0.001
Stroke risk factors						
Diabetes mellitus	991(34.6)	414(29.3)	50(35.5)	418(38.9)	109(41.8)	<0.001
Hypertension	2238(78.1)	1056(76.1)	105(74.5)	866(80.6)	211(80.8)	0.02
Hyperlipidemia	2173(75.9)	1042(75.1)	119(84.4)	807(75.1)	205(78.5)	0.05
Family history of stroke	296(10.3)	122(8.8)	16(11.4)	112(10.4)	46(17.6)	<0.001
History of cerebral ischemia	2018(70.5)	930(67.0)	117(83.0)	772(71.9)	199(76.3)	<0.001
History of hemorrhagic stroke	54(1.9)	29(2.1)	3(2.1)	19(1.8)	3(1.2)	0.73
Coronary heart disease	228(8.0)	102(7.4)	17(12.1)	88(8.2)	21(8.1)	0.30
Heavy drinking	142(5.0)	66(4.8)	9(6.4)	51(4.8)	16(6.1)	0.66
Smoking status						<0.001
Never smoker	1568(54.8)	774(55.8)	53(37.6)	623 (58.0)	118 (45.2)	
Former smoker	247(8.6)	118(8.5)	17(12.1)	84 (7.8)	28 (10.7)	
Current smoker	1049(36.6)	496(35.7)	71(50.4)	367 (34.2)	115 (40.1)	
Comorbidities						
COPD	12(0.4)	8(0.6)	1(0.7)	2(0.2)	1(0.4)	0.47
Hepatic cirrhosis	7(0.2)	1(0.1)	0(0.0)	5(0.5)	1(0.4)	0.22
Peptic ulcer or previous GIB	80(2.8)	43(3.1)	6(4.3)	23(2.1)	8(3.1)	0.34
Arthritis	46(1.6)	16(1.2)	3(2.1)	26(2.4)	1(0.4)	0.03
Dementia	19(0.7)	8(0.6)	1(0.7)	9(0.8)	1(0.4)	0.81
Cancer	48(1.7)	23(1.7)	5(3.6)	17(1.6)	3(1.2)	0.32
Peripheral angiopathy	21(0.7)	9(0.7)	1(0.7)	7(0.7)	4(1.5)	0.47
Index event						0.01
Transient ischemic attack	208(7.3)	106(7.6)	19(13.5)	62(5.8)	21(8.1)	
Acute ischemic stroke	2656(92.7)	1282(92.4)	122(86.5)	1012(94.2))	240(92.0)	
SBP at admission, mm Hg (median, IQR)	150(135–167)	150(136–165)	150(130–165)	150(135–170)	150(135–162)	0.31
DBP at admission, mm Hg (median, IQR)	88(80–95)	89(80–96)	85(80–90)	87(80–95)	85(80–95)	0.23
NIHSS at admission (median, IQR)	4(1–7)	3(1–5)	3(1–5)	4(2–8)	5(2–10)	<0.001
Fasting blood glucose, mmol/L (median, IQR)	5.4(4.8–6.8)	5.3(4.7–6.6)	5.3(4.8–6.2)	5.7(4.9–7.2)	5.8(4.8–7.1)	<0.001
TG, mmol/L (median, IQR)	1.5(1.1–2.1)	1.5(1.1–2.2)	1.6(1.1–2.1)	1.5(1.1–2.1)	1.4(1.1–2.0)	0.15
TC, mmol/L (median, IQR)	4.66(4.00–5.38)	4.67(4.06–5.40)	4.58(3.87–5.33)	4.68(3.98–5.38)	4.50(3.95–5.35)	0.15
HDL, mmol/L (median, IQR)	1.12(0.96–1.32)	1.15(0.98–1.36)	1.08(0.95–1.29)	1.09(0.95–1.29)	1.08(0.91–1.27)	<0.001
LDL, mmol/L (median, IQR)	2.82(2.27–3.45)	2.83(2.26–3.43)	2.74(2.28–3.40)	2.84(2.28–3.47)	2.82(2.25–3.49)	0.91

Abbreviations: *ICAS* indicates intracranial atherosclerotic stenosis, *ECAS* extracranial atherosclerotic stenosis, *SD* standard deviation, *COPD* chronic obstructive pulmonary disease, *GIB* gastrointestinal bleeding, *SBP* systolic blood pressure, *DBP* diastolic blood pressure, *IQR* interquartile range, *NIHSS* National Institutes of Health Stroke Scale, *TG* triglyceride, *TC* cholesterol, *HDL* high density lipoprotein, *LDL* low density lipoprotein

However, no significant association was found between time duration of smoking and the occurrence of ICAS or specific location of ICAS (intracranial ICA, MCA, ACA, PCA and BA) (Additional file 1: Table S2).

Association between extent of smoking and ECAS or ICAS

Association between extent of smoking and the occurrence of ECAS or ICAS was investigated in the subgroup of patients who were with never and current smoking (n = 2617). The risk of ECAS increased steadily with larger amount of cigarette smoked per day (Fig. 1b). After adjusting for all potential confounders, significant association was found between the number of cigarette smoked per day and the occurrence of ECAS. With one cigarette smoked per day increment, the risk of developing ECAS increased by 1.0% (adjusted OR = 1.010; 95% CI = 1.001–1.020; P = 0.03).

Table 2 Association between smoking status and ECAS and ICAS in all enrolled patients (N = 2864)

Arterial stenosis	Category	Unadjusted OR	P value	Adjusted OR_1	P value	Adjusted OR_2	P value	Adjusted OR_3	P value
ECAS	Previous smoking vs. never	1.82(1.27–2.61)	0.001	1.57(1.07–2.30)	0.02	1.49(1.01–2.09)	0.04	1.42(0.92–2.18)	0.11
	Current smoking vs. never	1.76(1.41–2.20)	<0.001	1.82(1.39–2.38)	<0.001	1.74(1.33–2.27)	<0.001	1.47(1.09–1.99)	<0.01
	Smoking vs. never	1.77(1.43–2.19)	<0.001	1.76(1.36–2.26)	<0.001	1.67(1.30–2.16)	<0.001	1.46(1.09–1.94)	<0.01
ICAS	Previous smoking vs. never	0.93(0.71–1.21)	0.58	0.94(0.71–1.25)	0.66	0.91(0.69–1.22)	0.54	1.01(0.71–1.44)	0.95
	Current smoking vs. never	0.95(0.81–1.11)	0.51	1.01(0.84–1.22)	0.91	0.99(0.82–1.20)	0.93	0.92(0.73–1.15)	0.45
	Smoking vs. never	0.94(0.82–1.10)	0.45	1.00(0.83–1.19)	0.95	0.97(0.82–1.17)	0.77	0.93(0.75–1.16)	0.53
Intra-ICA	Previous smoking vs. never	1.61(0.96–2.72)	0.07	1.42(0.98–2.11)	0.21	1.39(0.80–2.42)	0.25	1.26(0.65–2.45)	0.50
	Current smoking vs. never	1.58(1.14–2.18)	0.005	1.44(0.82–2.47)	0.06	1.34(0.91–1.98)	0.14	1.13(0.71–1.79)	0.61
	Smoking vs. never	1.58(1.16–2.16)	0.003	1.43(0.99–2.07)	0.05	1.35(0.94–1.95)	0.11	1.15(0.74–1.79)	0.52
MCA	Previous smoking vs. never	1.01(0.75–1.36)	0.94	1.01(0.74–1.37)	0.97	0.99(0.73–1.36)	0.97	1.05(0.72–1.53)	0.79
	Current smoking vs. never	1.03(0.87–1.23)	0.70	1.02(0.83–1.25)	0.86	1.01(0.82–1.24)	0.94	0.89(0.70–1.14)	0.36
	Smoking vs. never	1.03(0.88–1.21)	0.73	1.02(0.84–1.23)	0.87	1.01(0.83–1.22)	0.96	0.92(0.73–1.16)	0.50
ACA	Previous smoking vs. never	1.01(0.62–1.65)	0.97	1.17(0.69–1.97)	0.56	1.12(0.66–1.89)	0.69	0.93(0.49–1.76)	0.83
	Current smoking vs. never	0.86(0.63–1.16)	0.31	1.09(0.76–1.56)	0.64	1.04(0.73–1.50)	0.82	1.00(0.65–1.54)	0.99
	Smoking vs. never	0.89(0.67–1.17)	0.39	1.11(0.79–1.55)	0.56	1.06(0.75–1.49)	0.74	0.99(0.66–1.48)	0.94
PCA	Previous smoking vs. never	1.16(0.84–1.60)	0.37	1.29(0.92–1.83)	0.14	1.24(0.88–1.76)	0.22	1.40(0.93–2.11)	0.10
	Current smoking vs. never	0.71(0.58–0.88)	0.001	0.91(0.71–1.16)	0.45	0.88(0.68–1.13)	0.32	0.92(0.68–1.23)	0.57
	Smoking vs. never	0.79(0.65–0.96)	0.01	0.99(0.79–1.25)	0.94	0.96(0.76–1.21)	0.72	1.02(0.77–1.34)	0.90
BA	Previous smoking vs. never	0.91(0.53–1.56)	0.73	0.90(0.51–1.60)	0.73	0.83(0.47–1.47)	0.52	0.79(0.40–1.53)	0.48
	Current smoking vs. never	0.71(0.51–1.00)	0.05	0.81(0.55–1.20)	0.30	0.81(0.54–1.20)	0.28	0.88(0.56–1.40)	0.59
	Smoking vs. never	0.75(0.55–1.02)	0.07	0.83(0.58–1.20)	0.33	0.81(0.56–1.17)	0.26	0.86(0.56–1.32)	0.48

Abbreviations: *ICAS* indicates intracranial atherosclerotic stenosis, *ECAS* extracranial atherosclerotic stenosis, *OR* odds ration, *Intra-ICA* intracranial internal carotid artery, *MCA* middle cerebral artery, *ACA* anterior cerebral artery, *PCA* posterior cerebral artery, *BA* basilar artery

OR_1 adjusted for demographics (age and gender). OR_2 adjusted for demographics (age and gender) and stroke risk factors (diabetes mellitus, hypertension, dyslipidemia, family history of stroke, history of cerebral ischemia, history of hemorrhagic stroke, heart disease). OR_3 adjusted for all potential confounders including demographics, (age and gender), stroke risk factors (diabetes mellitus, hypertension, dyslipidemia, family history of stroke, history of cerebral ischemia, history of hemorrhagic stroke, heart disease), comorbidities (COPD, hepatic cirrhosis, peptic ulcer or previous GIB, arthritis, dementia, cancer and peripheral angiopathy), admission NIHSS, admission SBP and DBP, and admission blood tests (fasting blood glucose, TG, TC, HDL and LDL)

However, no significant association was found between extent of smoking and the occurrence of ICAS or specific location of ICAS (intracranial ICA, MCA, ACA, PCA and BA) (Additional file 1: Table S3).

Association between pack years of smoking and ECAS or ICAS

Association between pack years of smoking and the occurrence of ECAS or ICAS was investigated in the subgroup of patients who were with never and current smoking (n = 2617). The risk of ECAS increased steadily with larger number of pack years of smoking (Fig. 1c). After adjusting for all potential confounders, significant association was found between pack years of smoking and the occurrence of ECAS. With one pack year of smoking increment, the risk of developing ECAS increased by 0.7% (adjusted OR = 1.007; 95% CI = 1.002–1.012; P < 0.01). However, no significant association was found between pack years of smoking and the occurrence of ICAS or specific location of ICAS (intracranial ICA, MCA, ACA, PCA and BA) (Additional file 1: Table S4).

Discussion

In the present study, we systematically investigated the relationship between cigarette smoking and the occurrence of ECAS and ICAS. It was found that cigarette smoking was significantly associated with the occurrence of ECAS. In addition, dose–response relationship between time duration, extent and pack years of cigarette smoking and the occurrence of ECAS was identified. However, no similar association was found between cigarette smoking and the occurrence of ICAS or specific location of ICAS (intracranial ICA, MCA, ACA, PCA, and BA).

The evidence linking cigarette smoking to stroke is extremely convincing and dose–response relationship has been well established [4, 5, 12–14]. However, the mechanisms through which cigarette smoking affects stroke risk are not well understood and have been a topic of interest over the last decades. Cigarette smoking likely contributes to increased stroke risk through both short-term effect on thrombus generation in atherosclerotic arteries and long-term effect on the development of

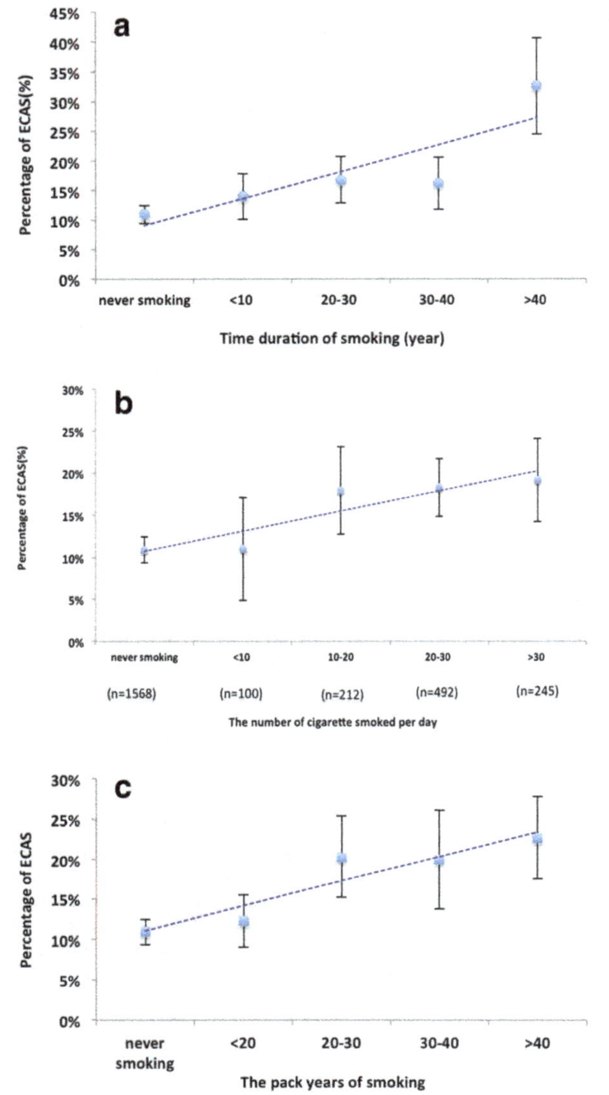

Fig. 1 relationship between cigarette smoking the development of extracranial atherosclerotic stenosis (ECAS). The risk of ECAS increased steadily with longer time duration (**a**), larger amount of cigarette smoked per day (**b**), and larger number of pack years (**c**) of smoking

atherosclerotic stenosis. Thus far, several studies have investigated the relationship between cigarette smoking and the occurrence of extracranial or intracranial atherosclerosis. To evaluate the prevalence and risk factors of asymptomatic carotid artery disease, Dr. Willeit and Kiechl analyzed a sample drawn from the community-based Study and found that pack years of smoking was the leading risk factor of carotid atherosclerosis in men [15]. In a cross-sectional study carried out in patients attending a lipid clinic, Dr. Baldassarre and his colleagues found that carotid intima-media thickness was significantly associated with pack years of smoking in both former and current smokers [14]. In the Atherosclerosis Risk in Communities (ARIC) Study, Dr. Howard and his colleagues found that exposure to cigarette smoking was associated with progression of atherosclerosis. Relative to never smokers, current cigarette smoking was associated with 50% increase and past smoking was associated with 25% increase in intimal-medial thickness of carotid artery over 3 years follow-up [16]. By using transcranial Doppler ultrasonography in patients who had at least one vascular risk factor of hypertension, diabetes, or hyperlipidemia, Dr. Wong and his colleagues found that age, hypertension, diabetes, and hyperlipidemia were associated with the occurrence of MCA stenosis; however, cigarette smoking was not significant [17]. Based on data from a consecutive series of subjects aged more than 40 years and without history of stroke, Dr. Bae and his colleagues found that age, hypertension, and diabetes were significantly associated with the occurrence of ICAS; however, no significant association was observed with regard to male gender, cigarette smoking and hyperlipidemia [18]. In a meta analysis including 15 Asian studies, Dr. Ding and his colleagues found that female or patients with metabolic syndrome were more likely to suffer from ICAS than ECAS; whereas, the smoker or patients with dyslipidemia were more likely to suffer from ECAS than ICAS [19]. Similar with these findings, our study verified that cigarette smoking was more associated with ECAS than ICAS. In addition, our study provided further evidence to indicate a dose–response relationship between cigarette smoking and the occurrence of ECAS. It was shown that with 1 year of smoking, one cigarette smoked per day, and one pack year of smoking increment, the risk of developing ECAS increased by 1.0, 1.1 and 0.7%, respectively. These numbers not only quantitatively showed the detrimental effect of cigarette smoking on cerebral atherosclerosis, but also suggested the potential effect of smoking cessation on stroke prevention. If we assumes an attributable risk of stroke as associated with ECAS of 0.4% per year [20] and the mean direct medical cost of ischemic stroke during acute hospitalization of 10,000 RMB (≈1548.25 US dollar with the exchange rate of 6.4589), taken in conjunction with the 350,000,000 smokers in China, then, if all Chinese stopped smoking, there would be 3,500,000 fewer ECAS and 14,000 fewer strokes every year. The cost benefits alone would be enormous, potentially saving 140,000,000 RMB (≈21,675,517.50 US dollar) per year spent on acute stroke care in China.

Although a clear association between smoking and health risk has long been established, the prevalence of smoking in our society remains alarmingly high. Smoking can be potentially reduced by population and individual-related measures. Smoke-free laws in certain areas have already been shown to be effective in reducing heart disease [21], declining in heart disease death [22], and improving health outcomes [23]. In addition, nowadays, smokers have more help than ever before to quit successfully [24, 25]. Given the clear evidence that intervention can lead to healthy change, clinicians, researchers, policymaker, social workers, smokers and their relatives should be organized together to establish reliable, feasible, and cost-effective networks and pathways to create an environment in which smoking is unacceptable and to decrease the burden of smoking on health continuously.

Indeed, limited is known about the molecular mechanisms underlying the paradoxical relationship between cigarette smoking and the development of ECAS and ICAS. Previous studies have shown that cigarette smoke exposure had complex and extensive roles in vasomotor dysfunction, inflammation, oxidative stress and modification of lipids [26–28], which are integral components for initiation and progression of atherosclerosis. Due to sorts of difference in anatomical structure and local hemodynamics, these intermediate factors induced by cigarette smoking might have different role in the development of intracranial and extracranial atherosclerosis. Further studies on molecular mechanisms are warranted.

Our study has limitations that deserve mention. First, like all observational studies, we cannot rule out the possibility that additional variable (unmeasured confounders, e.g. medications used before hospitalization) might have some impact on ECAS and ICAS. Second, our study included only hospitalized patients and those patients died in emergency room, treated in outpatient clinics and asymptomatic patients were not included. In addition, our study required informed consent and selection bias was inevitable [29]. Third, in our study, intracranial artery stenosis was evaluated with 3-D time-of-flight MRA. Currently, digital subtract angiography (DSA) remains the gold standard for the diagnosis of arterial stenosis. Although MRA is noninvasive and more easily accessible compared with DSA [30], time-of-flight MRA is prone to artifacts because of flow abnormalities [31]. Finally, information on environmental tobacco smoke was not collected. Evidence has shown that exposure to environmental tobacco smoke is an established risk factor for heart disease [32, 33]. Meanwhile, we did not collect relevant information on the type of cigarette smoked by the subjects. With these kinds of information included in the study, we would have more convincing conclusion.

Conclusion

We found a paradoxical dose–response relationship between cigarette smoking and the occurrence of ECAS and ICAS. Our study would encourage further studies to clarify molecular mechanisms underlying the different role of cigarette smoking in the development of ECAS and ICAS, as hopefully would pave ways to develop different acute care and preventive strategies for stroke patients with different smoking status.

Additional file

Additional file 1: Table S1. Proportion of intracranial and extracranial atherosclerotic stenosis. Showed the proportion of intracranial and extracranial atherosclerotic stenosis (n = 2864). **Table S2.** Association between time duration of smoking and ECAS and ICAS in subgroup of patients with never and current smoking. Showed the association between time duration of smoking and ECAS and ICAS in subgroup of patients with never and current smoking (n = 2617). **Table S3.** Association between extent of smoking and ECAS and ICAS in subgroup of patients with never and current smoking. Showed the Association between extent of smoking and ECAS and ICAS in subgroup of patients with never and current smoking (n = 2617).

Abbreviations

ACA: Anterior cerebral artery; AIS: Acute ischemic stroke; BA: Basilar artery; CICAS study: the Chinese intracranial atherosclerosis (CICAS) study; COPD: Chronic obstructive pulmonary disease; CRF: Case Report Form; CT: Computerized tomography; DBP: Diastolic blood pressure; DSA: Digital subtract angiography; DWI: Diffusion-weighted imaging; ECAS: Extracranial atherosclerotic stenosis; FLAIR: Fluid-attenuated inversion recovery sequences; GIB: Gastrointestinal bleeding; HDL: High density lipoprotein; ICA: Internal carotid artery; ICAS: Intracranial atherosclerotic stenosis; IQR: Interquartile range; IRB: Institutional Review Board; LDL: Low density lipoprotein; MCA: Middle cerebral artery; MRI: Magnetic resonance imaging; mRS: modified Rankin Scale; NIHSS: National Institutes of Health Stroke Scale; PCA: Posterior cerebral artery; SBP: Systolic blood pressure; SD: Standard deviation; TC: Cholesterol; TG: Triglyceride; TIA: Transient ischemic attack

Funding

This study was funded by the Ministry of Science and Technology and the Ministry of Health of the People's Republic of China, National S&T Major Project of China (2008ZX09312–008), State Key Development Program of Basic Research of China (2009CB521905), and partially supported by the Nova Program of Beijing Science and Technology Commission (Dr. Ji, 2008B30), National Natural Science Foundation of China (Dr. Ji, 81,471,208, 81,641,162) and Beijing high-level healthy human resource project (215 Project) (Dr. Ji, 2014–3- 033).

Authors' contributions

RJ and YW (Yongjun Wang) conceived of the study, participated in its design, and drafted the manuscript. HY and YP carried out statistical analysis. RJ, YP, HY, RH, GL, PW, YW (Yilong Wang), HL, XZ, YW (Yongjun Wang) participated in analysis or interpretation of data, and revised the manuscript for important intellectual content. All authors read and approved the final manuscript.

Competing interests

The authors declare that they have no competing interests.

Ethics approval and consent to participate

This study was based on the Chinese intracranial atherosclerosis (CICAS) study, which had been approved by the institutional review board (IRB) of all participating hospital (IRB at Beijing Tiantan Hospital of Capital Medical University, Beijing;; IRB at Beijing Tongren Hospital of Capital Medical University, Beijing; IRB at Shanghai Sixth People's Hospital, Shanghai; IRB at Tianjin Huanhu Hosptial, Tianjin; IRB at Shanxi Provincial People's Hospital, Xi'an, Shanxi; IRB at The First Affiliated Hospital of Xiamen University, Xiamen, Fujian; IRB at Xiangya Hospital Central South University, Changsha, Hunan; IRB at No. 3 People's Hospital of Chengdu, Chengdu, Sichuan; IRB at The First Affiliated Hospital of Jinan University (Guangzhou Overseas Hospital), Guangzhou, Guangdong; IRB at Handan Central Hospital, Handan, Heibei; IRB at Handan First People's Hospital, Handan, Heibei; IRB at Qingdao Municipal Hospital, Qingdao, Shandong; IRB at The First Affiliated Hospital of Zhengzhou University, Zhengzhou, Henan; IRB at The First Affiliated Hospital of Wenzhou Medical College (the First Provincial Wenzhou Hospital of Zhejiang), Wenzhou, Zhejiang; IRB at

The Affiliated Kailuan Hospital, North China Coal Medical College, Tangshan, Hebei; IRB at The First Affiliated Hospital of Beifang Medical College, Zhangjiakou, Hebei; and IRB at Shijiazhuang Center Hospital, Shijiazhuang, Hebei). All participants provided written informed consent.

Author details
[1]Department of Neurology, Tiantan Comprehensive Stroke Center, Tiantan Hospital, Capital Medical University, Beijing, China. [2]China National Clinical Research Center for Neurological Diseases, Beijing, China. [3]Center of Stroke, Beijing Institute for Brain Disorders, Beijing, China. [4]Beijing Key Laboratory of Translational Medicine for Cerebrovascular Disease, Beijing, China. [5]Beijing Key Laboratory of Brain Function Reconstruction, Beijing, China. [6]Tiantan Comprehensive Stroke Center, Beijing Tiantan Hospital, Capital Medical University, No.6 Tiantanxili, Dongcheng District, Beijing 100050, China.

References

1. Schroeder SA. New evidence that cigarette smoking remains the most important health hazard. N Engl J Med. 2013;368:389–90.
2. Jha P, Ramasundarahettige C, Landsman V, Rostron B, Thun M, Anderson RN, et al. 21st-century hazards of smoking and benefits of cessation in the united states. N Engl J Med. 2013;368:341–50.
3. Thun MJ, Carter BD, Feskanich D, Freedman ND, Prentice R, Lopez AD, et al. 50-year trends in smoking-related mortality in the united states. N Engl J Med. 2013;368:351–64.
4. Meschia JF, Bushnell C, Boden-Albala B, Braun LT, Bravata DM, Chaturvedi S, et al. Guidelines for the primary prevention of stroke: a statement for healthcare professionals from the american heart association/american stroke association. Stroke. 2014;45:3754–832.
5. Kernan WN, Ovbiagele B, Black HR, Bravata DM, Chimowitz MI, Ezekowitz MD, et al. Guidelines for the prevention of stroke in patients with stroke and transient ischemic attack: a guideline for healthcare professionals from the american heart association/american stroke association. Stroke. 2014;45: 2160–236.
6. Kaplan RC, Tirschwell DL, Longstreth WT Jr, Manolio TA, Heckbert SR, Lefkowitz D, et al. Vascular events, mortality, and preventive therapy following ischemic stroke in the elderly. Neurology. 2005;65:835–42.
7. Burns DM. Epidemiology of smoking-induced cardiovascular disease. Prog Cardiovasc Dis. 2003;46:11–29.
8. Gorelick PB, Wong KS, Bae HJ, Pandey DK. Large artery intracranial occlusive disease: a large worldwide burden but a relatively neglected frontier. Stroke. 2008;39:2396–9.
9. Wang Y, Zhao X, Liu L, Soo YO, Pu Y, Pan Y, et al. Prevalence and outcomes of symptomatic intracranial large artery stenoses and occlusions in china: the chinese intracranial atherosclerosis (cicas) study. Stroke. 2014;45:663–9.
10. Samuels OB, Joseph GJ, Lynn MJ, Smith HA, Chimowitz MI. A standardized method for measuring intracranial arterial stenosis. AJNR Am J Neuroradiol. 2000;21:643–6.
11. Grant EG, Benson CB, Moneta GL, Alexandrov AV, Baker JD, Bluth EI, et al. Carotid artery stenosis: grayscale and doppler ultrasound diagnosis–society of radiologists in ultrasound consensus conference. Ultrasound Q. 2003;19: 190–8.
12. Shah RS, Cole JW. Smoking and stroke: the more you smoke the more you stroke. Expert Rev Cardiovasc Ther. 2010;8:917–32.
13. Bhat VM, Cole JW, Sorkin JD, Wozniak MA, Malarcher AM, Giles WH, et al. Dose–response relationship between cigarette smoking and risk of ischemic stroke in young women. Stroke. 2008;39:2439–43.
14. Baldassarre D, Castelnuovo S, Frigerio B, Amato M, Werba JP, De Jong A, et al. Effects of timing and extent of smoking, type of cigarettes, and concomitant risk factors on the association between smoking and subclinical atherosclerosis. Stroke. 2009;40:1991–8.
15. Willeit J, Kiechl S. Prevalence and risk factors of asymptomatic extracranial carotid artery atherosclerosis. A population-based study. Arterioscler Thromb. 1993;13:661–8.
16. Howard G, Wagenknecht LE, Burke GL, Diez-Roux A, Evans GW, McGovern P, et al. Cigarette smoking and progression of atherosclerosis: the atherosclerosis risk in communities (aric) study. JAMA. 1998;279:119–24.
17. Wong KS, Ng PW, Tang A, Liu R, Yeung V, Tomlinson B. Prevalence of asymptomatic intracranial atherosclerosis in high-risk patients. Neurology. 2007;68:2035–8.
18. Bae HJ, Lee J, Park JM, Kwon O, Koo JS, Kim BK, et al. Risk factors of intracranial cerebral atherosclerosis among asymptomatics. Cerebrovasc Dis. 2007;24:355–60.
19. Ding X, Li C, Yu K, Gao A, Xiao L, Peng F, et al. Different risk factors between intracranial and extracranial atherosclerotic stenosis in asian population: a systematic review and meta-analysis. Int. J. Neurosci. 2014;124:834–40.
20. den Hartog AG, Achterberg S, Moll FL, Kappelle LJ, Visseren FL, van der Graaf Y, et al. Asymptomatic carotid artery stenosis and the risk of ischemic stroke according to subtype in patients with clinical manifest arterial disease. Stroke. 2013;44:1002–7.
21. Lin H, Wang H, Wu W, Lang L, Wang Q, Tian L. The effects of smoke-free legislation on acute myocardial infarction: a systematic review and meta-analysis. BMC Public Health. 2013;13:529.
22. Fichtenberg CM, Glantz SA. Association of the california tobacco control program with declines in cigarette consumption and mortality from heart disease. N Engl J Med. 2000;343:1772–7.
23. Song AV, Dutra LM, Neilands TB, Glantz SA. Association of smoke-free laws with lower percentages of new and current smokers among adolescents and young adults: an 11-year longitudinal study. JAMA Pediatr. 2015;169: e152285.
24. Rigotti NA, Clair C, Munafo MR, Stead LF. Interventions for smoking cessation in hospitalised patients. Cochrane Database Syst Rev. 2012;16(5):CD001837.
25. Stead LF, Lancaster T. Combined pharmacotherapy and behavioural interventions for smoking cessation. Cochrane Database Syst. Rev. 2012;10: CD008286.
26. Arnson Y, Shoenfeld Y, Amital H. Effects of tobacco smoke on immunity, inflammation and autoimmunity. J Autoimmun. 2010;34:J258–65.
27. Weber C, Noels H. Atherosclerosis: current pathogenesis and therapeutic options. Nat Med. 2011;17:1410–22.
28. Starke RM, Ali MS, Jabbour PM, Tjoumakaris SI, Gonzalez F, Hasan DM, et al. Cigarette smoke modulates vascular smooth muscle phenotype: implications for carotid and cerebrovascular disease. PLoS One. 2013;8:e71954.
29. Tu JV, Willison DJ, Silver FL, Fang J, Richards JA, Laupacis A, et al. Impracticability of informed consent in the registry of the canadian stroke network. N Engl J Med. 2004;350:1414–21.
30. Man BL, Fu YP, Chan YY, Lam W, Hui CF, Leung WH, et al. Use of magnetic resonance angiography to predict long-term outcomes of ischemic stroke patients with concurrent stenoses in hong kong. Cerebrovasc Dis. 2009;28:112–8.
31. Nederkoorn PJ, Elgersma OE, Mali WP, Eikelboom BC, Kappelle LJ, van der Graaf Y. Overestimation of carotid artery stenosis with magnetic resonance angiography compared with digital subtraction angiography. J Vasc Surg. 2002;36:806–13.
32. Barnoya J, Glantz SA. Cardiovascular effects of secondhand smoke: nearly as large as smoking. Circulation. 2005;111:2684–98.
33. Awawdi K, Steiner H, Green MS, Zelber-Sagi S. Association between second-hand smoking and acute coronary heart disease among arab women with multiple risk factors. Eur J Pub Health. 2016;26:141–5.

4

Greater periventricular white matter hyperintensity severity in basilar artery branch atheromatous disease

Po-Chen Lin[1,2], Feng-Chi Chang[2,3], Hui-Chi Huang[1,4], Jui-Yao Tsai[1,4], Yung-Yang Lin[1,2] and Chih-Ping Chung[1,2*]

Abstract

Background: Basilar artery branch atheromatous disease (BABAD), in which basilar artery atheroma occludes penetrating arteries at their origin, is a common etiology of posterior circulation stroke (PCS). It is currently unknown whether white matter hyperintensity(WMH), a marker of small vessel disease(SVD), is associated with BABAD.

Methods: The present study analyzed data from patients with PCS who were enrolled in the Taipei Veterans General Hospital Stroke Registry between January 1, 2010 and February 28, 2014. WMH severity was rated using the Scheltens scale. We used multivariate analyses to: (1) compare the severity of WMH between patients with BABAD, patients with large-artery > 50% atherosclerotic stenosis-related PCS(LAA), and non-stroke subjects(NS); and (2) evaluate the relationship between WMH severity and the 3-month prognosis of patients with BABAD.

Results: The study pool included 151 BABAD, 97 LAA, and 78 non-stroke patients. Multivariate analyses adjusting for age, sex, and vascular risk factors showed that compared to patients with LAA [Odds ratio(OR) = 0.51, $p = 0.037$] and NS (OR = 0.40, $p = 0.004$), patients with BABAD (OR = 1) had greater WMH severity (score ≥ 50th percentile) in periventricular, but not subcortical, regions. Moreover, greater periventricular WMH severity predicted poor 3-month functional outcomes (modified Rankin Scale > 3) with an OR of 3.21 ($p = 0.028$) in BABAD patients.

Conclusions: We are the first to show a significant association between WMH and BABAD that is independent of vascular risk factors and atherosclerotic large-artery disease. Our results suggest that small vessel abnormalities other than lipohyalinosis may be involved in BABAD pathophysiology. A future management strategy should include both large and small vessel protection.

Keywords: White matter hyperintensity, Branch atheromatous disease, Posterior circulation ischemic stroke, Basilar artery

Background

The two types of posterior circulation stroke (PCS) that are associated with atherosclerotic large-artery disease are (1) ischemic stroke with associated large-artery (vertebrobasilar artery, VBA) > 50% atherosclerotic stenosis (LAA) and (2) branch atheromatous disease (BAD) [1, 2]. In BAD, small vessels (i.e., penetrating arteries) are occluded at their origin by microatheroma or plaque within large parent arteries (e.g., basilar artery). We recently showed that basilar artery BAD (BABAD) was the most common etiology of PCS in our stroke registry [2]. BABAD typically causes small infarcts within the paramedian pons without significant VBA stenosis. Consequently, BABAD may be misdiagnosed as lacunar infarction, which is caused by the occlusion of small vessels resulting from lipohyalinosis [3, 4]. The seminal pathological studies of Fisher and Caplan [3] first described BABAD and distinguished it from lacunar infarction caused by small vessel lipohyalinotic degeneration. Decades later, high-resolution MRI is available to examine microatheromas or shallow plaques within the BA that occlude penetrating arteries at their origin and cause small infarcts

* Correspondence: pin324pin324@gmail.com
[1]Department of Neurology, Taipei Veterans General Hospital, No. 201 Sec.2, Shihpai Road, Peitou, Taipei 11217, Taiwan
[2]National Yang Ming University, Taipei, Taiwan
Full list of author information is available at the end of the article

within the paramedian brainstem [5, 6]. However, it is currently unknown whether small vessel abnormalities other than lipohyalinosis are involved in BAD mechanisms.

White matter hyperintensity (WMH) is commonly found in brain MR images of the elderly [7, 8]. Several small vessel abnormalities, including impaired cerebrovascular vasoreactivity, endothelial dysfunction, decreased blood flow to cerebral white matter, collagenosis of cerebral venules, and blood-brain-barrier (BBB) impairment, have been observed in subjects with WMH [7–13]. WMH has been classified as a marker of small vessel disease (SVD). The association between WMH and BAD has not been previously studied. Thus, the present study aimed to (1) compare the severity of WMH between patients with BABAD, patients with LAA, and non-stroke subjects (NS) and (2) examine the relationship between WMH severity and the 3-month prognosis of patients with BABAD. We hypothesized that in addition to large-artery atherosclerosis, BAD pathophysiology may also involve small vessel abnormalities, which would be reflected by (1) greater WMH severity in the BABAD group compared to the NS and LAA groups or (2) an association between WMH severity and the 3-month functional outcome of the BABAD group.

Methods

Stroke registry and stroke etiology

Since February 2009, the Taipei Veterans General Hospital Stroke Registry (TVGHSR) has collected data for all patients with acute stroke admitted to the emergency room or Neurology Department wards. Two specialized nurses, who were supervised by physicians specializing in stroke medicine, managed the patient data registry and followed up on patient outcomes. Registry data included: (1) demographic information and risk factors; (2) stroke severity at admission; (3) neurological, vascular, or cardiological assessment results acquired during hospitalization; and (4) outcomes at discharge and 3-month follow-up (via telephone). The TVGHSR data were analyzed for the present study.

Patient data were reviewed and a consensus concerning their stroke etiologies was reached by two neurologists (Drs. Chung and Lin) and one radiologist (Dr. Chang) who specialize in stroke medicine. The stroke etiology of patients with adequate investigations including brain MRI and MRA, duplex ultrasound of neck arteries, color-coded transcranial Doppler imaging, 24-h Holter monitor recording, and echocardiography, was determined. The following standardized criteria were used to classify stroke etiology LAA and BABAD [1, 2]:

(1) BABAD. Vascular and cardiological studies showed the absence of large artery occlusion or severe stenosis (> 50%) in the BA or vertebral arteries (VAs) as well as cardioembolic risks. BA showed atheroma or plaque by MRI T1 (isointense) or/and T2/FLAIR (hypointense) sequence at the level of cerebral infarct. Clinical and brain imaging study were compatible with paramedian pontine/midbrain/upper medulla infarct (usually were basal-brainstem involved and wedge-shaped) due to several penetrating vessels occlusion.

(2) LAA. Vascular studies showed occlusion or severe stenosis (>50%) of the relevant large artery. There should be multiple or diffusely atherosclerotic changes in the other large arteries. Abrupt cut-off of vessels was considered more likely due to embolism and was not considered for this category. Cerebral infarcts were in the territory of the large artery stenosis/occlusion larger than that of a single branch artery territory, or in distal fields.

Study population

We retrieved data from patients who were registered in the TVGHSR between January 1, 2010 and February 28, 2014. The following inclusion criteria were applied to the selected subjects: (1) presence of acute cerebral infarcts in the territory of posterior circulation with BABAD or LAA etiology; and (2) an adequate amount of supporting assessments during admission, including brain MRI. Patients with (1) malignancy, (2) autoimmune diseases, (3) hematological diseases, or (4) simultaneous acute cerebral infarcts in the territory of anterior circulation were excluded. We also excluded patients with posterior cerebral artery territory (i.e., supratentorial) infarct to avoid difficulties with WMH grading.

NS from our outpatient clinics who received brain MRI during physical examinations were invited to join the present study. Subjects with (1) dementia, (2) severe heart disease, and (3) malignancy were not enrolled. NS demographic and vascular risk factor information was obtained from patient history records or laboratory data. All participants provided informed consent. The Institutional Review Board of Taipei Veterans General Hospital approved the present study.

WMH assessment

All study participants (i.e., NS and patients with BABAD or LAA) were imaged with a 1.5 T MRI scanner (Excite II; GE Medical Systems, Milwaukee, WI, USA). Whole brain axial T1- and T2-weighted sequences and fluid-attenuated inversion recovery (FLAIR) pulse sequences were performed. WMHs were defined as lesions that appeared hyperintense on T2-weighted and FLAIR images and mildly hypointense or normal on T1-weighted images. Some patients with BABAD underwent both standard and high-resolution MRI examination to evaluate BA plaque. Only standard MRI datasets were used to determine the WMH rating.

To assess WMH severity and anatomical distribution, we used the semiquantitative Scheltens scale to rate WMH in periventricular and subcortical regions [14]. For this scale, the severity of hyperintensities in different brain areas is scored separately. These brain areas include three periventricular regions (i.e., frontal caps, bands, and occipital caps) and four areas of deep subcortical white matter (i.e., frontal, parietal, temporal, and occipital). The periventricular WMH rating was determined with scores of 0 = absent, 1 = ≤ 5 mm, and 2 = > 5 mm in each of the three periventricular regions, resulting in a maximum rating of 6 points. The subcortical WMH rating was determined using a 0–6-point scale related to lesion size and number. If the largest lesion in a region was <4 mm, then a score of 1 was given if there were ≤ five lesions, whereas a score of 2 was given if there were > five lesions. If the largest lesion was 4–10 mm, a score of 3 was given if there were ≤ five lesions, whereas a score of 4 was given if there were > five lesions. A score of 5 was given for very large lesions (≥ 10 mm) and a score of 6 was given for confluent lesions. Thus, in subcortical regions, the scale could produce a maximum score of 24 points. Analysis of MRI datasets was performed to determine WMH ratings by one neurologists (Dr Lin) who was well-trained in neuroimaging interpretation and blinded to the clinical characteristics of the subjects while MRI WMH rating. Intra-rater reliability was tested using a subset of 20 consecutive study subjects. The Kappa (κ) coefficient for periventricular and subcortical WMH ratings were 0.93 and 0.90, respectively.

Statistical analyses

Analyses were performed with SPSS software (version 22.0; IBM, USA). All data are presented as mean [standard deviation (SD)] for continuous variables and number (percentage) for discrete variables. Group comparisons were made using a nonparametric Kruskal-Wallis test. Bonferroni correction was applied for pairwise group comparisons. When appropriate, a chi-square ($\chi 2$) test or Fisher's exact test was performed for categorical variables. Multivariate analyses were used to adjust for confounding factors, such as age, sex, and vascular risk factors. Statistical significance was reached when $P < 0.05$. To adjust for confounding factors (age, sex and vascular risk factors including hypertension, diabetes mellitus, hyperlipidemia and cigarette smoking), we performed multivariate analyses. We used the 50th percentile of the WMH score as the cutoff point. To respectively compare the severity of WMH between BABAD group and NS and LAA group, we analyzed the odds ratio (OR) of greater WMH (>50th percentile of the WMH score) in NS and LAA group versus BABAD respectively.

Results

For this study, we analyzed data from 151 patients with BABAD, 97 patients with LAA, and 78 NS. Table 1 shows infarct locations and vascular involvement in the BABAD and LAA groups. The pons was the most common location involved in BABAD and LAA (93.4% versus 50.5%). The only other BABAD infarct locations were the midbrain (4.0%) and medulla (2.6%). All BABAD-associated PCS subjects exhibited a single lesion. In the BABAD group, severe VBA stenosis (> 50%) was not present; however, severe internal carotid artery (ICA) and middle cerebral artery (MCA) stenosis were present in 43.0% and 24.5% of the subjects, respectively.

Table 2 presents demographic and WMH comparisons between the BABAD, LAA, and NS groups. The frequency of vascular risk factors was significantly different between groups. The BABAD and LAA groups had greater frequencies of hypertension, diabetes mellitus, and hyperlipidemia compared to the NS group, whereas the NS group had a greater frequency of cigarette smoking.

The mean WMH score for the whole study population was 3.0 [2.0 (SD); 0–6 (range); 1 (1st quartile); 3 (2nd quartile); 5 (3rd quartile)] for the periventricular region and 2.9 (3.1; 0–14; 0; 2; 5) for the subcortical region. The group comparison showed that WMH severity was higher in the BABAD group; however, this difference was only statistically significant for the periventricular region (Table 2). *Post-hoc* Bonferroni analysis revealed that the BABAD group had a higher periventricular WMH score than the NS group.

To adjust for confounding factors, we performed multivariate analyses (Table 3). We used the 50th percentile of

Table 1 The location of brain infarcts and presence of >50% atherosclerotic stenosis in the large arteries of patients with BABAD and LAA

	BABAD (*n* = 151)	LAA (*n* = 97)
Infarct locations		
Midbrain	6 (4.0%)	5 (5.2%)
Pons	141 (93.4%)	49 (50.5%)
Medulla	4 (2.6%)	12 (12.4%)
Cerebellum	0	23 (23.7%)
> 50% atherosclerotic stenosis		
VA	0	70 (89.7%)
BA	0	57 (73.1%)
ICA	65 (43.0%)	51 (65.4%)
MCA	37 (24.5%)	38 (48.7%)
Admission NIHSS	4.7 (3.9)	5.9 (6.8)

Data are presented as mean (SD) or number of patients (percentage)
BABAD basilar artery branch atheromatous disease; *LAA* large-artery >50% atherosclerotic stenosis; *VA* vertebral artery; *BA* basilar artery; *ICA* internal carotid artery; *MCA* middle cerebral artery; *NIHSS* NIH Stroke Scale

Table 2 Demographic and white matter hyperintensity comparisons between NS and patients with BABAD and LAA

	BABAD (n = 151)	LAA (n = 97)	NS (n = 78)	p
Age (years)	72.3 (10.6)	73.2 (11.5)	72.6 (12.0)	0.786
Sex (men)	101 (66.9%)	54 (69.2%)	69 (71.1%)	0.790
Vascular risk factors				
Hypertension	121 (80.1%)	68 (87.2%)	51 (52.6%)	<0.001
Diabetes mellitus	72 (47.7%)	38 (48.7%)	18 (18.6%)	<0.001
Hyperlipidemia	32 (21.2%)	24 (30.8%)	14 (14.4%)	0.034
Cigarette Smoking	24 (15.9%)	20 (25.7%)	30 (30.9%)	0.008
Periventricular WMH				
Total score	3.3 (1.7)	2.9 (1.9)	2.4 (2.4)	0.001[a]
Score ≥ 3 (50th percentile)	99 (65.6%)	43 (44.3%)	43 (55.1%)	0.003
Subcortical WMH				
Total score	3.2 (3.1)	2.5 (2.8)	2.6 (3.4)	0.044
Score ≥ 2 (50th percentile)	84 (55.6%)	36 (37.1%)	47 (60.3%)	0.292

BABAD basilar artery branch atheromatous disease; *LAA* large-artery >50% atherosclerotic stenosis; *NS* non-stroke subjects; *WMH* white matter hyperintensity
[a]*Post-hoc* Bonferroni analysis revealed that the BABAD group had a higher periventricular WMH score than the NS group

the WMH score as the cutoff point. To respectively compare the severity of WMH between BABAD group and NS and LAA group, we analyzed the odds ratio (OR) of greater WMH (>50th percentile of the WMH score) in NS and LAA group versus BABAD respectively. Multivariate analysis revealed that greater periventricular WMH severity was associated with age and the presence of hypertension. It also showed that the BABAD group had a higher likelihood of greater periventricular WMH severity compared to the NS and LAA groups. Subcortical WMH was only associated with aging. Although the BABAD group showed a tendency for greater subcortical WMH severity compared to the other two groups, this finding was not statistically significant.

Finally, we investigated whether greater WMH severity in patients with BABAD was associated with poor 3-month functional outcomes [modified Rankin Scale (mRS) > 3; Table 4]. In BABAD-associated PCS, periventricular WMH severity was associated with poor functional outcome; however, subcortical WMH did not exhibit the same relationship. Moreover, greater periventricular WMH severity (score ≥ 50th percentile) at admission could predict a poor 3-month functional outcome with an odds ratio (OR) of 3.21.

Discussion

The main finding of the present study was that patients with BABAD had greater periventricular WMH severity than patients with LAA and NS. Moreover, the greater

Table 3 cFactors associated with severe white matter hyperintensity revealed by multivariate analyses

	Periventricular WMH ≥ 3			Subcortical WMH ≥ 2		
	OR	95% CI	p	OR	95% CI	p
Age (per year increase)	1.08	1.05–1.11	<0.001	1.04	1.02–1.07	<0.001
Sex (men versus women)	0.89	0.51–1.57	0.692	0.75	0.44–1.26	0.274
Hypertension (yes versus no)	2.66	1.46–4.82	0.001	1.30	0.75–2.26	0.352
Diabetes mellitus (yes versus no)	0.96	0.56–1.65	0.878	1.10	0.68–1.83	0.679
Hyperlipidemia (yes versus no)	0.99	0.54–1.82	0.964	0.88	0.50–1.54	0.646
Cigarette Smoking (yes versus no)	1.67	0.15–18.76	0.666	0.83	0.11–6.24	0.856
Etiology (LAA/NS versus BABAD)						
BABAD	1			1		
LAA	0.51	0.28–0.96	0.037	0.63	0.36–1.12	0.302
NS	0.40	0.21–0.74	0.004	0.74	0.42–1.31	0.302

BABAD basilar artery branch atheromatous disease; *LAA* large-artery >50% atherosclerotic stenosis; *NS* non-stroke subjects; *WMH* white matter hyperintensity; *OR* odds ratio; *95% CI* 95% confidence interval

Table 4 Association between the severity of white matter hyperintensity and poor functional outcomes in patients with BABAD

	Model 1			Model 2		
	OR	95% CI	*p*	OR	95% CI	*p*
Periventricular WMH score ≥ 3	3.10	1.14–8.47	0.027	3.21	1.13–9.12	0.028
Subcortical WMH score ≥ 2	1.14	0.43–3.04	0.791	0.94	0.34–2.63	0.909

Model 1 = adjusted for age, sex, and stroke severity at admission (NIH Stroke Scale). Model 2 = adjusted for age, sex, stroke severity at admission, and vascular risk factors (i.e., hypertension, diabetes mellitus, hyperlipidemia, and cigarette smoking)
WMH white matter hyperintensity; *OR* odds ratio; *95% CI* 95% confidence interval

periventricular WMH severity of patients with BABAD was associated with poor 3-month functional outcomes. Following Fisher and Caplan's pathological reports [3, 4], few studies investigated the mechanisms of BABAD. Consequently, it is currently unknown whether small vessel abnormalities other than lipohyalinosis are involved in BABAD mechanisms. Our results have provided new insights into the pathophysiology of BABAD.

In agreement with our findings, a previous study of a Chinese population revealed a very high frequency of WMH (96.4%) in patients with BABAD [15]. However, this study did not consider confounding factors, such as vascular risk factors and atherosclerotic large-artery disease, when evaluating the relationship between WMH and BABAD. WMH is associated with several vascular risk factors [7, 8, 13] and has been frequently reported in atherosclerotic large-artery disease [16, 17]. Thus, in order to validate the association between WMH and BABAD, we controlled for vascular risk factors and recruited patients with LAA for WMH comparisons. Moreover, the reduced frequency of severe atherosclerotic large-artery stenosis in patients with BABAD (Table 1) suggests that the greater periventricular WMH severity of these patients compared to patients with LAA could be attributed to other factors besides atherosclerotic large-artery disease.

Consistent with the pathological and clinical evidence for atherosclerotic large-artery disease involvement in BABAD [3, 4, 18], we also found a high frequency of severe large artery atherosclerotic stenosis (ICA and MCA) in BABAD patients. Considering WMH is a commonly used SVD marker [7–13], the vascular risk factor-adjusted finding of greater WMH severity in the BABAD group compared to the NS and LAA groups implies that SVD is also involvement in the pathophysiology of BABAD. Here we propose a "double-hit" theory concerning BABAD mechanisms. In BABAD, atheroma in the large parent artery (i.e., BA) at the opening of small penetrating vessels causes blood flow decrement (i.e., ischemia) in brainstem regions supplied by these penetrating vessels. Thus, BABAD-induced brainstem stroke may be facilitated by underlying SVD. In response to ischemia caused by large artery atheroma, penetrating vessels affected by SVD may be unable to dilate due to poor autoregulation ability. An accompany BBB damage with edema, another small vascular dysfunction, might also be involved.

Additional evidence suggests that small vessel abnormality may play a role in BABAD mechanisms. Clinical worsening (i.e., early neurological deterioration) following acute stroke, a common feature associated with lacunar infarction (i.e., small vessel occlusion infarction) [19], is also frequently reported in BABAD [18]. A recent trial found that Cilostazol, an anti-platelet drug that protects small vessel endothelium and the BBB [20], can reduce clinical worsening in BABAD [21]. This finding suggests that small vessel dysfunction may contribute to clinical worsening in BABAD. SVD involvement in BABAD pathophysiology is also supported by our finding that greater WMH severity predicts poor 3-month functional outcomes in patients with BABAD.

It is unclear why there was a difference in severity between periventricular and subcortical WMH in patients with BABAD. Different small vessel pathophysiologies have been reported for WMH in different brain regions [22]. Subcortical WMH is associated with lacunar infarction caused by small vessel lipohyalinosis [23], whereas periventricular WMH is associated with the other small vessel abnormalities such as arteriosclerosis, venous collagenosis, and perivascular edema [22, 24]. Region-specific small vessel pathophysiology again suggests that small vessel dysfunction caused by pathology other than lipohyalinotic degeneration may be involved in BABAD.

The present study has some limitations that merit discussion. Since most of our patients had brainstem infarcts, WMH rating in this region was difficult. Thus, we did not evaluate brainstem WMH, which would have been more representative of SVD in posterior circulation. Second, we did not investigate other SVD markers or small vessel function in BABAD. Future studies are needed to evaluate the role of small vessels in the pathophysiology of BABAD.

The strengths of the present study include a large patient population and validated BABAD diagnostic criteria, which were used to assess infarct location and detected plaque in the BA. Moreover, we are the first to show an association between WMH and BABAD. Greater periventricular WMH severity in patients with BABAD compared to patients with LAA and NS indicates SVD involvement in BABAD. Furthermore, greater periventricular WMH severity was an independent predictor of poor functional outcomes at 3 months after BABAD-associated PCS.

Conclusions

We are the first to reveal a relationship between WMH and BABAD-related PCS which findings have provided insights into BABAD pathophysiology. Management strategies for BABAD should consider both large and small vessel protection.

Abbreviations

BA: basilar artery; BABAD: basilar artery branch atheromatous disease; BAD: branch atheromatous disease; BBB: blood brain barrier; LAA: large artery atherosclerotic stenosis; mRS: modified Rankin Scale; NS: non-stroke subjects; PCS: posterior circulation stroke; SVD: small vessel disease; VBA: vertebrobasilar artery; WMH: white matter hyperintensity

Acknowledgements

None.

Funding

Dr. Chung received grants from Taiwan Ministry of Science and Technology (MOST 104-2314-B-075-MY3) and Taipei Veterans General Hospital, Taiwan (VGH V105C-055).

Authors' contributions

All authors have read and approve of the final version of the manuscript. Conceptualization: CPC, PCL. Data curation: CPC, PCL, FCC, HCH, JYT, YYL. Formal analysis: CPC, PCL. Writing: CPC, PCL. Supervision: CPC, FCC.

Competing interests

The authors declare that they have no competing interests.

Author details

[1]Department of Neurology, Taipei Veterans General Hospital, No. 201 Sec.2, Shihpai Road, Peitou, Taipei 11217, Taiwan. [2]National Yang Ming University, Taipei, Taiwan. [3]Department of Radiology, Taipei Veterans General Hospital, Taipei, Taiwan. [4]National Taipei University of Nursing and Health Sciences, Taipei, Taiwan.

References

1. Caplan LR, Wityk RJ, Glass TA, Tapia J, Pazdera L, Chang HM, Teal P, Dashe JF, Chaves CJ, Breen JC, Vemmos K, Amarenco P, Tettenborn B, Leary M, Estol C, Dewitt LD, Pessin MS. New England Medical Center posterior circulation registry. Ann Neurol. 2004;56(3):389–98.
2. Chung CP, Yong CS, Chang FC, Sheng WY, Huang HC, Tsai JY, Hsu HY, Hu HH. Stroke etiology is associated with outcome in posterior circulation stroke. Ann Clin Transl Neurol. 2015;2:510–7.
3. Fisher CM, Caplan LR. Basilar artery branch occlusion: a cause of pontine infarction. Neurology. 1971;21:900–5.
4. Caplan LR. Intracranial branch atheromatous disease: a neglected, understudied, and underused concept. Neurology. 1989;39:1246–50.
5. Klein IF, Lavallée PC, Schouman-Claeys E, Amarenco P. High-resolution MRI identifies basilar artery plaques in paramedian pontine infarct. Neurology. 2005;64:551–2.
6. Klein IF, Lavallée PC, Mazighi M, Schouman-Claeys E, Labreuche J, Amarenco P. Basilar artery atherosclerotic plaques in paramedian and lacunar pontine infarctions: a high-resolution MRI study. Stroke. 2010;41:1405–9.
7. Hachinski VC, Potter P, Merskey H. Leuko-araiosis. Arch Neurol. 1987;44:21–3.
8. Pantoni L, Garcia JH. Pathogenesis of leukoaraiosis: a review. Stroke. 1997;28:652–9.
9. Terborg C, Gora F, Weiller C, Röther J. Reduced vasomotor reactivity in cerebral microangiopathy: a study with near-infrared spectroscopy and transcranial Doppler sonography. Stroke. 2000;31:924–9.
10. Hassan A, Hunt BJ, O'Sullivan M, Parmar K, Bamford JM, Briley D, Brown MM, Thomas DJ, Markus HS. Markers of endothelial dysfunction in lacunar infarction and ischaemic leukoaraiosis. Brain. 2003;126:424–32.
11. Wardlaw JM, Valdés Hernández MC, Muñoz-Maniega S. What are white matter hyperintensities made of? Relevance to vascular cognitive impairment. J Am Heart Assoc. 2015;4:001140.
12. Moody DM, Brown WR, Challa VR, Anderson RL. Periventricular venous collagenosis: association with leukoaraiosis. Radiology. 1995;194:469–76.
13. Wardlaw JM, Smith C, Dichgans M. Mechanisms of sporadic cerebral small vessel disease: insights from neuroimaging. Lancet Neurol. 2013;12:483–97.
14. Scheltens P, Barkhof F, Leys D, Pruvo JP, Nauta JJ, Vermersch P, Steinling M, Valk J. A semiquantative rating scale for the assessment of signal hyperintensities on magnetic resonance imaging. J Neurol Sci. 1993;114:7–12.
15. Men X, Wu A, Zhang B, Li H, Zhang L, Chen S, Lin Y, Lu Z. Leukoaraiosis and NIHSS score help to differentiate subtypes of intracranial branch atheromatous disease in southern Han Chinese patients with stroke. Neurol Sci. 2013;34:1727–33.
16. de Leeuw FE, de Groot JC, Bots ML, Witteman JC, Oudkerk M, Hofman A, van Gijn J, Breteler MM. Carotid atherosclerosis and cerebral white matter lesions in a population based magnetic resonance imaging study. J Neurol. 2000;247:291–6.
17. Kwon HM, Lynn MJ, Turan TN, Derdeyn CP. Fiorella D, lane BF, Montgomery J, Janis LS, Rumboldt Z, Chimowitz MI; SAMMPRIS investigators. Frequency, risk factors, and outcome of coexistent small vessel disease and intracranial arterial stenosis: results from the stenting and aggressive medical Management for Preventing Recurrent Stroke in intracranial stenosis (SAMMPRIS) trial. JAMA Neurol. 2016;73:36–42.
18. Petrone L, Nannoni S, Del Bene A, Palumbo V, Inzitari D. Branch Atheromatous disease: a clinically meaningful. Yet Unproven Concept Cerebrovasc Dis. 2016;41:87–95.
19. Steinke W, Ley SC. Lacunar stroke is the major cause of progressive motor deficits. Stroke. 2002;33:1510–6.
20. Mok V, Kim JS. Prevention and Management of Cerebral Small Vessel Disease. J Stroke. 2015;17:111–22.
21. Kimura T, Tucker A, Sugimura T, Seki T, Fukuda S, Takeuchi S, Miyata S, Fujita T, Hashizume A, Izumi N, Kawasaki K, Katsuno M, Hashimoto M, Sako K. Ultra-early combination antiplatelet therapy with Cilostazol for the prevention of branch Atheromatous disease: a multicenter prospective study. Cerebrovasc Dis Extra. 2016;6:84–95.
22. Kim KW, MacFall JR, Payne ME. Classification of white matter lesions on magnetic resonance imaging in elderly persons. Biol Psychiatry. 2008;64:273–80.
23. Mäntylä R, Aronen HJ, Salonen O, Pohjasvaara T, Korpelainen M, Peltonen T, Standertskjöld-Nordenstam CG, Kaste M, Erkinjuntti T. Magnetic resonance imaging white matter hyperintensities and mechanism of ischemic stroke. Stroke. 1999;30:2053–8.
24. Farkas E, de Vos RA, Donka G, Jansen Steur EN, Mihály A, Luiten PG. Age-related microvascular degeneration in the human cerebral periventricular white matter. Acta Neuropathol. 2006;111:150–7.

5

Prevalence of and risk factors for enlarged perivascular spaces in adult patients with moyamoya disease

Tomoyoshi Kuribara[1], Takeshi Mikami[1*], Katsuya Komatsu[1], Hime Suzuki[1], Hirofumi Ohnishi[2], Kiyohiro Houkin[3] and Nobuhiro Mikuni[1]

Abstract

Background: Enlarged perivascular spaces (EPVS) are often observed with magnetic resonance imaging in patients with small vessel disease. However, the risk factors, radiological features, and clinical relevance of EPVS in patients with moyamoya disease are poorly understood. The purpose of this study was to evaluate EPVS, the risk factors of many EPVS, and the pathophysiology of EPVS in adult patients with moyamoya disease.

Methods: One hundred cerebral hemispheres of 50 adult patients with moyamoya disease were examined. The control group consisted of 50 age/sex-matched patients without ischemic disease. The numbers of EPVS at the level of the centrum semiovale per hemisphere were compared between the moyamoya disease and control groups. In each hemisphere, the total numbers of EPVS were categorized into five grades (0–4), and the clinical and radiological characteristics of the predictive factors in patients in the high EPVS grade group (EPVS grade = 4) were assessed.

Results: The EPVS counts and grades were significantly higher in the moyamoya disease group. Analyses of the background characteristics of the patients with moyamoya disease revealed that significantly higher prevalence of high EPVS grades were associated with the female sex, hypertension, high magnetic resonance angiography scores, high numbers of flow voids in the basal ganglia, high brain atrophy scores, ivy signs, and white matter lesions. A logistic multivariate analysis of the patients with high EPVS grades revealed significant associations with the female sex, hypertension, and flow voids in the basal ganglia.

Conclusions: Increased EPVS were confirmed in adult patients with moyamoya disease, and the associated clinical and radiological factors were identified. The presence of hypertension, the female sex, and flow voids in the basal ganglia were important for predicting high EPVS grades in patients with moyamoya disease. Reductions in arterial pulsations with steno-occlusive changes can inhibit the flow of interstitial fluid, which can increase the number of EPVS in patients with moyamoya disease. Other clinical factors, such as the female sex and hypertension, may promote secondary brain damage in patients with moyamoya disease. Further evaluations of EPVS in patients with moyamoya disease are needed to better understand their pathophysiological importance.

Keywords: Moyamoya disease, Small vessel disease, Leukoaraiosis, Hypertension

* Correspondence: tmikami@sapmed.ac.jp
[1]Department of Neurosurgery, Sapporo Medical University, South1 West16, Chuo-ku, Sapporo 060-8543, Japan
Full list of author information is available at the end of the article

Background

Moyamoya disease is a cerebrovascular disease that is characterized by chronic progressive stenosis of the terminal portion of the internal carotid artery (ICA) on both sides of the brain, which results in an abnormal vascular network of the collateral pathways at the base of the brain [1, 2]. Therefore, patients with moyamoya disease have decreased cerebral blood flow and reduced cerebral perfusion pressure [3], which can result in ischemic and/or hemorrhagic strokes. In patients with chronic hypoperfusion, ischemic injury to the white matter causes axonal destruction and glial proliferation [4]. As a result, white matter lesions are observed in these patients on T2-weighted magnetic resonance imaging (MRI) and fluid-attenuated inversion recovery (FLAIR) imaging [5]. Similarly, hemodynamic stress can induce microbleeds [6]. Thus, the deep white matter imaging findings in patients with moyamoya disease resemble those associated with patients with small vessel disease [7].

Perivascular spaces, which are also known as Virchow-Robin spaces, surround the walls of perforating arterioles and venules as they course from the subarachnoid space through the brain parenchyma [8]. Enlarged perivascular spaces (EPVS) are commonly detected on T2-weighted MRI as dot-like or linear hyperintensities in the basal ganglia and the centrum semiovale, and this is thought to be one of the radiological features of small vessel disease [9, 10]. EPVS are more numerous in patients with greater age [11–13], hypertension [11, 13, 14], vascular dementia [15], lacunar stroke [10, 11], and white matter lesions [10–12], and EPVS are considered markers of small vessel disease. Although EPVS have been observed in patients with moyamoya disease, their characteristics in patients with moyamoya disease have never been described. In this study, EPVS were compared between patients with moyamoya disease and those in the control group, and the risk factors for increased numbers of EPVS in moyamoya disease were identified.

Methods

Patients

Between August 2008 and April 2016, consecutive patients with moyamoya disease who were diagnosed at our hospital were enrolled in this study. The patients were diagnosed with moyamoya disease with MRI, magnetic resonance angiography (MRA), and/or digital subtraction angiography. Patients under 15 were excluded. One hundred 100 hemispheres of 50 patients (14 males and 36 females) with moyamoya disease were examined. The characteristics of the patients are presented in Table 1. The median age (interquartile range: IQR) of the patients was 41.5 (31.0-51.0) years (range, 20–74 years). In this moyamoya disease group, 18 hypertension patients, 1 type 2 diabetes mellitus patient, and 8 hyperlipidemia patients were included. Of these 50 individuals, 25 had ischemic onsets, 6 had hemorrhagic onsets, 2 had epileptic onsets, and the remaining 17 were asymptomatic or reported only headaches. The median MRA score was 4.0 (3.0-7.0) (range, 0–10). Five patients with unilateral involvement were included in the study. Because patients with quasi-moyamoya disease were excluded from the study, none of the patients had any concomitant diseases. For the control group, 50 age- and sex-matched patients (14 males and 36 females) who were treated at our hospital during the same period were recruited. The control group included 17 patients with cerebral aneurysms, 4 migraine patients, 2 patients with cerebral hemorrhages, 5 patients with brain arteriovenous malformations, 5 patients with epilepsy, 7 brain tumor patients, and 10 patients with other issues. The patients in the control group did not have ischemic cerebrovascular disease. Therefore, these were without TIA or previous ischemic stroke, and without intracranial and extracranial stenotic lesions. The median age of the control group was 40.5 (33.8-50.3) years (range, 15–69 years). In this control group, 9 hypertension patients, 1 type 2 diabetes mellitus patient, and 7 hyperlipidemia patients were included. Compared with the moyamoya disease group, the clinical characteristics of the control group were not significantly different except for hypertension.

In this study, the numbers and grades of EPVS were compared between the moyamoya disease and control groups. Interobserver discrepancies were also assessed. The 100 hemispheres that were analyzed in this study were divided into the following two groups according to their EPVS grades: high EPVS grade group (EPVS grade = 4) and low EPVS grade group (EPVS grade = 0–3). First, the following clinical and radiological characteristics were compared between the moyamoya disease group and the control group for assessing selection bias: age, sex, hypertension, diabetes, hyperlipidemia, disease subtype, presence or absence of stroke lesions, microbleeds, and white matter lesions. Stroke lesions were defined as follows: lacnar stroke (maximum diameter ≤ 1.5 cm), large ischemic stroke (maximum diameter > 1.5 cm), and hemorrhagic stroke. Next, the following clinical and radiological characteristics were compared between the high EPVS grade group and the low EPVS grade group in the moyamoya disease group for assessing risk factors of high EPVS in moyamoya disease: age, sex, hypertension, diabetes, hyperlipidemia, disease subtype, MRA score, number of flow voids in the basal ganglia, brain atrophy score, presence or absence of stroke lesions (lacnar stroke, large ischemic stroke, and hemorrhagic stroke), ivy signs, microbleeds, and white matter lesions.

Table 1 Clinical characteristics of the moyamoya disease and control groups

	Moyamoya disease group	Control group	*p* value
n, patients (hemisphere)	50 (100)	50 (100)	
Age, median (IQR), y	41.5 (31.0-51.0)	40.5 (33.8-50.3)	0.629
Sex, male/female	14/36	14/36	1.000
Total number of EPVS, median (IQR)	43.8 (26.0-52.9)	23.8 (15.1-33.0)	<0.001
EPVS Grade, median (IQR)	4.0 (3.0-4.0)	3.0 (2.0-3.0)	<0.001
Grade 0/1/2/3/4, n	0/2/12/33/53	0/8/30/44/18	
Interobserver discrepancy, n, median (IQR)	13, 0.0 (0.0-0.0)	25, 0.0 (0.0-0.8)	
Hypertension, presence/absence	18/32	9/41	0.043
Diabetes mellitus, presence/absence	1/49	1/49	1.000
Hyperlipidemia, presence/absence	8/42	7/43	0.779
Stroke lesions (total), presence/absence	32/68	6/94	<0.001
Lacnar stroke, presence/absence	15/84	4/96	0.008
Large ischemic stroke, presence/absence	13/88	0/100	<0.001
Hemorrhagic stroke, presence/absence	4/96	2/98	0.683
Microbleeds, presence/absence	15/83	4/96	0.007
White matter lesions, presence/absence	57/43	34/66	0.001
Disease subtype	Ischemic stroke: 10	Cerebral aneurysm: 17	
	TIA: 15	Migraine: 4	
	Hemorrhagic stroke: 6	Cerebral hemorrhage: 2	
	Epilepsy: 2	Brain AVM: 5	
	Other: 17	Epilepsy: 5	
		Brain tumor: 7	
		Other: 10	

IQR interquartile range, *TIA* transient ischemic attack, *AVM* arteriovenous malformation

MRI and MRA examinations

The MRI examinations, including T2-weighted MRI, FLAIR MRI, T2*-weighted MRI, and three-dimensional time-of-flight spoiled gradient-recalled echo sequence (3D TOF SPGR), were performed with a 3.0-T magnetic resonance system (Signa Excite, Ver. 11; GE Healthcare, Milwaukee, WI, USA) The imaging parameters were as previously described [5, 16]. Volume rendering and maximum intensity projection were applied as postprocessing techniques to aid in the evaluation.

All MRI and MRA data were independently evaluated in each hemisphere of each subject by two independent observers (T.K. and T.M.), and the mean of the observers' values was calculated for the assessment. EPVS was measured on presurgical T2-weighted imaging at the level of the centrum semiovale as shown in Fig. 1. EPVS were defined as <3 mm round or linear cerebrospinal fluid-isointense lesions (hyperintense on T2-weighted and hypointense on FLAIR imaging with respect to brain) along the courses of penetrating arteries [9, 10]. Hemispheres were scored according to the mean number of EPVS as follows: 0 = none, 1 = 1–10, 2 = 11–20, 3 = 21–40, and 4 = > 40 EPVS per side [17]. In this study, EPVS in the basal ganglia could not be evaluated because of the characteristic flow voids in the basal ganglia in moyamoya disease. The number of flow voids in the basal ganglia was determined with three-dimensional time-of-flight spoiled gradient-recalled echo sequence imaging of a slice of the basal ganglia as previously described [18]. The brain atrophy scores were assessed in deep lesions (enlargement of the ventricles) and superficial lesions (enlargement of the gyri) and rated on a validated scale of 0 to 3 (normal, slight, moderate, and severe) against a reference MRI brain template of normal subjects [19, 20]. The MRA scores were based on Houkin et al.'s classification [21]. Depending on the severity of the steno-occlusive changes, MRA scores were assigned to each of the following: C1 portion of the ICA, M2 portion of the middle cerebral artery (MCA), A1 portion of the anterior cerebral artery (ACA), and P2 portion of the posterior cerebral artery (PCA). The smallest score was 0, and the largest was 10 (ICA3 + MCA3 + ACA2 + PCA2 = 10). The total score was calculated for each hemisphere. The presence of stroke lesions, ivy signs, and white matter lesions was evaluated with T2-weighted and FLAIR imaging, and the

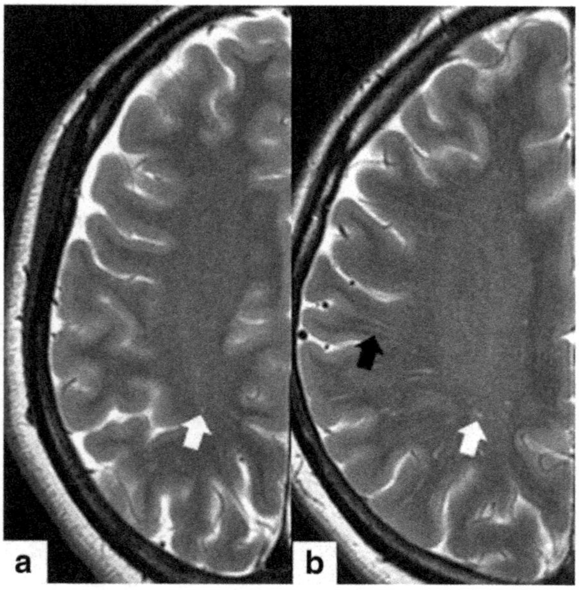

Fig. 1 This figure shows hemispheres from a patient in the low EPVS group (**a**) and a patient in the high EPVS group (**b**). In the left hemisphere of the patient with a low EPVS grade (a 38-year-old female), the mean number of EPVS was 10.5, and the hemisphere was categorized as a grade 1 (**a**). In the left hemisphere of the patient with a high EPVS grade (a 36-year-old female), the mean number of EPVS was 83, and the hemisphere was categorized as a grade 4 (**b**). The white arrow shows dot-like EPVS, and the black arrow shows linear EPVS

presence of microbleeds was determined with T2*-weighted imaging.

Statistical analysis

The data are expressed as median (IQR). Mann–Whitney U tests and Chi-squared test were used to compare the moyamoya and control groups and the high EPVS grade and low EPVS grade groups. For tests that resulted in p values less than 0.10 in the Mann–Whitney U tests and Chi-squared test, a simple logistic regression was used in the univariate analyses of the EPVS in the moyamoya group. Odds ratios (ORs) and 95% confidence intervals (CIs) were obtained with these models. Each item was selected with stepwise methods (model selection criterion: $\alpha = 0.10$), and multivariate analyses were performed on all potential predictive factors that were associated with EPVS in the univariate analysis. The statistical analyses were performed with SPSS software (version 22; IBM Corporation, Armonk, NY, USA). p values less than 0.05 indicated statistical significance.

Results

The characteristics of the patients comparing the moyamoya disease group and the control group are presented in Table 1. The median ages and the percentage of females did not significantly differ, meaning that the median ages and sex tended to be similar in the groups. The median number of EPVS was significantly increased ($p < 0.001$) in the moyamoya group (43.8 [26.0-52.9]) compared with the control group (23.8 [15.1-33.0]). The median EPVS grade was significantly higher ($p < 0.001$) in the moyamoya group (4.0 [3.0-4.0]) compared with the control group (3.0 [2.0-3.0]). The distribution of the EPVS grades was as follows: grade 0 = 0, grade 1 = 2, grade 2 = 12, grade 3 = 33, and grade 4 = 53 in the moyamoya group and grade 0 = 0, grade 1 = 8, grade 2 = 30, grade 3 = 44, and grade 4 = 18 in the control group. The median interobserver discrepancies in the reported EPVS grades were 0.0 (0.0-0.0) in the moyamoya group and 0.0 (0.0-0.8) in the control group. Comparing the moyamoya disease group and the control group, the prevalence of hypertension was significantly higher in the high EPVS grade group ($p = 0.043$), though the prevalence of type 2 diabetes mellitus and hyperlipidemia was not significant. Presence of stroke lesions was significantly higher in the moyamoya disease group ($p < 0.001$). Of these, the presence of lacnar stroke was significantly higher in the moyamoya disease group ($p = 0.008$), and the presence of large ischemic stroke was significantly higher in the moyamoya disease group ($p < 0.001$). There was also significant difference between the moyamoya disease group and the control group in terms of the presence of microbleeds ($p = 0.007$) and the presence of white matter lesions ($p = 0.001$). Based on this data, multivariate analysis was performed to assess selection bias (Table 2). For tests that resulted in p values less than 0.10 in the

Table 2 Univariate and multivariate analysis concerning background characteristics

	Univariate analysis		Multivariate analysis	
Characteristics	Odds ratio (95% CI)	p value	Odds ratio (95% CI)	p value
Moyamoya disease	5.51 (2.87-10.58)	<0.001	4.84 (2.48-9.43)	<0.001
Hypertension	2.67 (1.40-5.07)	0.003		
Lacnar stroke	2.84 (1.09-7.44)	0.033		
Large ischemic stroke	3.23 (1.01-10.27)	0.047		
Microbleeds	2.87 (1.10-7.51)	0.032		
White matter lesions	2.69 (1.48-4.89)	0.001	2.01 (1.05-3.82)	0.034

EPVS enlarged perivascular spaces, *SD* standard deviation

Mann–Whitney U tests and Chi-squared test, a simple logistic regression was used. In the univariate analysis, moyamoya disease had higher EPVS grades (OR, 5.51; 95% CI, 2.87-10.58; $p < 0.001$). High EPVS grades in a particular hemisphere were associated with a higher prevalence of hypertension (OR, 2.67; 95% CI, 1.40-5.07; $p = 0.003$), lacnar stroke (OR, 2.84; 95% CI, 1.09-7.44; $p = 0.033$), large ischemic stroke (OR, 3.23; 95% CI, 1.01-10.27; $p = 0.047$), microbleeds (OR, 2.87; 95% CI, 1.10-7.51; $p = 0.032$), and white matter lesions (OR, 2.69; 95% CI, 1.48-4.89; $p = 0.001$). Two items (moyamoya disease and white matter lesions) were selected with stepwise methods, and the following significant differences were noted in the multivariate analysis: High EPVS grades in hemispheres were associated with moyamoya disease (OR, 4.84; 95% CI, 2.48-9.43; $p < 0.001$) and white matter lesions (OR, 2.01; 95% CI, 1.05-3.82; $p = 0.034$).

In the moyamoya disease group, the characteristics of the patients when comparing the high and low EPVS grade groups are presented in Table 3. The group with high EPVS grades included 53 hemispheres, while the low EPVS grade group included 47 hemispheres. The median number of EPVS was significantly increased ($p < 0.001$) in the group with high EPVS grades (52.0 [46.0-70.0]) compared with the group with low EPVS grades (25.0 [18.0-31.5]). The median ages were 42.0 (32.0-51.5) years in the high EPVS grade group and 41.0 (31.0-50.0) years in the low EPVS grade group, which did not significantly differ ($p = 0.516$). Thus, the median ages tended to be similar in the groups. The percentage of females was significantly higher ($p = 0.026$) in the group with high EPVS grades (81.1%; 43/53) compared with the group with low EPVS grades (61.7%; 29/47). The prevalence of hypertension was significantly higher in the high EPVS grade group ($p = 0.040$), though the prevalence of type 2 diabetes mellitus and hyperlipidemia was not significant. The median MRA score was significantly higher ($p = 0.021$) in the high EPVS grade group (5.0 [3.5-7.0]) compared with the low EPVS grade group (3.0 [2.0-6.0]). The median number of flow voids in the basal ganglia was significantly higher ($p < 0.001$) in the group with high EPVS grades (2.0 [1.5-3.5]) compared with the group with low EPVS grades (1.0 [0.0-2.0]). The brain atrophy score was significantly higher ($p = 0.004$) in the group with high EPVS grades (4.0 [3.0-5.0]) compared with the group with low EPVS grades (2.0 [1.0-4.0]). There was also significant difference between the high EPVS group and the low EPVS group in terms of the prevalence of ivy signs ($p = 0.005$) and white matter lesions ($p = 0.006$). However, the group did not significantly differ for disease subtype or the prevalence of stroke lesions and microbleeds.

Table 3 Clinical characteristics of the patients with high EPVS grades on T2-imaging

	High EPVS grade (4)	Low EPVS grade (0–3)	*p* value
n, hemisphere	53	47	
Total number of EPVS, median (IQR)	52.0 (46.0-70.0)	25.0 (18.0-31.5)	<0.001
Age, median (IQR)	42.0 (32.0-51.5)	41.0 (31.0-50.0)	0.516
Sex, male/female	10/43	18/29	0.026
Hypertension, presence/absence	24/29	12/35	0.040
Diabetes mellitus, presence/absence	2/51	0/47	0.497
Hyperlipidemia, presence/absence	11/42	5/42	0.168
Disease subtype	Ischemic stroke: 29	Ischemic stroke: 23	
	Hemorrhagic stroke: 5	Hemorrhagic stroke: 7	0.677
	Other: 19	Other: 17	
MRA score, median (IQR)	5.0 (3.5-7.0)	3.0 (2.0-6.0)	0.021
Flow voids in the basal ganglia, median (IQR)	2.0 (1.5-3.5)	1.0 (0.0-2.0)	<0.001
Brain atrophy score, median (IQR)	4.0 (3.0-5.0)	2.0 (1.0-4.0)	0.004
Ivy sign, presence/absence	34/19	17/30	0.005
Stroke lesions (total), presence/absence	20/33	12/35	0.192
Lacnar stroke, presence/absence	10/43	5/42	0.250
Large ischemic stroke, presence/absence	8/45	5/42	0.508
Hemorrhagic stroke, presence/absence	2/51	2/45	1.000
Microbleeds, presence/absence	9/43	6/40	0.558
White matter lesions, presence/absence	37/16	20/27	0.006

EPVS enlarged perivascular spaces, *SD* standard deviation, *MRA* magnetic resonance angiography

The predictive factors that were associated with EPVS in the patients with moyamoya disease are presented in Table 4. In the univariate analysis, females had higher EPVS grades (OR, 2.67; 95% CI, 1.08-6.60; p = 0.034). High EPVS grades in a particular hemisphere were associated with higher prevalence of hypertension (OR, 2.41; 95% CI, 1.03-5.65; p = 0.042), higher MRA scores (OR, 1.22; 95% CI, 1.03-1.44; p = 0.020), higher numbers of flow voids in the basal ganglia (OR, 1.53; 95% CI, 1.18-1.99; p = 0.001), higher brain atrophy scores (OR, 1.40; 95% CI, 1.10-1.78; p = 0.007), ivy signs (OR, 3.16; 95% CI, 1.39-7.16; p = 0.006), and white matter lesions (OR, 3.12; 95% CI, 1.37-7.11; p = 0.007). Three items (female sex, hypertension, and flow voids in the basal ganglia) were selected with stepwise methods, and the following significant differences were noted in the multivariate analysis. High EPVS grades in hemispheres were associated with the female sex (OR, 3.03; 95% CI, 1.04-8.84; p = 0.042), prevalence of hypertension (OR, 3.32; 95% CI, 1.23-9.00; p = 0.018), and higher number of flow voids in the basal ganglia (OR, 1.51; 95% CI, 1.16-1.97; p = 0.003).

Discussion

Pathophysiology of EPVS in the patients with moyamoya disease

This study confirmed that the patients with moyamoya disease tended to have higher numbers of EPVS, which are characteristic findings in patients with moyamoya disease due to chronic ischemic changes. The perivascular spaces are thought to constitute a perivascular lymphatic drainage pathway for interstitial fluid and solutes, such as amyloid-beta, from the brain parenchyma. Interstitial fluid and solutes drain along narrow basement membranes in the walls of arterioles to the lymph nodes in the neck [22, 23]. This system, which is largely separate from the cerebrospinal fluid system known as the glymphatic system [22, 23], is powered by vascular pulsations [24, 25]. When the system is inhibited by reduced pulsations, interstitial fluid and solutes, such as amyloid-beta, can accumulate. The accumulation of amyloid-beta causes Alzheimer's disease [26, 27], and the accumulation of interstitial fluid induces EPVS [13]. In moyamoya disease, chronic progressive stenosis of the terminal portion of the bilateral ICA results in an abnormal vascular network that is composed of collateral pathways at the base of the brain [1, 2]. The vessels that are derived from the collateral circulation are expected to have weak arterial pulsations compared with normal circulation, which can reduce the arterial pulsations and thereby inhibit the glymphatic system and increased EPVS counts in patients with moyamoya disease.

Risk factors of EPVS in patients with moyamoya disease

In the multivariate analysis, hypertension, female sex, and flow voids in the basal ganglia were selected for examination because of their association with high EPVS grades in the patients with moyamoya disease.

A relationship between EPVS and hypertension has been reported in previous studies of patients with lacunar strokes and normal subjects [11, 13]. This was confirmed in the patients with moyamoya disease. Two biological mechanisms are thought to underlie the hypertension-related increase in EPVS. The first mechanism involves arteriosclerosis, which van Swieten et al. have suggested is related to EPVS [28]. Arteriosclerosis might result in a reduction in the pulsations of the arterioles and, subsequently, more EPVS. The second involves impairments in the arteriole dilatation in the brain. Patients with moyamoya disease have lower cerebral blood flow and reduced cerebral perfusion pressure due to chronic progressive steno-occlusive changes in the ICA in both hemispheres. The arterioles dilate to maintain normal cerebral perfusion, and the cerebral blood volume increases [3, 29]. As a result, the impairments in the arteriole pulsation inhibit the glymphatic system, and the subsequent accumulation of interstitial fluid results in EPVS. In other words, hypertension might promote an increase in EPVS. On the other hand, the prevalence of hypertension in the moyamoya disease group was significantly higher than that in the control group, as shown in Table 1. Moyamoya disease is often

Table 4 Predictive factors of high EPVS in patients with moyamoya disease

	Univariate analysis		Multivariate analysis	
Characteristics	Odds ratio (95% CI)	p value	Odds ratio (95% CI)	p value
Female sex	2.67 (1.08-6.60)	0.034	3.03 (1.04-8.84)	0.042
Hypertension	2.41 (1.03-5.65)	0.042	3.32 (1.23-9.00)	0.018
MRA score	1.22 (1.03-1.44)	0.020		
Flow voids in the basal ganglia	1.53 (1.18-1.99)	0.001	1.51 (1.16-1.97)	0.003
Brain atrophy score	1.40 (1.10-1.78)	0.007		
Ivy sign	3.16 (1.39-7.16)	0.006		
White matter lesions	3.12 (1.37-7.11)	0.007		

EPVS enlarged perivascular space, *MRA* magnetic resonance angiography, *CI* confidence interval

accompanied by hypertension [30, 31], and a recent study suggested that a polymorphism of RNF213 is also associated with systolic blood pressure [32]. The prevalence of hypertension is higher than that in the age-sex matched control group. Although there is a possibility that hypertension might have a statistical influence in the comparison of clinical characteristics of high EPVS grade, hypertension was not selected as a confounding factor in the multivariate analysis comparing the moyamoya disease group and the control group. Therefore, the selection bias will not be high for evaluating high EPVS.

In this study, the female sex was associated with high EPVS grades. In elderly patients and patients with cerebral autosomal-dominant arteriopathy with subcortical infarcts and leukoencephalopathy (CADASIL) syndrome, no associations between sex and EPVS counts in the central semiovale have been observed [10, 11], while the male sex has been associated with high EPVS grades in the basal ganglia [12, 13]. Our observation of a female dominancy for the EPVS was thought to be characteristic of moyamoya disease. A previous study has shown that female patients with moyamoya disease are more susceptible to the development of preoperative transient ischemic attacks and have higher risks of adverse postoperative events, despite successful revascularizations [33]. In addition, unilateral moyamoya disease is less common in female patients with moyamoya disease [33, 34], which suggests that the disease might be more aggressive in female patients, perhaps because of specific sex-related factors that affect the pathophysiology and clinical course of the moyamoya disease. Similar sex-specific differences have been described in patients with symptomatic atherosclerotic intracranial arterial stenosis [35, 36]. In those studies, sex-specific differences in coagulation and fibrinolytic pathways, which occur due to the effects of estrogen on the endothelial wall and surrounding connective tissue, X-linked genetic differences, and methylation patterns have all been suggested to explain these sex differences. Whether these or other factors that specifically influence the pathophysiology of moyamoya disease are the cause of our observed sex differences remain unclear. Because there are few cases, further observations are needed before conclusions can be made.

From the viewpoint of MRI findings, disease stage and degree of ischemia should be associated with high EPVS grade. An association between flow voids in the basal ganglia and high EPVS grades was also confirmed, even though the ORs were not strong. The development of deep parenchymal collaterals is associated with the progression of moyamoya disease [18]. The deep parenchymal collaterals and the degree of steno-occlusive changes partially affect EPVS in adult patients with moyamoya disease. Although ivy sign and white matter lesions were not selected in multivariate analysis, the odds ratio revealed high values that were significant. The ivy sign is associated with low cerebral perfusion or misery perfusion [37, 38]; therefore, high EPVS might be associated with lower cerebral blood flow. However, this is not true in pediatric cases with moyamoya disease, which can exhibit linear hyperintensities that extend into the perivascular space of the deep white matter in FLAIR imaging [39]. These linear hyperintensities, which have been called medullary streaks, are thought to be associated with vasculature [40] or might result in a stagnation of cerebrospinal fluid of the perivascular spaces [41]. Because of this difference in adult and pediatric patients with moyamoya disease, pediatric patients were not included in this study. To confirm this observation, EPVS studies that use different methods must be conducted on pediatric patients with moyamoya disease.

In terms of lacnar stroke and microbleeds, their prevalence values were higher in the high EPVS grade group than in the low EPVS grade group though it was not significant. From the viewpoint of small vessel disease, high EPVS is associated with other morphological features, such as white matter hyperintensities and lacnar stroke [8, 10, 42]. In this study, these items could not be included in the multivariate analysis because their p values were less than 0.10 in the Mann–Whitney U tests and Chi-squared test. Although their sample size and prevalence were small in this study, their interaction might be apparent with a greater number of cases.

Study limitations

This study had several limitations. First, the EPVS assessments were performed with 3.0-T MRI at the level of the centrum semiovale. Therefore, the EPVS counts were relatively large, especially in the patients with high EPVS grades. Subsequently, interobserver discrepancies cannot be ruled out. In this study, two observers independently counted the EPVS and assigned each hemisphere an EPVS grade (0–4), which was undertaken in order to try to decrease the interobserver discrepancy shown in Table 2. Second, this study was a retrospective case–control study, and it did not track the progress of the EPVS in the studied hemispheres over time. The control group might not have been sufficiently rigorous in this study. Because we could not perform MRI on the normal volunteers in this study, we enrolled patients with nonischemic small lesions as controls because we considered them almost identical to normal volunteers for our purposes. The association between EPVS and the progression of the symptoms of moyamoya disease is still unclear. The pathophysiological significance of EPVS in moyamoya disease should be analyzed in future prospective cohort studies. Finally, because moyamoya disease is rare, the sample size was necessarily relatively small. Studies with larger sample sizes are needed to confirm our observations.

Conclusions

Adult patients with moyamoya disease exhibited increased numbers of EPVS. Hypertension, the female sex, and flow voids in the basal ganglia were found to be the most important factors for predicting high EPVS grades in patients with moyamoya disease. Reductions of arterial pulsations due to steno-occlusive changes might have inhibited the flow of interstitial fluid in the patients with moyamoya disease, which would increase the number of EPVS in these patients. Other clinical factors, such as female sex and hypertension, might also promote secondary brain damage in moyamoya disease. Further evaluations of EPVS in patients with moyamoya disease are needed to better understand their pathophysiological importance.

Abbreviations

ACA: Anterior cerebral artery; EPVS: Enlarged perivascular spaces; FLAIR: Fluid-attenuated inversion recovery; ICA: Internal carotid artery; MCA: Middle cerebral artery; MRA: Magnetic resonance angiography; MRI: Magnetic resonance imaging; PCA: Posterior cerebral artery

Acknowledgements

None.

Funding

This work was supported in part by JSPS KAKENHI grant Number 16 K10732 (to T.M.).

Authors' contributions

Conceptualization: TK and TM. Data curation: TK, TM, KK, HS, and KH. Formal analysis: TK, TM, KK, and HO. Writing: TK and TM. Supervision: TM and NM. All authors have read and approved the final version of the manuscript.

Competing interests

The authors declare that they have no competing interests.

Author details

[1]Department of Neurosurgery, Sapporo Medical University, South1 West16, Chuo-ku, Sapporo 060-8543, Japan. [2]Department of Public Health, Sapporo Medical University, Sapporo, Japan. [3]Department of Neurosurgery, Hokkaido University Graduate School of Medicine, Sapporo, Japan.

References

1. Nishimoto A, Takeuchi S. Abnormal cerebrovascular network related to the internal cartoid arteries. J Neurosurg. 1968;29(3):255–60.
2. Suzuki J, Takaku A. Cerebrovascular "moyamoya" disease. Disease showing abnormal net-like vessels in base of brain. Arch Neurol. 1969;20(3):288–99.
3. Ogawa A, Yoshimoto T, Suzuki J, Sakurai Y. Cerebral blood flow in moyamoya disease. Part 1: Correlation with age and regional distribution. Acta Neurochir. 1990;105(1–2):30–4.
4. Pantoni L, Garcia JH. Pathogenesis of leukoaraiosis: a review. Stroke. 1997;28(3):652–9.
5. Komatsu K, Mikami T, Noshiro S, Miyata K, Wanibuchi M, Mikuni N. Reversibility of White Matter Hyperintensity by Revascularization Surgery in Moyamoya Disease. J Stroke Cerebrovasc Dis. 2016;25(6):1495–502.
6. Kikuta K, Takagi Y, Nozaki K, Hanakawa T, Okada T, Mikuni N, Miki Y, Fushmi Y, Yamamoto A, Yamada K, et al. Asymptomatic microbleeds in moyamoya disease: T2*-weighted gradient-echo magnetic resonance imaging study. J Neurosurg. 2005;102(3):470–5.
7. Inzitari D. Leukoaraiosis: an independent risk factor for stroke? Stroke. 2003;34(8):2067–71.
8. Kwee RM, Kwee TC. Virchow-Robin spaces at MR imaging. Radiographics. 2007;27(4):1071–86.
9. Potter GM, Chappell FM, Morris Z, Wardlaw JM. Cerebral perivascular spaces visible on magnetic resonance imaging: development of a qualitative rating scale and its observer reliability. Cerebrovasc Dis. 2015;39(3–4):224–31.
10. Doubal FN, MacLullich AM, Ferguson KJ, Dennis MS, Wardlaw JM. Enlarged perivascular spaces on MRI are a feature of cerebral small vessel disease. Stroke. 2010;41(3):450–4.
11. Rouhl RP, van Oostenbrugge RJ, Knottnerus IL, Staals JE, Lodder J. Virchow-Robin spaces relate to cerebral small vessel disease severity. J Neurol. 2008; 255(5):692–6.
12. Yao M, Herve D, Jouvent E, Duering M, Reyes S, Godin O, Guichard JP, Dichgans M, Chabriat H. Dilated perivascular spaces in small-vessel disease: a study in CADASIL. Cerebrovasc Dis. 2014;37(3):155–63.
13. Zhu YC, Tzourio C, Soumare A, Mazoyer B, Dufouil C, Chabriat H. Severity of dilated Virchow-Robin spaces is associated with age, blood pressure, and MRI markers of small vessel disease: a population-based study. Stroke. 2010;41(11):2483–90.
14. Hiroki M, Miyashita K. Linear hyperintensity objects on magnetic resonance imaging related to hypertension. Cerebrovasc Dis. 2001;11(3):164–8.
15. Patankar TF, Mitra D, Varma A, Snowden J, Neary D, Jackson A. Dilatation of the Virchow-Robin space is a sensitive indicator of cerebral microvascular disease: study in elderly patients with dementia. AJNR Am J Neuroradiol. 2005;26(6):1512–20.
16. Suzuki H, Mikami T, Komatsu K, Noshiro S, Miyata K, Hirano T, Wanibuchi M, Mikuni N. Assessment of the cortical artery using computed tomography angiography for bypass surgery in moyamoya disease. Neurosurg Rev. 2017; 40(2):299–307.
17. Maclullich AM, Wardlaw JM, Ferguson KJ, Starr JM, Seckl JR, Deary IJ. Enlarged perivascular spaces are associated with cognitive function in healthy elderly men. J Neurol Neurosurg Psychiatry. 2004;75(11):1519–23.
18. Mikami T, Sugino T, Ohtaki S, Houkin K, Mikuni N. Diagnosis of moyamoya disease on magnetic resonance imaging: are flow voids in the basal ganglia an essential criterion for definitive diagnosis? Journal of stroke and cerebrovascular diseases : the official journal of National Stroke Association. 2013;22(6):862–8.
19. Zhang X, Ding L, Yang L, Qin W, Yuan J, Li S, Hu W. Brain Atrophy Correlates with Severe Enlarged Perivascular Spaces in Basal Ganglia among Lacunar Stroke Patients. PLoS One. 2016;11(2):e0149593.
20. Farrell C, Chappell F, Armitage PA, Keston P, Maclullich A, Shenkin S, Wardlaw JM. Development and initial testing of normal reference MR images for the brain at ages 65–70 and 75–80 years. Eur Radiol. 2009;19(1):177–83.
21. Houkin K, Nakayama N, Kuroda S, Nonaka T, Shonai T, Yoshimoto T. Novel magnetic resonance angiography stage grading for moyamoya disease. Cerebrovasc Dis. 2005;20(5):347–54.
22. Weller RO, Djuanda E, Yow HY, Carare RO. Lymphatic drainage of the brain and the pathophysiology of neurological disease. Acta Neuropathol. 2009;117(1):1–14.
23. Carare RO, Bernardes-Silva M, Newman TA, Page AM, Nicoll JA, Perry VH, Weller RO. Solutes, but not cells, drain from the brain parenchyma along basement membranes of capillaries and arteries: significance for cerebral amyloid angiopathy and neuroimmunology. Neuropathol Appl Neurobiol. 2008;34(2):131–44.
24. Schley D, Carare-Nnadi R, Please CP, Perry VH, Weller RO. Mechanisms to explain the reverse perivascular transport of solutes out of the brain. J Theor Biol. 2006;238(4):962–74.
25. Iliff JJ, Wang M, Zeppenfeld DM, Venkataraman A, Plog BA, Liao Y, Deane R, Nedergaard M. Cerebral arterial pulsation drives paravascular CSF-interstitial fluid exchange in the murine brain. The Journal of neuroscience: the official journal of the Society for Neuroscience. 2013;33(46):18190–9.
26. Weller RO, Preston SD, Subash M, Carare RO. Cerebral amyloid angiopathy in the aetiology and immunotherapy of Alzheimer disease. Alzheimers Res Ther. 2009;1(2):6.
27. Kyrtsos CR, Baras JS. Modeling the Role of the Glymphatic Pathway and Cerebral Blood Vessel Properties in Alzheimer's Disease Pathogenesis. PLoS One. 2015;10(10):e0139574.

28. van Swieten JC, van den Hout JH, van Ketel BA, Hijdra A, Wokke JH, van Gijn J. Periventricular lesions in the white matter on magnetic resonance imaging in the elderly. A morphometric correlation with arteriolosclerosis and dilated perivascular spaces. Brain J Neurol. 1991;114(Pt 2):761–74.
29. Kuroda S, Houkin K, Kamiyama H, Abe H, Mitsumori K. Regional cerebral hemodynamics in childhood moyamoya disease. Child's nervous system : ChNS. 1995;11(10):584–90.
30. Yamada I, Himeno Y, Matsushima Y, Shibuya H. Renal artery lesions in patients with moyamoya disease: angiographic findings. Stroke. 2000;31(3):733–7.
31. Togao O, Mihara F, Yoshiura T, Tanaka A, Kuwabara Y, Morioka T, Matsushima T, Sasaki T, Honda H. Prevalence of stenoocclusive lesions in the renal and abdominal arteries in moyamoya disease. AJR Am J Roentgenol. 2004;183(1):119–22.
32. Koizumi A, Kobayashi H, Liu W, Fujii Y, Senevirathna ST, Nanayakkara S, Okuda H, Hitomi T, Harada KH, Takenaka K, et al. P.R4810K, a polymorphism of RNF213, the susceptibility gene for moyamoya disease, is associated with blood pressure. Environ Health Prev Med. 2013;18(2):121–9.
33. Khan N, Achrol AS, Guzman R, Burns TC, Dodd R, Bell-Stephens T, Steinberg GK. Sex differences in clinical presentation and treatment outcomes in Moyamoya disease. Neurosurgery. 2012;71(3):587–93. discussion 593
34. Hallemeier CL, Rich KM, Grubb RL Jr, Chicoine MR, Moran CJ, Cross DT 3rd, Zipfel GJ, Dacey RG Jr, Derdeyn CP. Clinical features and outcome in North American adults with moyamoya phenomenon. Stroke. 2006;37(6):1490–6.
35. Barrett KM, Worrall BB. Sex and stroke: are they really different in midlife? Neurology. 2007;69(20):1894–5.
36. Williams JE, Chimowitz MI, Cotsonis GA, Lynn MJ, Waddy SP. Gender differences in outcomes among patients with symptomatic intracranial arterial stenosis. Stroke. 2007;38(7):2055–62.
37. Kaku Y, Iihara K, Nakajima N, Kataoka H, Fukushima K, Iida H, Hashimoto N. The leptomeningeal ivy sign on fluid-attenuated inversion recovery images in moyamoya disease: positron emission tomography study. Cerebrovasc Dis. 2013;36(1):19–25.
38. Vuignier S, Ito M, Kurisu K, Kazumata K, Nakayama N, Shichinohe H, Shiga T, Kiss JZ, Tamaki N, Houkin K. Ivy sign, misery perfusion, and asymptomatic moyamoya disease: FLAIR imaging and (15)O-gas positron emission tomography. Acta Neurochir. 2013;155(11):2097–104.
39. Maeda M, Tsuchida C. "Ivy sign" on fluid-attenuated inversion-recovery images in childhood moyamoya disease. AJNR Am J Neuroradiol. 1999;20(10):1836–8.
40. Takanashi J, Suzuki H, Barkovich AJ, Sugita K, Saeki N, Kobayashi E, Fujii K, Kohno Y. Medullary streaks: dilated medullary vessels in chronic ischemia in children. Neurology. 2003;61(4):583–4.
41. Suzuki H, Mikami T, Kuribara T, Yoshifuji K, Komatsu K, Akiyama Y, Ohnishi H, Houkin K, Mikuni N. Pathophysiological consideration of medullary streaks on FLAIR imaging in pediatric moyamoya disease. J Neurosurg Pediatr. 2017;19(5):560–6.
42. Charidimou A, Boulouis G, Pasi M, Auriel E, van Etten ES, Haley K, Ayres A, Schwab KM, Martinez-Ramirez S, Goldstein JN, et al. MRI-visible perivascular spaces in cerebral amyloid angiopathy and hypertensive arteriopathy. Neurology. 2017;88(12):1157–64.

6

Stroke caused by an inflammatory thrombus

Kai Shan and Wei Guo*

Abstract

Background: Stroke is the leading cause of mortality and disability worldwide. Several definite risk factors have been identified for stroke, although infectious factors might also contribute to stroke episodes through increased susceptibility or direct induction.

Case presentation: A 46-year-old Chinese male initially presented with fever, headache, and impaired memory and developed disturbance of consciousness after admission. A clinical diagnosis of *Staphylococcus aureus* sepsis, massive cerebral infarction and haemorrhagic transformation (left internal carotid arterial system, inflammatory thrombus) were made based on brain radiography, blood culture and postoperative pathological examinations. These symptoms improved following antibiotic therapy with vancomycin and conventional treatments for stroke.

Conclusion: For stroke patients without traditional cerebrovascular risk factors but with signs of infection, infectious causes should be considered.

Keywords: Stroke, Infection, *Staphylococcus aureus*, Inflammatory thrombus, Haemorrhagic transformation

Background

Stroke is the leading cause of mortality and disability worldwide [1], and several definite risk factors have been identified for stroke. As shown by the INTERSTROKE study, approximately 90% of stroke episodes are associated with hypertension, smoking, heart disease, diabetes and six additional risk factors [2]. However, infectious factors might also contribute to stroke episodes through increased susceptibility or direct induction [3]. In this paper, one case admitted to our hospital due to stroke induced by *Staphylococcus aureus* sepsis is described with the purpose of increasing clinicians' understanding of infectious stroke.

Case presentation

A 46-year-old male visited the emergency department of our hospital on April 23, 2015 due to fever and headache for three days and impaired memory for half a day. The patient had experienced fever three days before, with a peak body temperature of 38.5 °C. No other discomfort was described. He had visited other hospitals before and was diagnosed with an upper respiratory infection based on haematological findings. However, his condition did not improve after treatment with intravenous levofloxacin. Within a half a day, he developed impaired memory, concomitant with speech disturbance, poor response, no significant limb movements and convulsions before being referred to the emergency department of our hospital. The patient had no medical history. No histories of food and drug allergies were obtained. The patient denied any prior history of smoking, heavy drinking or drug abuse. On arrival, the initial physical examination revealed the following: body temperature 38.0 °C, pulse 100 beats/min, respirations 26 breaths/min, blood pressure 144/76 mmHg, delirium, speech disturbance, equal size and round shape of bilateral pupils with diameters of approximately 3.0 mm, sensitive to light reflex, basically normal cranial nerve examination, limb muscle strength Grade V, negative bilateral pathological signs, and no ataxia. The patient's neck was soft, and there were no signs of meningeal irritation. No significant findings were found on the cardiopulmonary and abdominal examinations. No skin rashes or bleeding sites were observed after examining the entire body. The laboratory test results were the following: haematology: white blood cells (WBC), 12.5×10^9/L, neutrophil percentage, 87.6%; C-reactive protein (CRP), 56 mg/L;

* Correspondence: guowei1010@126.com
Emergency Department, Beijing Tiantan Hospital, Capital Medical University, Beijing 100050, China

procalcitonin (PCT), 2.8 ng/mL; and D-dimer, 3.2 μg/mL. A chemistry panel and screens for infectious diseases and cardiac markers were generally normal. No abnormal findings were observed on chest X-ray or electrocardiogram. Brain computed tomography (CT) showed a curved high-density mass at the left sylvian fissure area and an ischemic lesion of the left temporal lobe (Fig. 1).

As an emergency diagnosis, massive cerebral infarction (probable atherosclerosis of the left internal carotid artery system) was considered, and intracranial infection could not be excluded; appropriate treatments included aspirin for anti-platelet aggregation, atorvastatin for lipid regulation and plaque stabilization, and cefuroxime and acyclovir for anti-infection.

The patient experienced aggravated unconsciousness after two hours of admission, and physical examination showed the following: lethargy, aphasia, equal size and round shape of bilateral pupils with diameters of approximately 3.0 mm, sensitive to light reflex, shallow right nasolabial folds, immobilization of right limbs upon orbital pressure, movable left limbs, positive right pathological signs and negative left pathological signs. Further revascularization therapy was considered, and the patient was immediately transferred to undergo brain magnetic resonance imaging (MRI). On the way to the radiology department, the patient experienced further aggravation of unconsciousness and entered a light coma, concomitant with limb seizure, gazing to the left of bilateral eyes, equal size and round shape of bilateral pupils with diameters of approximately 2.0 mm, and disappearance of the light reflex. Appropriate treatments included midazolam for epilepsy, mannitol for dehydration and intracranial hypotension. After termination of the seizure, re-examination of the brain CT showed a curved high-density mass at the left sylvian fissure area and a massive low-density area in the left temporal lobe with many high-density plot areas scattered within it. CT images also showed compressed deformation of the left ventricle and a shift of the brain midline to the right (Fig. 2). Considering that the patient developed haemorrhagic transformation, he was admitted to the emergency intensive care unit for further management.

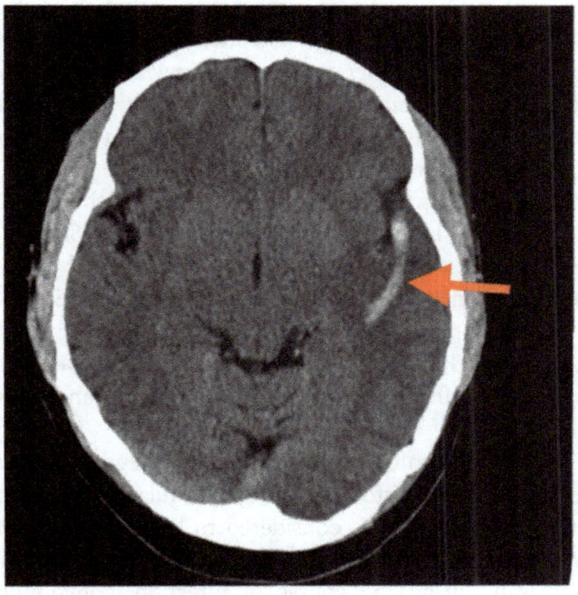

Fig. 1 A brain computed tomography image showing the thrombus in the left middle cerebral artery (arrow)

Eighteen hours after admission, the patient experienced further aggravation of unconsciousness and entered a moderate coma, concomitant with high fever (body temperature 39.9 °C), bilateral pupils: left versus right = 5.0 mm versus 3.0 mm, respectively, disappearance of the light reflex, increased muscle tone of the right limbs, and positive pathological signs of bilateral limbs. The brain CT re-examination showed expansion of the bleeding area, with overt signs of brain herniation. The patient underwent emergency left frontal temporal craniotomy, removal of the intracranial hematoma and a decompressed craniotomy performed by neurosurgeons. The intraoperative findings were as follows: dark red appearance of the left temporal brain tissue, concomitant with subarachnoid haemorrhage (SAH); an ostomy of approximately 0.2 cm was created along the left temporal sulcus; a visible purple blood clot was observed, concomitant with surrounding contused brain tissues; and a large vascular embolization could be observed in the hematoma cavity. Approximately 10 mL of the hematoma and contused brain tissues were removed and sampled for pathological evaluation. Histopathological examination showed haemorrhage, oedema and inflammatory changes in brain tissues, neutrophil infiltration into the vascular walls and surrounding tissues, and microvascular purulent thrombosis (Figs. 3–4). The patient was transferred to the neurologic intensive care unit for further treatment after the operation. During the course of the treatment, negative findings were found for *Chlamydia pneumoniae*, mycopsslasma, influenza, tuberculosis, the TORCH panel, hepatitis B, hepatitis C, syphilis and human immunodeficiency virus (HIV); the sputum culture was negative, and the blood culture suggested *Staphylococcus aureus*. No abnormal findings were found on chest X-ray or ultrasound. In addition, two transthoracic echocardiography (TTE) examinations were normal, and there were no observations of valvular dysfunction or neoplasm. The following final diagnosis was considered: massive cerebral infarction, consistent with haemorrhagic transformation (the left internal carotid artery system, inflammatory thrombus), *Staphylococcus aureus* sepsis and symptomatic epilepsy. After two months of vancomycin anti-infective treatments and supportive and symptomatic treatment, the consciousness of the patient improved gradually, and several blood cultures were negative. He

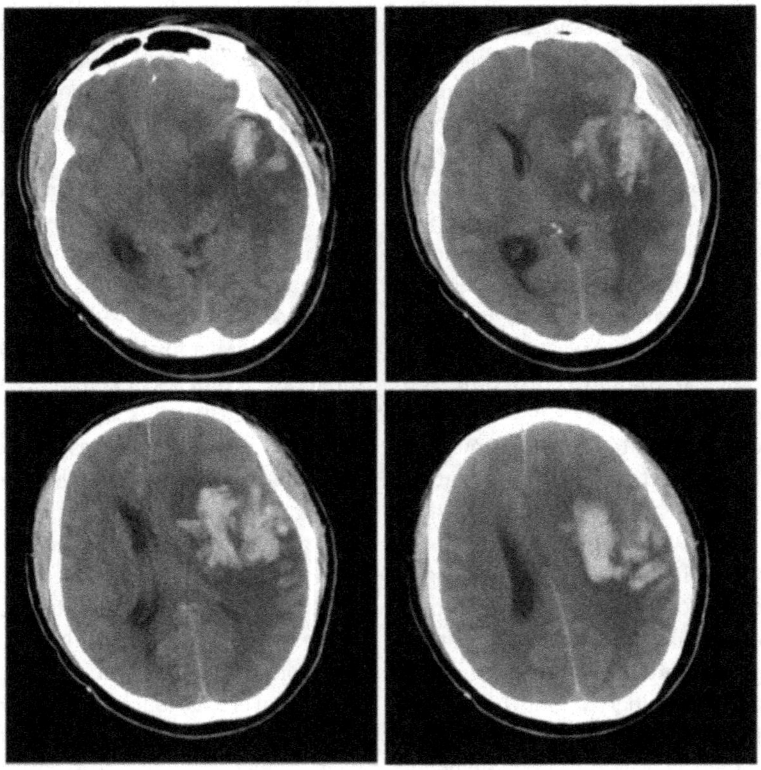

Fig. 2 Brain computed tomography images showing left temporal lobe insular lobe infarction and haemorrhagic transformation

underwent rehabilitation and was discharged from the hospital on the 72nd postoperative day (POD). At discharge, his Glasgow Coma Scale (GCS) was E4V4M6, and the modified Rankin scale score was 3.

Discussion

The patient described herein was middle-aged and healthy; although no stroke risk factors were identified, a rapid onset of disease was observed. After admission, the brain CT suggested cerebral infarction, subsequently followed by haemorrhagic transformation. After craniotomy, the pathological examination indicated that the cerebral infarction was induced by inflammatory thrombosis. Additionally, the patient also experienced fever, shortness of breath and unconsciousness. Laboratory examinations suggested abnormal elevations of haematological variables, CRP, PCT and D-dimer. *Staphylococcus aureus* was indicated by blood culture. This condition responded well to vancomycin treatment. Therefore, the sepsis was considered to be induced by *Staphylococcus aureus* infection.

Although there were definite risk factors for stroke, all episodes of this disease could not be fully explained by the factors currently identified. Indeed, many patients who develop stroke do not have any risk factors, and no definite aetiologies are identified for approximately one-third of stroke cases. As shown by several studies, there might be a correlation between systemic infection and episodes of stroke [4]. Indeed, relevant case–control studies have confirmed this correlation between systemic infection and stroke. In patients with stroke, the odds ratio of a precursor infection was in the range of 2–14.5 [5–10].

A wide range of pathogens has been found to be associated with an elevation of stroke risk, including viruses, bacteria, fungi and parasites. The most investigated pathogens include *Helicobacter pylori, Chlamydia pneumoniae, Mycoplasma pneumoniae, Haemophilus influenzae,* Epstein-Barr virus (EBV), herpes simplex virus (HSV)-1, HSV-2 and cytomegalovirus [3, 11].

Staphylococcus aureus is a major human pathogen that causes a wide range of clinical infections [12]. *Staphylococcus aureus* bacteraemia (SAB) is associated with a short-term increased risk of stroke, and the risk can persist for up to 180 days. The risk factors for stroke after SAB include old age, prior arterial thromboembolic events, atrial flutter/fibrillation, hypertension and endocarditis [13].

The mechanism of stroke induced by infection remains incompletely understood, although stimulation of the inflammatory response is considered to be the main driver for stroke [14–16]. Pathogens may directly invade the vascular wall during the course of infection, concomitant with an increase in smooth muscle cell proliferation or inflammatory cytokine production. Additionally, regions far

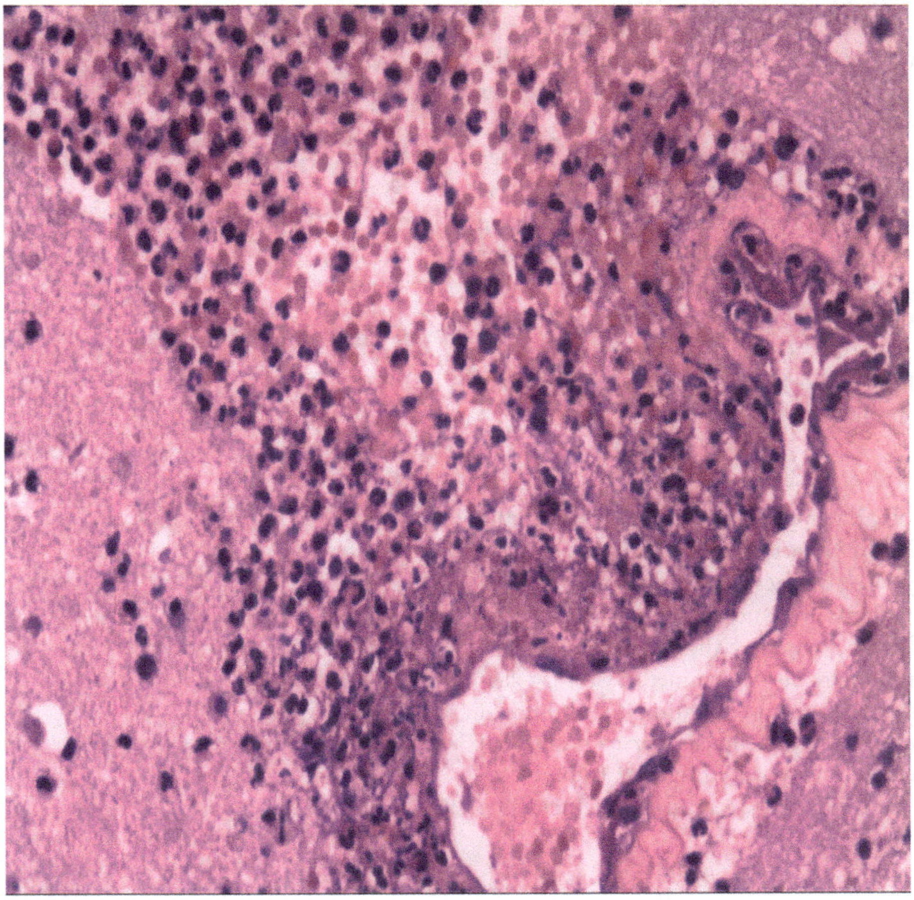

Fig. 3 Postoperative histopathological examination showing vasculitis and perivascular inflammatory exudates (hematoxylin-eosin staining, ×200)

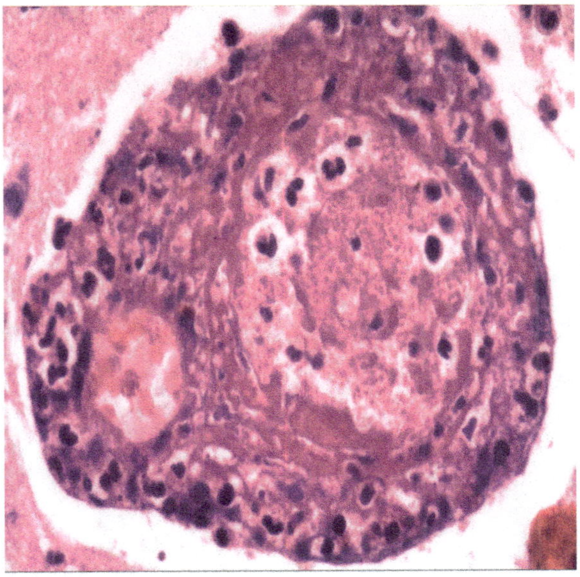

Fig. 4 Postoperative pathological examination showing the inflammatory thrombus in the artery (hematoxylin-eosin staining, ×400)

away from the primary infected loci might also be affected, and this secondary impairment might also lead to damage of the arterial wall. Furthermore, the inflammatory response induced by infection could stimulate enhancement of platelet aggregation and dysfunction of vasodilation [15]. It has been described that blood levels of high-sensitivity CRP (HS-CRP) may be considered an independent predictor for ischemic stroke, although the exact correlation remains unclear [17, 18].

Based on the current patient's medical history, physical examination, and laboratory, radiology and pathological examinations, the aetiology of stroke was considered to be embolic stroke and subsequent haemorrhagic transformation as a result of migration of the septic emboli induced by systematic *Staphylococcus aureus* infection to the left internal carotid artery system. *Staphylococcus aureus* is a common pathogen of acute infective endocarditis, and infective endocarditis has been identified as an important cause of cardioembolic stroke [19–21]. However, two TTE examinations showed no abnormal findings. A diagnosis of infective endocarditis was still possible for this case because one major and one minor criterion of the modified Duke criteria were met [22].

Further cardiac evaluation, such as a transoesophageal echocardiography (TEE), should have been considered. Unfortunately, due to the serious condition of the patient and the unavailability of bedside TEE in our hospital, TEE was not performed in this case.

Additionally, post-operational pathological findings suggested inflammatory changes of brain tissues, consistent with purulent thrombosis. However, a culture of brain tissue was not obtained because of the poor communication between the emergency physicians and neurosurgeons during such an urgent situation. If the same strain were identified between this culture and the blood culture, the aetiological diagnosis of this case would be further confirmed.

Conclusion

Appropriate aetiological judgment is critical for the treatment of stroke. In clinical practice, the possibility of stroke induced by infective factors should be considered with caution for patients with no traditional risk factors of stroke and infective signs. For these patients, an appropriate regimen should be determined based on targeted anti-infective therapies in addition to traditional treatments for stroke. Additionally, similar to traditional risk factors, preventive interventions against some infections might also contribute to decreasing the incidence of stroke in some cases.

Abbreviations

CRP: C-reactive protein; CT: Computed tomography; EBV: Epstein-Barr virus; GCS: Glasgow coma scale; HIV: Human immunodeficiency virus; HS-CRP: High-sensitivity C-reactive protein; HSV: Herpes simplex virus; MRI: Magnetic resonance imaging; PCT: Procalcitonin; POD: Postoperative day; SAB: *Staphylococcus aureus* bacteraemia; SAH: Subarachnoid haemorrhage; TORCH: Toxoplasmosis other infections, rubella, cytomegalovirus, and herpes simplex virus; WBC: White blood cell

Acknowledgements

The authors would like to thank Dr. Jun-Mei Wang, a neuropathologist at the Laboratory of Pathology, Beijing Institute of Neurosurgery, China, for her valuable advice on interpreting the pathological findings.

Funding

No funding was obtained.

Authors' contributions

KS examined the patient and drafted the manuscript. WG participated in the design of the case report and helped to draft the manuscript. Both authors read and approved the final manuscript.

Competing interests

The authors declare that they have no competing interests.

References

1. Murray CJ, Vos T, Lozano R, Naghavi M, Flaxman AD, Michaud C, et al. Disability-adjusted life years (DALYs) for 291 diseases and injuries in 21 regions, 1990–2010: a systematic analysis for the Global Burden of Disease Study 2010. Lancet. 2012;380:2197–223.
2. O'Donnell MJ, Chin SL, Rangarajan S, Xavier D, Liu L, Zhang H, et al. Global and regional effects of potentially modifiable risk factors associated with acute stroke in 32 countries (INTERSTROKE): a case-control study. Lancet. 2016;388:761–75.
3. Fugate JE, Lyons JL, Thakur KT, Smith BR, Hedley-whyte ET, Mateen FJ. Infectious causes of stroke. Lancet Infect Dis. 2014;14:869–80.
4. Grau AJ, Urbanek C, Palm F. Common infections and the risk of stroke. Nat Rev Neurol. 2010;6:681–94.
5. Grau AJ, Buggle F, Heindl S, Steichen-Wiehn C, Banerjee T, Maiwald M, et al. Recent infection as a risk factor for cerebrovascular ischemia. Stroke. 1995; 26:373–9.
6. Bova IY, Bornstein NM, Korczyn AD. Acute infection as a risk factor for ischemic stroke. Stroke. 1996;27:2204–6.
7. Syrjänen J, Valtonen V, Livanainen M, Kaste M, Huttunen JK. Preceding infection as an important risk factor for ischaemic brain infarction in young and middle aged patients. BMJ (Clin Res Ed). 1988;296:1156–60.
8. Clayton TC, Thompson M, Meade TW. Recent respiratory infection and risk of cardiovascular disease: case-control study through a general practice database. Eur Heart J. 2008;29:96–103.
9. Nencini P, Sarti C, Innocenti R, Pracucci G, Inzitari D. Acute inflammatory events and ischemic stroke subtypes. Cerebrovasc Dis. 2003;15:215–21.
10. Paganini-Hill A, Lozano E, Fischberg G, Barreto MP, Rajamani K, Ameriso SF, et al. Infection and risk of ischemic stroke: differences among stroke subtypes. Stroke. 2003;34:452–7.
11. Miller E, Elkind MS. Infection and Stroke: an Update on Recent Progress. Curr Neurol Neurosci Rep. 2016;16:1–10.
12. Tong SY, Davis JS, Eichenberger E, Holland TL, Fowler Jr VG. Staphylococcus aureus Infections: Epidemiology, Pathophysiology, Clinical Manifestations, and Management. Clin Microbiol Rev. 2015;28:603–61.
13. Mejer N, Gotland N, Uhre ML, Westh H, Schonheyder HC, Petersen A, et al. Increased risk of arterial thromboembolic events after Staphylococcus aureus bacteremia: A matched cohort study. J Infect. 2015;71:167–78.
14. Elkind MS, Ramakrishnan P, Moon YP, Bodenalbala B, Liu K, Rundek T, et al. Infectious burden and risk of stroke: the northern Manhattan study. Arch Neurol. 2010;67:33–8.
15. Epstein SE, Zhou YF, Zhu J. Infection and atherosclerosis: emerging mechanistic paradigms. Circulation. 1999;100:e20–8.
16. Lindsberg PJ, Grau AJ. Inflammation and infections as risk factors for ischemic stroke. Stroke. 2003;34:2518–32.
17. Elkind MS. Inflammatory mechanisms of stroke. Stroke. 2010;41:S3–8.
18. DA E, Lowe GD, Thompson S, Collins R, Danesh J, Nissinen A, et al. C-reactive protein concentration and risk of coronary heart disease, stroke, and mortality: an individual participant meta-analysis. Lancet. 2010;375:132–40.
19. Dickerman SA, Abrutyn E, Barsic B, Bouza E, Cecchi E, Moreno A, et al. The relationship between the initiation of antimicrobial therapy and the incidence of stroke in infective endocarditis: an analysis from the ICE Prospective Cohort Study (ICE-PCS). Am Heart J. 2007;154:1086–94.
20. Duval X. lung B, Klein I, Brochet E, Thabut G, Arnoult F, et al. Effect of early cerebral magnetic resonance imaging on clinical decisions in infective endocarditis: A prospective study. Ann Intern Med. 2010;152:497–504.
21. Chow FC, Marra CM, Cho TA. Cerebrovascular disease in central nervous system infections. Semin Neurol. 2011;31:286–306.
22. Hoen B, Duval X. Infective endocarditis. N Engl J Med. 2013;368:1425–33.

Are the anomalous vertebral arteries more hypoplastic? Retrospective linear mixed model approach

Chulho Kim, Jong-Hee Sohn* and Hui-Chul Choi

Abstract

Background: Small or hypoplastic vertebral artery (VA) is one of the risk factor for posterior circulation stroke. We assess whether various types of VA anomaly contribute to its diameter.

Methods: We screened 238 patients who underwent neck CT and MR angiography within 1 month. A V1 anomaly was defined as the abnormal origin of the VA on a three-dimensional MR angiography and a V2 anomaly was defined as the VA not passing through the 6th cervical transverse foramen (TF) on an axial CT image. A linear mixed model was used to evaluate the determinants of VA size.

Results: Among participants, 24 (10.1%) subjects exhibited an anomalous VA and, of the 476 VAs examined, 11 (2.3%) had an aortic origin and 27 (5.7%) had an abnormal entrance into the C6 TF. Presence of the V1 anomaly was positively associated with the V2 anomaly (P for chi-square < 0.001) and a linear mixed model revealed that being male (0.2 mm larger, $P = 0.015$), having a right VA anomaly (0.3 mm smaller, $P < 0.001$), having a V1 anomaly (0.9 mm smaller, $P < 0.001$), and having a V2 anomaly (0.7 mm smaller, $P < 0.001$) were significant predictor of VA diameter.

Conclusion: The diameters of VAs with an anomalous aortic origin or an abnormal entrance of the TF were significantly smaller than those of normal VAs. These findings suggest that anomalies of the VA detected in 3-dimensional CTA or MRA may be clues for vertebral artery hypoplasia.

Keywords: Vertebral artery, Abnormalities, Computed tomography angiography, Magnetic resonance angiography

Background

Vertebrobasilar atherosclerosis is a common etiology of posterior circulation strokes (PCS), which account for 20% of all ischemic strokes [1, 2]. Although there is a high prevalence of vertebral artery hypoplasia (VAH) among the normal population [3], VAH also greatly contributes to an increased risk of PCS [3–5]. However, the rates of VAH reported in the literature are quite variable because there is no standard definition for this disorder as of yet [4–8].

During embryological development, the vertebrobasilar artery forms from paired neural arteries that receive their blood supply from carotid-vertebrobasilar anastomoses such as the trigeminal, otic, hypoglossal, and proatlantal arteries [9, 10]. At the same time, the longitudinal anastomoses of the cervical intersegmental arteries contribute to the development of the vertebral artery (VA) which, in turn, is connected to the subclavian artery [11, 12]. The exact nature and precise underlying mechanisms of persistent carotid-vertebrobasilar anastomoses have yet to be fully characterized, but some researchers have suggested that these anastomoses remain unchanged to compensate for the delayed development of the vertebrobasilar artery [12, 13]. In other words, VAH is the product of the delayed development of the vertebrobasilar artery and might be associated with anomalies in posterior circulation.

It is important to distinguish between acquired narrowing and hypoplasia of the VA because each of these has different atherosclerotic burden. Even in the case of digital subtraction angiography, which is the gold standard method for assessing cerebral arterial pathology, it is difficult to distinguish between atherosclerotic narrowing and

* Correspondence: deepfoci@hallym.or.kr
Department of Neurology, Chuncheon Sacred Heart Hospital, Chuncheon-si, Gangwon-do 200-704, Republic of Korea

hypoplasia because it only evaluates internal lumen of the blood vessel. The present study hypothesized that certain vascular anomalies of the VA would be associated with a small or hypoplastic VA. For example, the VA usually arises from the subclavian artery (Fig. 1a) but 2-5% of all VAs originate directly from the aorta [14–17]. Additionally, the VA typically penetrates the transverse foramen (TF) of sixth cervical vertebra (C6) but approximately 5-10% of VAs do not pass through this area (Fig. 1b) [17–19]. These anomalies are relatively common, which account for ~5% of incidence in general [15, 19]. Thus, the present study aimed to determine whether an anomalous origin of the VA and/or its abnormal penetration of TF other than C6 would contribute to the VA diameter in hospital-based populations.

Methods

Participants

The present study was a single-center retrospective observational investigation. Inclusion criteria for this study were a subject who visited our neurology clinic and underwent computed tomography (CT) and magnetic resonance (MR) angiography from January 2012 to December 2015. Additionally, the CT and MR images of each subjects were taken within a 1-month interval ($n = 279$ subjects). We excluded subjects who had motion artifacts on the CT or MR images ($n = 12$), insufficient arterial enhancement on the CT image ($n = 23$), and missing clinical information ($n = 4$). Additionally, patients who had profound vertebral artery tortuosity ($n = 2$) were excluded because vascular tortuosity could affect the radiologic parameter measurement of the VA. Our study is retrospective in nature, therefore, written informed consent was not obtained. However, the design of this study was approved by our Institutional Review Board/Ethics Committee.

Definitions of anatomical variations

The VA usually originates from the subclavian artery and can be divided into four anatomical parts along the course of craniocervical area [20]. The V1 segment arises from the subclavian artery and extends to the proximal portion of the C6 TF, the V2 (transforaminal) segment extends from the C6 to the C1 TF, the V3 segment extends from the C1 to the dura, and the V4 segment extends from the dura to the vertebrobasilar junction. In the present study, the anomalous origin of the VA was referred to as a V1 anomaly and consisted of the VA directly originating from the aorta, as shown on a three-dimensional MRA (Fig. 1b). A V2 anomaly was defined as a VA that did not pass through the C6 TF (Fig. 1c and d) on an axial source CTA. A window level and a width setting of 400 and 1400 Hounsfield Units, respectively, were selected to optimally visualize the V2 segment anomalies on the CT images.

Measurements of the radiologic parameters

A 64-section multidetector CT scanner (Somatom Sensation 64, Siemens AG Medical Solutions; Erlangen, Germany) was used to identity V2 segment anomalies using the following settings: 120 kVp, 100 mA, slice thickness of 1.5 mm, and 512 × 512 matrix. All MR imaging

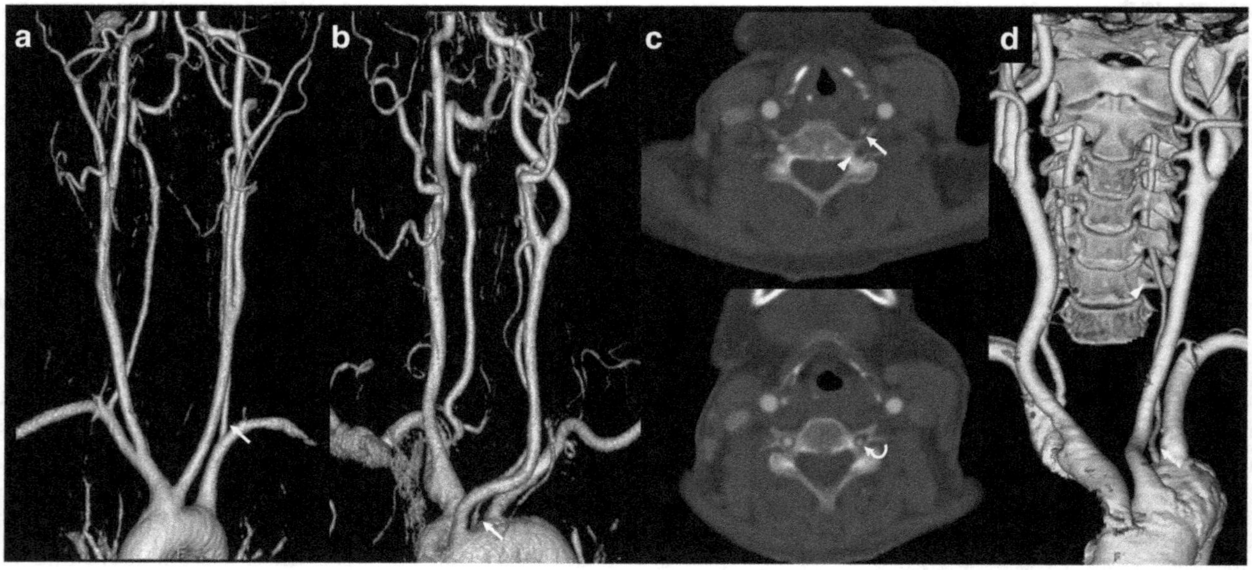

Fig. 1 Left VAs (*arrows*) originating from (**a**) the subclavian artery and (**b**) the aorta on a three-dimensional MR angiography. Axial source images (window level = 400 Hounsfield Units, width = 1400 Hounsfield Units) of the CT angiography showing that the left VA (**c**, *arrow*) did not penetrate the C6 transverse foramen (*arrow head*) but that it passed through the C5 transverse foramen (**c**, *curved arrow*). Three-dimensional reconstructed CT image (**d**) showing a left VA (*arrow*) with an aortic origin and an empty left C6 transverse foramen (*arrow head*)

was performed on a 1.5 T MRI system (Intera, Philips Medical Systems; Best, the Netherlands) with the following settings: slice thickness of 1.3 mm, TR = 3.5, TE = 1.2 ms, field of view = 70 × 70, flip angle = 40°, and acquisition matrix = 256 × 256. Additionally, real-time MRA was conducted to determine whether there was an anomalous origin of the VA (aortic origin) by administering a dynamic three-dimensional gadolinium injection at a rate of 4 ml/s. The identification of VA anomalies and the measurement of the VA diameters were performed in a pi-view workstation (Infinitt; Seoul, Korea) by two blinded investigators (C Kim and H-C Choi) Because there were many cases of stenotic narrowing and vascular tortuosity, which could augment stenotic degree of the VA, the VA diameter was measured at 1 cm above its origin on the MRA, and defined as the longest diameter perpendicular to the direction of the VA.

Statistical analysis

These data were freely available from the online (Additional file 1). The baseline characteristics of the patients were summarized using proportions for categorical variables and means ± standard deviations for numerical data. Descriptive comparisons between the anomalous VA and normal VA groups were assessed using the chi-square test or the Mann-Whitney U test for categorical variables and Student's t-test or paired t-test for continuous variables, as appropriate. The inter-rater reliability of the two blind investigators in terms of the VA diameter measurements was analyzed using the intra-class correlation value and the diameters of the VA were entered into dependent variable. Linear mixed models used to investigate the association of the diameters of the VA with anatomical and demographic characteristics, modeled as fixed effects (including age, sex [female vs. male], the side of the VA (right-sided vs. left-sided; within-subject variable), V1 anomaly [yes vs. no], and V2 anomaly [yes vs. no]). The compound symmetry of the variance-covariance matrix was used for the repeated measure analysis because the variance and correlation (covariance) between the right and the left VAs were constant.

Results

Patient characteristics

Of the 238 patients, the mean age (± standard deviation) of the population was 65.9 (± 12.1) years and the proportion of females was 41.6% (99 of 238 patients). Nearly half of the patients (45%) had experienced an ischemic stroke followed by headaches and/or dizziness with intracerebral hemorrhage (Table 1). Twenty four subjects (10.1%) exhibited either a V1 (aortic origin) or V2 (abnormal penetration of the TF) anomaly. Patients with an anomalous VA were significantly younger than patients who had a normal VA ($P < 0.030$) but there were no significant differences in terms of gender or comorbid conditions between these two groups.

Anomalies of the VA

Of the 476 VAs (from 238 patients) that were evaluated in the present study, 11 (2.3%) had an anomalous origin directly from the aorta and 27 (5.7%) did not have a normal penetration through the C6 TF (Table 2). Of the 11 VAs with an anomalous origin, nine (81.8%) had an aortic origin and were preferentially located on the left side. Of the 27 VAs with an abnormal entrance into the C6 TF, there were slightly more on the right side than on the left side (15 vs. 12, respectively) and the most frequent anomaly was a penetration of the C5 TF in the V2 segment ($n = 23$, 85.2%) followed by a penetration of the C4 ($n = 3$, 11.1%) and C3 ($n = 1$, 3.7%) TF. Additionally, eight of the VAs exhibited anomalies that included both an aortic origin and an abnormal entrance into the C6 TF. An anomalous origin of the VA was associated with an abnormal entrance into the C6 TF (chi-square test, $P < 0.001$; Table 3).

Relationships between VA diameter and anomalies of the VA

The inter-rater correlation coefficient for the measurement of the VA diameter was 0.91 (95% confidence interval [CI]: 0.85-0.94, $P < 0.001$). The diameters of the VAs with either type of anomaly were significantly smaller than those with a normal morphology (Fig. 2). In the case of a VA with an anomalous origin or an abnormal foraminal entrance, the diameters of the left VAs were significantly smaller than those of the right side. Additionally, eight of the VAs exhibited a combined aortic origin and abnormal foraminal entrance; these were exclusively located on left side and had the smallest diameter of all the measured VAs.

Table 4 illustrates the findings of the linear mixed model analysis regarding the diameters of the VAs. Age did not significantly predict VA diameter but the diameters of the VAs in males were 0.2 mm larger than those in females ($P = 0.015$) and the diameters of the right VAs were 0.3 mm smaller than those of the left VAs ($P < 0.001$). Moreover, the diameters of the VAs with either type of anomaly (V1 anomaly, 0.9 mm smaller, $P < 0.001$; V2 anomaly, 0.7 mm smaller, $P < 0.001$) were considerably smaller than those of normal VAs, respectively. The (anomalous origin)*(abnormal entrance) interaction term was also included in the present linear mixed model but it was not significant. Therefore, this term was removed from the final analysis.

A power analysis with a 0.05 alpha error was performed using the results of the linear mixed model to

Table 1 Clinical characteristics of the anomalous and non-anomalous VA groups

	Total (*n* = 238)	Anomalous (*n* = 24)	Non-anomalous (*n* = 214)	*P*
Female (%)	101 (42.4%)	12 (50%)	89 (41.6%)	0.429
Age, years (mean ± SD)	65.9 (±12.1)	60.8 (±12.1)	66.5 (±11.9)	0.030
Comorbidities				0.244[a]
Ischemic stroke	107 (45.0%)	8 (33.3%)	99 (46.3%)	
Headache/Dizziness	42 (17.7%)	8 (33.3%)	34 (15.9%)	
Intracerebral hemorrhage	31 (13.0%)	4 (16.7%)	27 (12.6%)	
Neoplasm	30 (12.6%)	2 (8.3%)	28 (13.1%)	
Others	28 (11.7%)	2 (8.3%)	26 (12.1%)	
V1 anomaly, number (%)[b]	11 (2.3%)	11 (22.9%)	-	-
V2 anomaly, number (%)[b]	27 (5.7%)	27 (56.3%)	-	-

SD Standard deviation, V1 anomaly = vertebral artery with an aortic origin; V2 anomaly = vertebral artery with an abnormal entrance to the transverse foramen
[a]Pearson's chi-square test
[b]proportions in a total of 476 vertebral arteries

evaluate differences in the diameters of the VAs between the anomalous V2 and normal V2 patients; the diameters of the anomalous VAs and the normal VAs were 2.4 and 3.48 mm, respectively. The actual power for the repeated measures analysis using G*Power 3.1 (Franz Faul, Christian-Albrechts-Universität Kiel; Kiel, Germany) was 0.93.

Discussion

In the present retrospective case-control study, the diameters of the VAs of patients with two types of VA anomaly were assessed from an anatomical perspective. A linear mixed model analysis revealed that VA diameter was associated with sex, laterality (right or left), and an anomalous origin and abnormal foraminal entrance of the VAs. Additionally, the prevalence of an anomaly in either the V1 or V2 segment was 10% (24 of 238 patients), and the diameters of the anomalous VAs were considerably smaller (~2 mm) than those of normal VAs. These findings suggest that V1 and V2 anomalies may be useful marker for small or hypoplastic VA.

Table 2 Incidence of anomalies of the VA according to laterality of the VA

	Right	Left	Total
V1 segment			
Normal	236	229	465
Anomalous	2	9	11
V2 segment			
Normal	223	226	449
Anomalous	15	12	27
C5[a]	14	9	2
C4[a]	1	2	3
C3[a]	0	1	1

Data are presented as number
[a]VA Entrance to the transverse foramen at each level. For example, C5 represents VAs not passing through C6 but C5 transverse foramen

Currently, there is a lack of optimal criteria with which to accurately define VAH; there may be several reasons for this. First, VAH is considered to be a clinically benign condition and [21], therefore, digital subtraction angiography cannot be used as a gold standard method of assessment due to the invasiveness of this procedure [22]. Second, previous studies have used various criteria to define VAH in different populations [3–6, 8, 21, 23]. Importantly, as the cutoff value for VAH diameter and the age of the studied population increase, there is an escalating probability of a higher incidence of VAH. Additionally, the definition of hypoplasia includes the meaning 'at birth' and its presence should not change based on the definition of VA diameter, participants' age, or the atherosclerotic burden of each patient. On the other hand, an anomalous origin of the VA and an abnormal entrance of the VA into the C6 TF are present at birth and do not change over time. Anomalous development of the VA is quite commonly accompanied by those of the adjacent bony structure such as an abnormal entrance of the vertebral artery not passing through the C6 TF [24–26]. Therefore, these characteristic

Table 3 Associations between an abnormal origin and an abnormal penetration of the VA into the transforamen

		MRA		Total
		V2 anomaly (+)	V2 anomaly (−)	
CTA	V1 anomaly (+)	8 (1.7%)	3 (0.6%)	11 (2.3%)
	V1 anomaly (−)	19 (4.0%)	446 (93.7%)	465 (97.7%)
Total		27 (5.7%)	449 (94.3%)	476 (100%)

P for chi-square < 0.001
V1 VA with aortic origin in V1 segment, *V2* VA with an abnormal entrance into the C6 transverse foramen

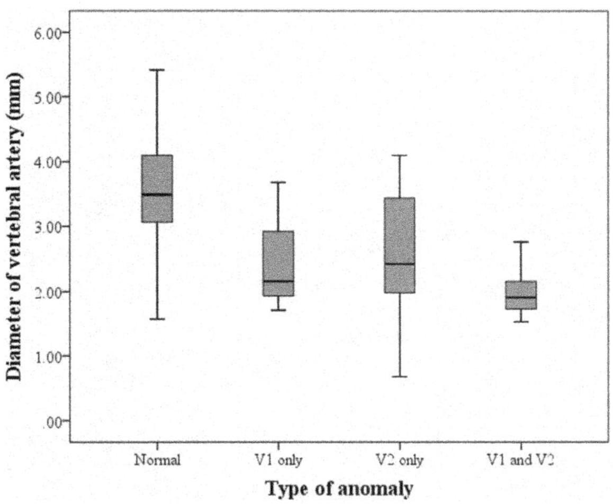

Fig. 2 *Box plots* showing the median and interquartile range values for the VA diameters. V1: VA with an aortic origin anomaly; V2: VA with an abnormal entrance into the transverse foramen

anomalies of the VA and the TF could be consistent markers for defining small or hypoplastic VA.

During embryological development, the VA develops from the longitudinal anastomosis of the intersegmental arteries [11, 12]. An abnormal development of the caudal portion of the intersegmental artery leads to the formation of a VA with an aortic origin which, in turn, may lead to an increased risk of developing VAH compared to a person with a normal VA [27, 28]. In an autopsy study, the prevalence of VAs with an aortic origin was reported to be 2-6% [14, 29]. A similar prevalence of VAs with an aortic origin was identified in the present study using MRA. Likewise, VAH is associated with the development of spontaneous VA dissection [30] and the present findings show that VAH was also closely related with the abnormal development or congenital vasculopathy of the VA.

Table 4 A linear mixed model analysis revealed associations between VA diameter and the clinico-anatomical characteristics of the patients

Predictor	B[a] (mm)	95% CI	*P*
Age, years	0.0004	−0.005 – 0.006	0.881
Female[b]	reference		
Male	0.174	0.033 – 0.315	0.015
Left VA[b]	reference		
Right VA	−0.351	−0.484 – −0.217	< 0.001
V1 normal[b]	reference		
V1 anomaly	−0.916	−1.420 – −0.412	< 0.001
V2 normal[b]	reference		
V2 anomaly	−0.783	−1.112 – −0.454	< 0.001

[a]Reference
[b]Estimates of fixed effects (VA diameter, mm)

A previous study of the association between the VA and the TF revealed a close relationship between the diameter of the TF and VA flow/diameter [19, 25, 26, 31]. Additionally, Hong et al. [19] reported that the incidence of an abnormal penetration of the VA into the TF (other than through C6) is approximately 5% and that the diameter of the TF significantly differs whether the VA passes through it or not. The present observations are in line with these previous findings. Taken together, these findings indicate that there is a close relationship between the VA and the TF.

In the present study, a linear mixed model analysis was used to estimate the diameter of the VA. A mixed model is a hierarchical model used to examine the associations among between-subject and within-subject variables [32]. As a rule, there are two VAs in the body, and the left VA tends to be larger than the right one. Therefore, a hierarchical linear mixed model is an optimal method to account for the repeated measures (two VAs) used in the present study. Additionally, patients with atretic or non-visualized VAs on vessel images were often excluded from the analyses of previous studies, which can lead to an underestimation of the prevalence of VAH because smaller arteries are more easily narrowed or occluded than larger ones [3, 4, 6]. Although atretic or non-visualized arteries are considered as a missing value, which in turn excluded in a traditional linear regression analysis, the mixed model can take account these missing data into the final statistical model [33]. Therefore, when using a linear mixed model, the data from patients with atretic or non-visualized VAs can be included in the estimation of VA diameter. Thus, in conjunction with the constant radiological characteristics of the VA anomalies, the use of a mixed model to assess the diameters of VAs strengthened the present results.

However, the present study has several limitations that must be considered. First, this study included only patients who were examined using CT and MR angiography simultaneously and this inclusion criterion may have led to an unintended selection bias. However, the proportions of comorbidities in the anomalous and non-anomalous VA groups did not differ significantly, particularly for patients with atherosclerotic diseases such as ischemic stroke. Second, although it is reasonable to assume that young patients would be included in the present study population based on the definition of VAH and there was an effort to focus on young patients free of cerebrovascular disease, a large number of older participants (65.9 ± 12.0 years of age) were included in the present analyses. However, it is unreasonable to perform the CT angiography procedure on normal individuals to screen for VA diseases due to the hazards associated with the radiation and contrast agents.Finally, some stroke patients were included ($n = 107$subjects) in this study. Because they are not all patient with posterior circulation infarct, we could not conclude the relationship between the VA anomalies and the occurrence of ischemic stroke. In addition, there is a sample size issue because small number of VA anomalies were not sufficient for subgroup analysis. Therefore, it is necessary to study whether the presence of vertebral artery variation is associated with the occurrence of posterior circulation stroke.

Conclusion

The present study demonstrated that the size of the VA was closely related with sex, laterality, and anomalies of the VA and that a linear mixed model was an optimal statistical method in assessing size of the VA.

Abbreviations

PCS: Posterior circulation stroke; TF: Transverse foramen; VA: Vertebral artery; VAH: Vertebral artery hypoplasia

Acknowledgements

None.

Funding

The authors received a fund from Hallym Specialization Fund (No. HRF-S-53).

Authors' contributions

CK: data collection, study design, interpretation of the data, statistical analysis and drafting of the manuscript; JHS, study design, technical comments, interpretation of the data and drafting the manuscript; HCC: data collection, interpretation of the data. All the authors have read and approved the final manuscript.

Competing interests

The authors declare that they have no competing interests.

References

1. Bogousslavsky J, Regli F, Maeder P, et al. The etiology of posterior circulation infarcts a prospective study using magnetic resonance imaging and magnetic resonance angiography. Neurology. 1993;43:1528–33.
2. Caplan L, Wityk R, Pazdera L, et al. New England Medical Center posterior circulation stroke registry II. Vascular lesions J Clin Neurol. 2005;1:31–49.
3. Park JH, Kim JM, Roh JK. Hypoplastic vertebral artery: frequency and associations with ischaemic stroke territory. J Neurol Neurosurg Psychiatry. 2007;78:954–8.
4. Chuang YM, Huang YC, Hu HH, et al. Toward a further elucidation: role of vertebral artery hypoplasia in acute ischemic stroke. Eur Neurol. 2005;55: 193–7.
5. Perren F, Poglia D, Landis T, et al. Vertebral artery hypoplasia a predisposing factor for posterior circulation stroke? Neurology. 2007;68:65–7.
6. Chen YY, Chao AC, Hsu HY, et al. Vertebral artery hypoplasia is associated with a decrease in net vertebral flow volume. Ultrasound Med Biol. 2010;36: 38–43.
7. Jeng JS, Yip PK. Evaluation of vertebral artery hypoplasia and asymmetry by color-coded duplex ultrasonography. Ultrasound Med Biol. 2004;30:605–9.
8. Thierfelder KM, Baumann AB, Sommer WH, et al. Vertebral artery hypoplasia frequency and effect on cerebellar blood flow characteristics. Stroke. 2014; 45:1363–8.
9. Caldemeyer KS, Carrico JB, Mathews VP. The radiology and embryology of anomalous arteries of the head and neck. AJR Am J Roentgenol. 1998;170: 197–203.
10. Menshawi K, Mohr JP, Gutierrez J. A functional perspective on the embryology and anatomy of the cerebral blood supply. J Stroke. 2015;17: 144–58.
11. Padget DH. The development of the cranial arteries in the human embryo. Contr Embryol. 1948;32:205–61.
12. Luh GY, Dean BL, Tomsick TA, et al. The persistent fetal carotid-vertebrobasilar anastomoses. AJR Am J Roentgenol. 1999;172:1427–32.
13. Van Overbeeke JJ, Hillen B, Tulleken CA. A comparative study of the circle of Willis in fetal and adult life. The configuration of the posterior bifurcation of the posterior communicating artery. J Anat. 1991;176:45–54.
14. Sartor K, Freckmann N, Böker DK. Related anomalies of origin of left vertebral and left inferior thyroid arteries. Neuroradiology. 1980;19:27–30.
15. Vorster W, du Plooy PT, Meiring JH. Abnormal origin of internal thoracic and vertebral arteries. Clin Anat. 1998;11:33–7.
16. Dudich K, Bhadelia R, Srinivasan J. Anomalous vertebral artery origin may be an independent risk factor for arterial dissection. Eur J Neurol. 2005;12:571–2.
17. Uchino A, Saito N, Takahashi M, et al. Variations in the origin of the vertebral artery and its level of entry into the transverse foramen diagnosed by CT angiography. Neuroradiology. 2013;55:585–94.
18. Yi ZQ, Li L, Mo DP, et al. Anomalous vertebral artery not passing through the transverse foramen of the atlas. Chin Med J. 2009;122:2675–7.
19. Hong JT, Park DK, Lee MJ, et al. Anatomical variations of the vertebral artery segment in the lower cervical spine: analysis by three-dimensional computed tomography angiography. Spine. 2008;33:2422–6.
20. Cloud GC, Markus HS. Diagnosis and management of vertebral artery stenosis. QJM. 2003;96:27–54.
21. Giannopoulos S, Markoula S, Kosmidou M, et al. Lateral medullary ischaemic events in young adults with hypoplastic vertebral artery. J Neurol Neurosurg Psychiatry. 2007;78:987–9.
22. Heiserman JE, Dean B, Hodak J, et al. Neurologic complications of cerebral angiography. AJNR Am J Neuroradiol. 1994;15:1401–7.
23. Sato K, Yoneya M, Otsuki A, et al. Anatomical vertebral artery hypoplasia and insufficiency impairs dynamic blood flow regulation. Clin Physiol Funct Imaging. 2015;35:485–9.
24. Meila D, Tysiac M, Petersen M, et al. Origin and course of the extracranial vertebral artery: CTA findings and embryologic considerations. Clin Neuroradiol. 2012;22:327–33.
25. Kim C, Lee SH, Park SS, et al. A quantitative comparison of the vertebral artery and transverse foramen using CT angiography. J Clin Neurol. 2012;8: 259–64.
26. Sanelli PC, Tong S, Gonzalez RG, et al. Normal variation of vertebral artery on CT angiography and its implications for diagnosis of acquired pathology. J Comput Assist Tomogr. 2002;26:462–70.
27. Panicker HK, Tarnekar A, Dhawane V, et al. Anomalous origin of left vertebral artery-embryological basis and applied aspects-a case report. J Anat Soc India. 2002;51:234–5.
28. Mishra A, Pendharkar H, Jayadaevan ER, et al. Anomalous origins of bilateral vertebral arteries in a child with down syndrome and Moyamoya disease. A case report. Interv Neuroradiol. 2012;18:259–63.
29. Lemke AJ, Benndorf G, Liebig T, et al. Anomalous origin of the right vertebral artery: review of the literature and case report of right vertebral artery origin distal to the left subclavian artery. AJNR Am J Neuroradiol. 1999;20:1318–21.
30. Zhou M, Zheng H, Gong S, et al. Vertebral artery hypoplasia and vertebral artery dissection a hospital-based cohort study. Neurology. 2015;84:818–24.
31. Kotil K, Kilincer C. Sizes of the transverse foramina correlate with blood flow and dominance of vertebral arteries. Spine J. 2014;14:933–7.
32. Edwards LJ. Modern statistical techniques for the analysis of longitudinal data in biomedical research. Pediatr Pulmonol. 2000;30:330–44.
33. Laird NM, Ware JH. Random-effects models for longitudinal data. Biometrics. 1982;38:963–74.

8

Hospital treatment costs and length of stay associated with hypertension and multimorbidity after hemorrhagic stroke

Adrian V. Specogna[1*], Tanvir C. Turin[2], Scott B. Patten[3] and Michael D. Hill[4]

Abstract

Background: Previous studies have identified various treatment and patient characteristics that may be associated with higher hospital cost after spontaneous intracerebral hemorrhage (ICH); a devastating type of stroke. Patient morbidity is perhaps the least understood of these cost-driving factors. We describe how hypertension and other patient morbidities affect length of stay, and hospital treatment costs after ICH using primary and simulated data. We also describe the relationship between cost and length of stay within these patients.

Methods: We used a cohort design; evaluating 987 consecutive ICH patients across one decade in a Canadian center. Economic, treatment, and patient data were obtained from clinical and administrative sources. Multimorbidity was defined as the presence of one or more diagnoses at hospital admission in addition to a primary diagnosis of ICH.

Results: Hypertension was the most frequent (67%) morbidity within these patients, as well as the strongest predictor of longer stay (adjusted RR for >7 days: 1.31, 95% CI: 1.07-1.60), and was significantly associated with higher cost per visit when accounting for other morbidities (adjusted cost increase for hypertension $8123.51, 95% CI: $4088.47 to $12,856.72 USD). A Monte Carlo simulation drawing one million samples of patients estimated for a generation (100 years) assuming 0.94% population growth per year, and a hospitalization rate of 12 per 100,000 inhabitants, supported these findings ($p = 0.516$ for the difference in unadjusted cost: simulated vs primary). Using a restricted cubic spline, we observed that the rate of change in overall cost for all patients was greatest for the first 3 weeks ($p < 0.001$) compared to subsequent weeks.

Conclusion: Patient multimorbidity, specifically hypertension, is a strong predictor of longer stay and cost after ICH. The non-linear relationship between cost and time should also be considered when forecasting healthcare spending in these patients.

Keywords: Intracerebral hemorrhage, Cost of care, Comorbidity, Hypertension, Critical care, Economics, Epidemiology

Background

Spontaneous intracerebral hemorrhage (ICH) is a devastating and costly condition with high mortality and morbidity. Previous studies have attempted to identify various patient or treatment characteristics that may be associated with higher hospital costs to assist in economic planning [1–3]. Patient comorbidity has been cited as an important cost-driving factor [2], however the details of its association with hospital resource use remains unclear.

Hypertension is arguably the strongest risk factor for the development of ICH and thus the most common secondary disease patients present with in the emergency department [4]. How specific comorbid or ICH-associated conditions, such as hypertension affect length of stay in hospital, or cost of specific services has yet to be reported and thus there little understanding of the extent of care for these patients, and thus little understanding of how new promising treatment strategies [5] for such conditions could affect hospital resource use once implemented. Further, identifying differences in

* Correspondence: adrian.specogna@ucf.edu
[1]Department of Health Professions, College of Health and Public Affairs, University of Central Florida, 12805 Pegasus Drive, Orlando, FL 32816, USA
Full list of author information is available at the end of the article

how specific morbidities are associated with specific costs could reveal differences in care amongst some patients. This cost information could provide insight into ICH care efficiency; both within and beyond emergency departments. The primary purpose of this study was to describe how patient morbidities, specifically hypertension, affect length of stay, and treatment cost after ICH. We also describe as a secondary objective, the relationship between cost and length of stay, and explore the potential relationship between stroke severity, clinical outcomes, and cost within these patients.

Methods

We used a cohort study design to evaluate the economic cost of ICH hospital care within one Canadian hospital between 1999 and 2008. This center is one of two dedicated stroke centers in the province of Alberta, and is located in a city with a population of approximately one million people overall. The cost of care was estimated retrospectively from the time of admission to the time of discharge using administrative data provided by the province and included both direct and indirect expenditures combined.

In order to ensure our economic estimates were precise and selection bias was minimized, we sought to obtain all financial data on all ICH cases treated during the decade. This center is one of several centers nationally that captures micro-costing data on all hospital admissions; thus detailed cost data were available from administrative sources. Capturing all economic data is particularly important for costing studies of ICH since the variability in ICH economic data is high [3], and if the number of ICH cases observed is low, cost estimates may be imprecise and uninformative. Thus, all adult (> = 18 years) hospitalized patients with a Most Responsible Diagnosis of ICH (ICD-9-CM and ICD-10-CA: 431, I61.0-I61.6, I61.8, and I61.9) were eligible for inclusion. Patients were excluded only if the cost of treatment could not be estimated or was not reported to the provincial government.

The provincial government follows national guidelines [6] for the collection, coding and quality assurance of patient demographic and comorbidity data, and provides the ability to link such data to information provided by different departments within its organization. In this study, the costs associated with hospital stays were provided by the provincial health-costing department and linked to an electronic patient record. Financial data were inflated to the year 2015 using the Consumer Price Index [7], to adjust for overall economic inflation.

Ordinary binomial regression was used to investigate the association between specific diseases recorded at hospital admission (yes vs. no), and length of stay (<= 7 days vs. >7 days), and calendar year. Ordinary linear regression was used to investigate the association between these diseases and inflation-adjusted cost overall, and within specific costed categories. For our primary morbidity of interest, hypertension, we explored the potential confounding effect of stroke severity, in-hospital mortality, and disability on its relationship with cost and length of stay using ordinary linear regression and stratified analysis. We also performed a Monte Carlo sensitivity analysis to investigate the association between cost and hypertension; which was informed using current ICH summary data from different centers.

All analyses were conducted using Stata statistical software [8] assuming alpha was equal to 0.05. For the purpose of this study, multimorbidity was defined as the presence of one or more diseases, which patients experienced, in addition to the index ICH [9]. Decisions for morbidity classification and stratification were informed from previous investigations [2, 10, 11] (Table 1). As expected, all cost data were right skewed thus they were log (ln) transformed for analysis. The significance of cost increases and decreases were determined using robust standard errors. Log costs were reported using smear retransformation [12] to provide realistic cost values from linear regression and reported per discharge in United States Dollars (USD) at December 31, 2015 to allow for international comparison. All those individuals who reported costs and measured clinical variables were blinded to the study objectives. We obtained approval and a waiver of written consent from the University of Calgary's Conjoint Health Research Ethics Board to conduct this study.

Results

One thousand and two ICH patients were treated at the center during the decade. Cost data were not available in 15 patients; thus they were excluded. The characteristics of the 987 patients included are described in Table 2. The median total inflation-adjusted cost of care per stay (discharge) was $10,202.73 ($351.76 [min] to $256,867.22 [max]). Two percent of patients had survived an ICH previous to their current admission, although recurrent ICH was not associated with overall cost ($p = 0.109$).

Morbidity, length of stay, and cost

The majority (81%) of patients had at least one additional diagnosis irrespective of their primary diagnosis of ICH at hospital admission (median: 1, 0 [min] to 6 [max]). Sixty-seven percent of all patients were hypertensive; which was the most frequent multimorbidity (Table 2). We felt it was reasonable to assume age could be associated with cost, and thus considered age as a confounder in all of our cost analyses. In contrast, sex was not associated with cost in our cohort. When adjusting for age, hypertension was significantly associated with higher cost (dollar increase in

Table 1 International Classification of Diseases codes (ICD-9-CM and ICD-10-CA) used to classify patient morbidity

Morbidity Category	ICD-9-CM and ICD-10-CA Codes
Hypertension	401.x, 402.x, 403.x, 404.x, 405.x, I10.x, I11.x, I12.x, I13.x, I15.x
Secondary Cerebrovascular Disease [a]	362.34, 430.x–438.x, G45.x, G46.x, H34.0, I60.x–I69.x
Diabetes	250.0–250.3, 250.4–250.7, 250.8, 250.9, E10.0–E10.9, E11.0–E11.9, E12.0- E12.9, E13.0–E13.9, E14.0-E14.9
Cardiac Disorders	398.91, 402.01, 402.11, 402.91, 404.01, 404.03, 404.11, 404.13, 404.91, 404.93, 410.x, 412.x, 425.4–425.9, 428.x, I09.9, I11.0, I13.0, I13.2, I25.5, I21.x, I22.x, I25.2, I42.0, I42.5–I42.9, I43.x, I50.x, P29.0
Chronic Pulmonary Disease	416.8, 416.9, 490.x–505.x, 506.4, 508.1, 508.8, I27.8, I27.9, J40.x–J47.x, J60.x–J67.x, J68.4, J70.1, J70.3
Malignancy or Tumour	140.x–172.x, 174.x–195.8, 196.x–199.x, 200.x–208.x, 238.6, C00.x–C26.x, C30.x–C34.x, C37.x–C41.x, C43.x, C45.x–C58.x, C60.x–C76.x, C77.x–C80.x, C81.x–C85.x, C88.x, C90.x–C97.x
Dementia	290.x, 294.1, 331.2, F00.x–F03.x, F05.1, G30.x, G31.1
Mood Disorders	296.x, 311.x, F30.x, F31.x, F32.x, F33.x, F34.x, F38.x, F39.x
Renal Disease	403.01, 403.11, 403.91, 404.02, 404.03, 404.12, 404.13, 404.92, 404.93, 582.x, 583.0–583.7, 585.x, 586.x, 588.0, I12.0, I13.1, N03.2–N03.7, N05.2–N05.7, N18.x, N19.x, N25.0, V42.0, V45.1, V56.x, Z49.0–Z49.2, Z94.0, Z99.2
Peripheral Vascular Disease	093.0, 437.3, 440.x, 441.x, 443.1–443.9, 447.1, 557.1, 557.9, I70.x, I71.x, I73.1, I73.8, I73.9, I77.1, I79.0, I79.2, K55.1, K55.8, K55.9, V43.4, Z95.8, Z95.9
Liver Disease	070.22, 070.23, 070.32, 070.33, 070.44, 070.54, 070.6, 070.9, 456.0–456.2, 570.x, 571.x, 572.2–572.8, 573.3, 573.4, 573.8, 573.9, B18.x, I85.0, I85.9, I86.4, I98.2, K70.0–K70.4, K70.9, K71.1, K72.1, K72.9, K76.5, K76.6, K76.7, K71.3–K71.5, K71.7, K73.x, K74.x, K76.0, K76.2–K76.4, K76.8, K76.9, V42.7, Z94.4
Rheumatic Disease	446.5, 710.0–710.4, 714.0–714.2, 714.8, 725.x, M05.x, M06.x, M31.5, M32.x–M34.x, M35.1, M35.3, M36.0
Peptic Ulcer Disease	531.x–534.x, K25.x–K28.x

[a]Patients with ICH in two or more locations were classified as having primary ICH with multimorbid secondary cerebrovascular disease

total cost per discharge: $10,324.56, 95% CI: $5586.55 to $15,862.53, Table 3). ICH patients with at least one additional disease were more likely to stay in hospital longer compared to those without any multimorbidity (RR for longer stay: 1.69, 95% CI: 1.36-2.10) and these patients were significantly more costly to treat at all stages of care (Table 3). When making the assumption that each morbidity contributed equally to cost, overall cost increased significantly for each added morbidity (age-adjusted cost increase per added morbidity: $4958.36, 95% CI: $3144.97 to $6907.00).

After adjusting for age and all other comorbid diagnoses listed in Table 3, to address the issue that some ICH patients may have multiple secondary diseases simultaneously, hypertension remained the strongest predictor of longer stay (age and additional morbidity adjusted RR: 1.31, 95% CI: 1.07-1.60) and, along with secondary cerebrovascular disease, remained significantly associated with higher cost overall (adjusted dollar increase for hypertension: $8123.51, 95% CI: $4088.47 to $12,856.72, and for secondary cerebrovascular disease: $6637.13, 95% CI: $2541.79 to $11,502.75).

Cost and length of stay

The relationship between overall cost and time spent in hospital is described in Fig. 1. As illustrated, the relationship between cost and time was not linear, thus we estimated the average change in cost over time using a restricted cubic spline function (model R^2: 0.73, Fig. 1). For ease of interpretation, we also estimated a linear spline function using weekly intervals; making the assumption that the association between cost and time was linear within each respective interval. According to this model, the rate of change in cost per day was significant for the first 3 weeks ($p < 0.001$ for linear slope for days 0-7, 8-14, and 15-21), but not significant compared to the previous interval for the rest of the follow-up period; suggesting that although cost continues to increase over time, the rate of this increase is not significant beyond 3 weeks after ICH. The median cost of care during the first week, first 2 weeks, and first 3 weeks were $4685.52 (interquartile range: $2761.84 to $7196.43), $6435.37 (interquartile range: $3592.59 to $11,248.09), and $8867.64 (interquartile range: $3867.85 to $13,612.64) respectively. Table 4 illustrates the median and average total cost for other commonly reported follow-up intervals.

Table 2 Sample characteristics

Patient Characteristic	Overall (n = 987)
Sex (% Males)	55
Age (Years)	72 (20-99)
Length of Stay in Hospital (Days)	8 (1-190)
Died in Hospital (%)	28*
Had Surgery (%)	18*
Accessed Diagnostic Services (%)	
Diagnostic Investigations	88
Laboratory Services	97
Overall	99
Accessed Acute Care Services (%)	
Ambulatory Care	3**
Clinical Nutrition	41*
Nursing	100
Pharmacy	85**
Overall	100
Accessed Rehabilitation Services (%)	
Audiology and Speech Therapy	38
Occupational Therapy	62**
Physiotherapy	70
Recreation Therapy	2
Respiratory Therapy	42*
Social Work	45
Overall	88
Morbidities at Admission (%)	
Hypertension	67
Secondary Cerebrovascular Disease	23
Diabetes	15
Cardiac Disorders	10*
Chronic Pulmonary Disease	6*
Malignancy or Tumour	5
Dementia	5
Mood Disorders	3*
Renal Disease	3
Peripheral Vascular Disease	2*
Liver Disease	1
Rheumatic Disease	1
Peptic Ulcer Disease	1*
Overall	81

Data are reported as median (min to max) unless otherwise noted. Percentages are rounded to the nearest whole number. Diseases were classified at hospital admission. Some patients may be classified in multiple categories. Overall morbidity indicates the percentage of patients who had at least one additional diagnosis irrespective of their primary diagnosis of ICH. Of the 15 patients who did not access diagnostic services; 8 died within the first 2 days, 3 were referred from other centers, 1 died with dementia within 5 days, 1 died within 6 days with no multimorbidity, 1 was discharged alive with a malignancy or tumour, and 1 was discharged alive with no multimorbidity
*Significant (p < 0.05) decrease over a decade
**Significant (p < 0.05) increase over a decade

Exploratory analysis of stroke severity, death, and disability

We ran additional regression analyses on a consecutive series of patients who had detailed clinical information (n = 148) obtained during routine care to investigate the potential affect of stroke severity, in-hospital mortality, and disability on the association between hypertension and cost, and length of stay; to determine whether these characteristics may be acting as confounders. The mean log total cost of this subgroup was not different than the entire sample of patients (p = 0.298) and hypertension, the most common multimorbidity, was significantly associated with length of stay in the subgroup (p = 0.032), and significantly associated with overall cost in the subgroup (p = 0.021), as it was in the entire cohort.

Admission National Institutes of Health Stroke Scale (NIHSS: > = 15 (poor) vs. <15 (good)), a commonly used scale to assess stroke severity, was significantly associated with higher overall cost in the subgroup (p < 0.001), and significantly associated with longer stay (unadjusted RR for longer stay: 1.41, 95% CI: 1.11 to 1.79), but was not associated with hypertension at admission (unadjusted RR for hypertension: 0.99, 95% CI: 0.78 to 1.24). Interestingly, hypertension was protective against in-hospital mortality in this subgroup (unadjusted RR for death: 0.23, 95% CI: 0.07 to 0.81) although there were only 9 patients who died in this group suggesting that these findings may be uninformative. However, it was noted that hypertension was also not associated with in-hospital mortality in the entire cohort (unadjusted RR for death: 0.90, 95% CI: 0.73 to 1.11).

Amongst those who survived in the subgroup (n = 139), Modified Rankin Scale (mRS: 3-5 (poor) vs 0-2 (good)), a commonly used measure of disability assessed at hospital discharge, was significantly associated with higher overall cost (p < 0.001) and longer length of stay (unadjusted RR for longer stay: 2.05, 95% CI: 1.46 to 2.88), although, like in-hospital mortality, was also not associated with hypertension (p = 0.256).

Sensitivity analysis with all ICH admissions across 100 years

To address the issue of potentially below-satisfactory (<90%) statistical power for the primary exposure of interest, hypertension, possibly due to an insufficient sample size given the variability of cost data and effect size we observed, we used Monte Carlo methods to predict the total cost of hypertension adjusted for age in a hypothetical

Table 3 Cost of patient morbidities measured at admission

Multimorbidity	RR for In-Hospital Mortality (95% CI)	Days Spent In Hospital	RR for Longer Stay (95% CI)	Dollar Change in Cost Diagnostic Services (95% CI)	Dollar Change in Cost Acute Care Services (95% CI)	Dollar Change in Cost Rehabilitation Services (95% CI)	Dollar Change in Cost Overall (95% CI)	*P*-Value for Dollar Change in Cost Overall
Hypertension	0.86 (0.69-1.06)	9 (4-20)	1.32* (1.14-1.53)	\$1846.01* (\$321.66 to \$3817.97)	\$6567.21* (\$3432.52 to \$10,296.64)	\$3426.76* (\$1621.76 to \$6667.09)	\$10,324.56* (\$5586.55 to \$15,862.53)	$p < 0.001$
Secondary Cerebrovascular Disease	1.41* (1.14-1.75)	9 (4-21)	1.08 (0.95-1.24)	\$2559.95* (\$1078.05 to \$4401.97)	\$4268.28* (\$1015.40 to \$8195.50)	\$1020.98* (\$187.84 to \$2477.67)	\$8675.26* (\$3557.60 to \$14,724.72)	$p < 0.001$
Diabetes	0.86 (0.64-1.17)	10 (5-26)	1.18* (1.02 to 1.36)	\$1127.79 (−\$662.19 to \$3586.67)	\$5658.97* (\$1220.92 to \$11,308.39)	\$2826.20* (\$1309.58 to \$5341.17)	\$7581.65* (\$7835.58 to \$15,357.99)	$p = 0.016$
Cardiac Disorders	1.40* (1.06-1.85)	12 (4-27)	1.14 (0.96-1.35)	\$3754.75* (\$1028.21 to \$7613.74)	\$4030.50 (−\$1004.88 to \$10,796.07)	\$1004.67 (−\$67.81 to \$3191.30)	\$8259.74* (\$531.06 to \$18,195.80)	$p = 0.034$
Chronic Pulmonary Disease	1.39 (0.99-1.96)	9 (4-20)	1.09 (0.87-1.36)	\$3005.11* (\$1183.36 to \$5317.47)	-\$2736.45 (\$7296.18 to \$4283.75)	\$2143.12* (\$573.89 to \$5172.46)	\$1069.32 (−\$6346.84 to \$11,195.36)	$p = 0.804$
Malignancy or Tumour	1.32 (0.87-1.99)	10 (3-43)	1.08 (0.83-1.40)	-\$1267.34 (−\$3801.80 to \$4622.35)	\$3830.40 (−\$3029.04 to \$14,479.19)	-\$97.25 (−\$831.66 to \$2529.73)	\$4521.52 (−\$5750.61 to \$19,924.11)	$p = 0.443$
Dementia	0.97 (0.64-1.49)	14 (5-26)	1.19 (0.97-1.46)	\$78.64 (−\$2260.05 to \$4060.67)	\$3840.99 (−\$2810.53 to \$13,882.24)	\$1249.18 (−\$20.97 to \$3929.90)	\$5346.22 (−\$3998.06 to \$18,509.50)	$p = 0.299$
Mood Disorders	1.07 (0.59-1.94)	17 (6-44)	1.37* (1.06-1.75)	\$3090.06* (\$719.04 to \$6364.49)	\$10,112.11 (−\$836.62 to \$29,273.87)	\$3440.20* (\$344.54 to \$13,369.57)	\$16,818.57* (\$1569.25 to \$40,450.14)	$p = 0.026$
Renal Disease	1.48 (0.96-2.28)	9 (5-42)	1.14 (0.84-1.54)	\$2610.50 (−\$177.15 to \$6873.98)	\$8763.22 (−\$1039.77 to \$25,357.48)	\$1520.56 (−\$353.38 to \$8403.06)	\$14,969.86* (\$69.12 to \$38,456.89)	$p = 0.049$
Peripheral Vascular Disease	1.16 (0.66-2.06)	10 (7-15)	1.24 (0.93-1.64)	\$6391.68* (\$3331.82 to \$10,504.63)	\$298.49 (−\$5061.45 to \$8352.73)	-\$544.78 (−\$988.97 to \$1578.40)	\$2218.22 (−\$6135.35 to \$13,973.98)	$p = 0.646$
Liver Disease	1.55 (0.76-3.16)	11 (8-18)	1.64* (1.21-2.23)	\$3181.54 (−\$128.61 to \$8541.41)	\$10,737.56 (−\$1195.32 to \$32,732.61)	\$4186.12 (−\$319.55 to \$37,111.26)	\$13,254.18 (−\$4186.59 to \$44,542.85)	$p = 0.169$
Rheumatic Disease	1.76 (0.78-3.95)	17 (5-45)	1.24 (0.71-2.18)	-\$406.54 (−\$4072.03 to \$12,134.32)	\$9393.44 (−\$3464.65 to \$35,755.59)	\$5273.28* (\$1630.79 to \$13,757.05)	\$10,184.51 (−\$9610.37 to \$53,007.91)	$p = 0.410$
Peptic Ulcer Disease	1.01 (0.32-3.24)	16 (9-39)	1.62* (1.18-2.24)	\$9010.32* (\$6377.15 to \$12,224.36)	\$14,473.14 (−\$1563.28 to \$48,733.45)	\$988.84 (−\$1033.07 to \$58,779.38)	\$21,867.99 (−\$544.05 to \$63,578.35)	$p = 0.058$
Overall	1.12 (0.85-1.49)	9 (4-21)	1.69* (1.36-2.10)	\$3701.07* (\$1500.94 to \$6854.65)	\$9777.19* (\$6156.57 to \$14,204.96)	\$4949.90* (\$2080.47 to \$11,239.82)	\$16,388.39* (\$10,772.65 to \$16,388.39)	$p < 0.001$

Days spent in hospital are reported as median (interquartile range). Longer stay is defined as <=7 days vs. >7 days. The relative risk (RR) for longer stay and in-hospital mortality is defined as the risk for those with the morbidity compared to those without. Cost estimates are for both direct and indirect expenditures combined. All estimates were adjusted for patient age as a continuous variable. CI denotes confidence interval. Confidence intervals which encompass zero suggest no evidence of a dollar change in cost

*Significant ($p < 0.05$)

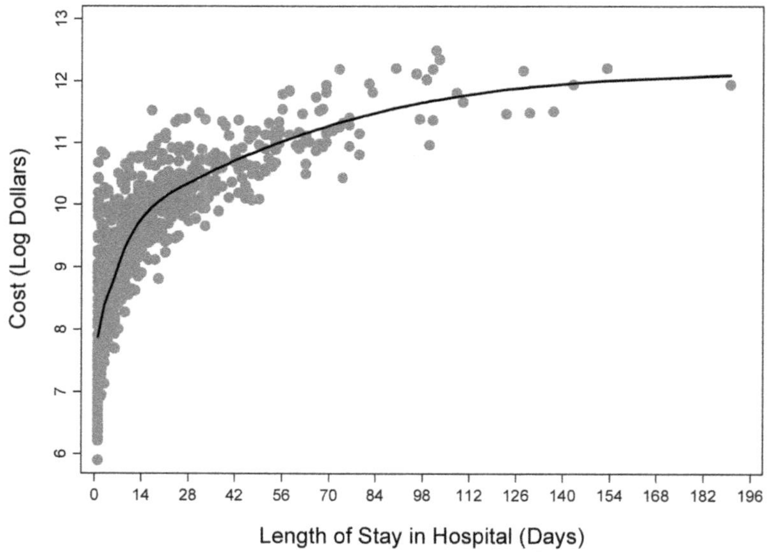

Fig. 1 Total treatment cost vs. length of stay in hospital. Scatter plot of log (ln) total inflation-adjusted cost of hospital care and days spent in hospital after ICH. The plot shows a non-linear relationship between log cost and length of stay with cost variability being the highest within the first few days after ICH. The shaded area represents the raw data and the solid line represents the average through the data using an unadjusted restricted cubic spline function

cohort of ICH patients over one generation (100 years) and compared this estimate to the estimate generated from our data.

To develop the cohort we assumed a theoretical random sample of 717,727 ICH patients over a 100-year period, which assumes a 0.94% population growth per year [13], and a hospitalization rate of 12 per 100,000 inhabitants per year within Canada which would be unchanged overall across the generation despite declines in some specific groups of patients [14, 15]. These estimates were assumed and entered into the simulation model based on previously published incidence rates within Canada [14], Canadian demographic data [13], as well as estimates derived from studies of large cohorts within North America [15]. For the purpose of the simulation, we assumed there was a real age-adjusted association between hypertension and total inflation-adjusted cost, but did not make an assumption as to the actual cost due to hypertension or its variability. The random sample of ICH patients were drawn from a normal population with an average age of 70 years, and standard deviation of 13 years [16]. All patients were between the ages of 18 and a theoretical human maximum of 126 years [17]. Hypertension occurred with an overall frequency of 77% in this group [15]. Like the primary analysis, all costs for the sensitivity analysis are reported in 2015 US Dollars for comparison.

One million unique samples of 717,727 ICH patients were drawn. Using these data, we estimated the average dollar increase per discharge for hypertension was $12,027.27; which was higher but not significantly different (p = 0.516; using a Welch's mean comparison test assuming unequal variances) from our estimate derived from primary data; $10,324.56 (Table 3).

Discussion

This study demonstrated that additional morbidities may be associated with longer stay and higher cost of hospital care overall after hemorrhagic stroke; with hypertension being the most frequent and costly multimorbidity. Patients with ICH arriving at hospital with hypertension were 31% more likely to stay in hospital beyond 1 week and cost an average of $8123.51 more per visit compared to non-hypertensive patients, when accounting for age and other morbidities. Most importantly, this cost increase was apparent at all stages of care from diagnosis

Table 4 Cost of hospital treatment during the first day, first week, first month, and first year after ICH

Length of Stay	No. of Patients	Median Cost	Mean Cost
0-1 Day after ICH	90	$1909.45 ($1085.58 to $5456.15)	$5457.47 ± $8144.59 ($351.76 to $42,090.59)
0-30 Days after ICH	850	$8397.25 ($4159.22 to $16,829.43)	$12,355.65 ± $12,168.34 ($351.76 to $98,207.53)
0-365 Days after ICH	987	$10,202.73 ($4821.50 to $22,905.50)	$20,165.14 ± $28,433.37 ($351.76 to $256,867.19)

Data are unadjusted and presented as median (interquartile range) and mean ± standard deviation (min to max)

to in-hospital rehabilitation. Although the data were collected for one time frame (one decade), analogous to a cross-sectional study design, we can assume the exposures (morbidity, length of stay, stroke severity, in-hospital mortality, disability) preceded the outcome (cost) in all cases; as patients cannot incur costs until they have been seen by a healthcare professional and received care.

As suggested in this study and others [18], it is reasonable to believe that the overall cost of ICH care increases as the total number of morbidities increases; since patients who are more sick would naturally require more care and additional resources. However, if the additive, equal-contribution assumption of multimorbidity were true, the adjusted cost increase for each multimorbidity would be the same across all multimorbidities. This study illustrates the contrary; suggesting that the adjusted cost to treat hypertension is different by $1486.38 on average per discharge compared to secondary cerebrovascular disease for example. Although this difference overall may not be statistically significant, owing to high cost variability, it may be clinically meaningful and exemplify differences in how these patients are cared for. Perhaps there are other treatment-process factors contributing to increasing costs in patients with specific multimorbidities beyond their overall number of additional diseases at admission which warrants further investigation.

We examined the risk of longer stay for different multimorbidities since length of stay in hospital is often cited as one of the most important predictors of treatment costs after ICH [19]; such that, those who stay longer in hospital may be significantly more costly to treat overall compared to those who stay for a shorter period of time. Often costs are assumed to fit normal parameters for these analyses; such that cost data are assumed to be normally distributed when compared to time spent in hospital. It would be inappropriate to compare raw costs to time if it were skewed as it was in our study, thus for this study all costs were transformed on the log scale prior to comparison to allow for a better examination of the relationship between cost and time.

When examining the association between length of stay and log cost we noted that these variables were not linearly related (Fig. 1). Further, the variability in cost appeared to be higher when hospital stay was short and lower when hospital stay was long, thus we did not assess this relationship using normal linear models. Previous authors have been less conservative and reported cost-per-day estimates overall for ICH and ischemic stroke patients [19–21]. These estimates assume cost data are normally distributed and linearly associated with time. Our data suggests that the greatest costs-per-day after ICH are likely incurred during the first day, conceivably due to high diagnostic resource use, and the magnitude of the increase in cost may decline as time progresses and is perhaps not significant after the third week of care; which is likely indicative of a curvilinear relationship. It should be noted that the significance of these findings is likely related to a reduction in sample size over time, such that, the probability of being discharged from hospital, and thus no longer contributing to cost, increases as time goes on; potentially affecting our ability to predict costs long after hospital admission.

Not surprisingly, in our exploratory analysis we illustrate that baseline stroke severity and disability was associated with overall cost and longer stay. One would expect that patients who are in serious condition when they arrive at hospital would likely be provided with the most aggressive, diverse, and potentially costly care overall compared to those with mild ICH. This analysis also suggested that stroke severity may not be acting as a confounder for the association between hypertension and cost since admission NIHSS was not associated with hypertension. Also, hypertension was not associated with in-hospital mortality or disability; suggesting that neither death nor disability could be acting as confounders in the hypertension-cost relationship. These exploratory analyses demonstrate a lack of clarity we have as to why costs are potentially higher for patients with stroke and hypertension. Despite this, it does shed light on an interesting health services phenomenon worth investigating in more detail in future studies. It is recommended the results from these analyses be used to generate discussion and guide future studies of this phenomena versus being interpreted as firm evidence to change practice as these observations, although interesting, are based on an exploratory analysis of a small subgroup of ICH patients in a single center without considering the impact of specific treatments.

Our study was limited in that we did not assess the association between clinical stroke severity or morbidity, and cost in the entire cohort as we only started recording this information in the latter half of the decade; and thus did not have complete data. Further, hypertension in this study was captured using ICD codes from administrative data and thus not defined using direct blood pressure measurements. Thus our definition of hypertension depended on the accurate diagnoses of responsible physicians. Further, as with all studies that use administrative data, we cannot rule out misclassification of diagnoses, and thus presume that patients classified as hypertensive are those presenting with hypertension and not those with only a history of hypertension. Although we attempted to identify patients with spontaneous ICH, we also cannot rule out the inclusion of some patients with other forms of primary intracranial hemorrhage due to the limitations of administrative data sources. As with nearly all centers, it is likely that many difficult to diagnose diseases, such as mood disorders, were under represented in our data which may affect the cost variability observed. Finally, we did not examine the impact of stroke physician fees on ICH costs as it was not possible to link patients with specific stroke physicians.

The primary cost data for this study was collected up to the year 2008 and inflated to the end of 2015. We believe our data is valid given the lack of meaningful changes in ICH care over the past several decades due to a lack of robust effective treatments available [4, 22, 23]. Despite this, we still took a conservative approach and assumed it could have been possible that patients may have changed over time, and thus informed our sensitivity analysis using current data collected at other centers. Using this approach, we found our data may in fact underestimate the impact of hypertension on cost; albeit not significantly.

Conclusion

Patient multimorbidity, specifically hypertension, is a strong predictor of cost after spontaneous ICH. The greatest costs after ICH are incurred during the first week and the magnitude of the increase in cost declines overtime, thus time and cost are not linearly related. These factors should be considered when forecasting health spending for stroke.

Acknowledgements
None.

Funding
This research was supported by the University of Calgary. This research did not receive any specific funding from granting agencies in the public, commercial, or not-for-profit sectors.

Authors' contributions
AVS conceived and designed the study, coordinated and collected the data, conducted all analyses, interpreted the results, wrote all the drafts, and submitted the paper for publication. TCT contributed to study design. TCT, SBP, MDH reviewed the final drafts and provided recommendations. All authors read and approved the final manuscript.

Competing interests
None of the authors have any competing interests.

Author details
[1]Department of Health Professions, College of Health and Public Affairs, University of Central Florida, 12805 Pegasus Drive, Orlando, FL 32816, USA. [2]Department of Family Medicine, Cumming School of Medicine, University of Calgary, 3330 Hospital Drive NW, Calgary, AB T2N 4N1, Canada. [3]Department of Community Health Sciences, Cumming School of Medicine, University of Calgary, 3280 Hospital Drive NW, Calgary, AB T2N 4Z6, Canada. [4]Department of Clinical Neurosciences, Cumming School of Medicine, Foothills Hospital, Room 1242A, 1403 29th Street NW, Calgary, AB T2N 2T9, Canada.

References
1. Russell MW, Joshi AV, Neumann PJ, Boulanger L, Menzin J. Predictors of hospital length of stay and cost in patients with intracerebral hemorrhage. Neurology. 2006;67:1279–81.
2. Specogna AV, Patten SB, Turin TC, Hill MD. Cost of spontaneous intracerebral hemorrhage in Canada during 1 decade. Stroke. 2014;45:284–6.
3. Qureshi AI, Suri MF, Nasar A, Kirmani JF, Ezzeddine MA, Divani AA, Giles WH. Changes in cost and outcome among US patients with stroke hospitalized in 1990 to 1991 and those hospitalized in 2000 to 2001. Stroke. 2007;38:2180–4.
4. Hemphill JC 3rd, Greenberg SM, Anderson CS, Becker K, Bendok BR, Cushman M, Fung GL, Goldstein JN, Macdonald RL, Mitchell PH, et al. Guidelines for the Management of Spontaneous Intracerebral Hemorrhage: a guideline for healthcare professionals from the American Heart Association/American Stroke Association. Stroke. 2015;46:2032–60.
5. Barber PA, Kleinig TJ. INTERACT2: a reason for optimism with spontaneous intracerebral hemorrhage? Int J Stroke. 2014;9:59–60.
6. Canadian Institute for Health Information [http://www.cihi.ca/]. Accessed 3 Aug 2017.
7. Table 326-0021. Consumer Price Index (CPI). In. Ottawa: Statistics Canada; 2016.
8. Stata Statistical Software. In., 9-13 edn. College Station: StataCorp.
9. Ording AG, Sorensen HT. Concepts of comorbidities, multiple morbidities, complications, and their clinical epidemiologic analogs. Clin Epidemiol. 2013;5:199–203.
10. Quan H, Khan N, Hemmelgarn BR, Tu K, Chen G, Campbell N, Hill MD, Ghali WA, McAlister FA. Validation of a case definition to define hypertension using administrative data. Hypertension. 2009;54:1423–8.
11. Quan H, Sundararajan V, Halfon P, Fong A, Burnand B, Luthi JC, Saunders LD, Beck CA, Feasby TE, Ghali WA. Coding algorithms for defining comorbidities in ICD-9-CM and ICD-10 administrative data. Med Care. 2005;43:1130–9.
12. Duan N. Smearing estimate: a nonparametric retransformation method. J Am Stat Assoc. 1983;78:605–10.
13. Table 051-0005. Estimates of population, Canada, provinces and territories quarterly (persons). In. Ottawa: Statistics Canada; 2016.
14. Health Indicators Interactive Tool [https://yourhealthsystem.cihi.ca/epub/]. Accessed 3 Aug 2017.
15. Mozaffarian D, Benjamin EJ, Go AS, Arnett DK, Blaha MJ, Cushman M, Das SR, de Ferranti S, Despres JP, Fullerton HJ, et al. Heart disease and stroke statistics-2016 update: a report from the American Heart Association. Circulation. 2016;133:e38–e360.
16. Zahuranec DB, Lisabeth LD, Sanchez BN, Smith MA, Brown DL, Garcia NM, Skolarus LE, Meurer WJ, Burke JF, Adelman EE, et al. Intracerebral hemorrhage mortality is not changing despite declining incidence. Neurology. 2014;82:2180–6.
17. Weon BM, Je JH. Theoretical estimation of maximum human lifespan. Biogerontology. 2009;10:65–71.
18. Bar B, Hemphill JC. Charlson comorbidity index adjustment in intracerebral hemorrhage. Stroke. 2011;42(10):2944–6.
19. Reed SD, Blough DK, Meyer K, Jarvik JG. Inpatient costs, length of stay, and mortality for cerebrovascular events in community hospitals. Neurology. 2001;57:305–14.
20. Holloway RG, Witter DM Jr, Lawton KB, Lipscomb J, Samsa G. Inpatient costs of specific cerebrovascular events at five academic medical centers. Neurology. 1996;46:854–60.
21. Mittmann N, Seung SJ, Hill MD, Phillips SJ, Hachinski V, Cote R, Buck BH, Mackey A, Gladstone DJ, Howse DC, et al. Impact of disability status on ischemic stroke costs in Canada in the first year. Can J Neurol Sci. 2012;39:793–800.
22. Broderick J, Connolly S, Feldmann E, Hanley D, Kase C, Krieger D, Mayberg M, Morgenstern L, Ogilvy CS, Vespa P, et al. Guidelines for the management of spontaneous intracerebral hemorrhage in adults: 2007 update: a guideline from the American Heart Association/American Stroke Association stroke council, high blood pressure research council, and the quality of care and outcomes in research interdisciplinary working group. Stroke. 2007;38:2001–23.
23. Morgenstern LB, Hemphill JC 3rd, Anderson C, Becker K, Broderick JP, Connolly ES Jr, Greenberg SM, Huang JN, MacDonald RL, Messe SR, et al. Guidelines for the management of spontaneous intracerebral hemorrhage: a guideline for healthcare professionals from the American Heart Association/American Stroke Association. Stroke. 2010;41:2108–29.

9

Predictors of early-onset post-ischemic stroke depression

Guilin Meng*, Xiaoye Ma, Lei Li, Yan Tan, Xiaohui Liu, Xueyuan Liu and Yanxin Zhao*

Abstract

Background: Post-stroke depression (PSD) seriously affects the rehabilitation of nerve function and quality of life. However, the pathogenesis of PSD is still not clear. This study aimed to investigate the demographic, clinical, and biochemical factors in patients with PSD.

Methods: Patients with an acute ischemic stroke, who met the inclusion criteria at Shanghai Tenth People's Hospital from April 2016 to September 2016, were recruited for this study. The stroke severity was assessed using the National Institutes of Health Stroke Scale (NIHSS), and the mental state was assessed using Mini-Mental State Examination (MMSE), Hamilton Depression Scale (HAMD), and Hamilton Anxiety Scale (HAMA) at 1 week of admission. The patients were divided into PSD and non-PSD groups. The demographic and clinical characteristics, as well as the biochemical factors, were compared between the two groups. A logistic regression analysis was performed to identify the risk factors for depression following stroke.

Results: A total of 83 patients with acute ischemic stroke were recruited. Of these, 36 (43.4%) developed depression. The multivariate logistic regression analysis indicated that high NIHSS [odds ratio (OR): 1.84, 95% confidence interval (CI): 1.09–3.12, $P = 0.023$] and high HAMD scores (OR: 2.38, 95% CI: 1.61–3.50, $P < 0.001$) were independent risk predictors for PSD and so were lower dopamine level (OR: 0.64, 95% CI: 0.45–0.91, $P = 0.014$), lower 5-hydroxytryptamine level (OR: 0.99, 95% CI: 0.98–1.00, $P = 0.046$), higher tumor necrosis factor-α level (OR: 1.05, 95% CI: 1.00–1.09, $P = 0.044$), and lower nerve growth factor level (OR: 0.06, 95% CI: 0.01–0.67, $P = 0.022$).

Conclusions: The identification of higher NIHSS scores, higher HAMD scores, lower dopamine level, lower 5-hydroxytryptamine level, higher tumor necrosis factor-α level, and lower nerve growth factor level might be useful for clinicians in recognizing and treating depression in patients after a stroke.

Keywords: Acute ischemic stroke, Inflammatory cytokine, Monoamine neurotransmitter, Nerve growth factor, Post-stroke depression

Background

Post-stroke depression (PSD) is a common mental disease after stroke onset, mainly manifested as depression, sleep disorders, decreased interest and worthlessness, and even suicidal tendencies, accounting for one third of all patients with stroke [1]. PSD can significantly affect the recovery of neurological function in patients with stroke, significantly reduce the quality of life, and increase mortality [2].

As a result, predicting the occurrence of PSD after primary treatment is important not only for counseling the patients about the disease prognosis but also for applying additional treatment.

However, it is hard to identify the consistent risk factors from the literature. Large studies have paid much attention to the vascular factors [3, 4] and socioeconomic risk factors [5], but minimal attention has been paid to the biological factors. Intracerebral neurotransmitters have been directly related to PSD, especially monoamine neurotransmitters including noradrenaline (NE), 5-hydroxytryptamine (5-HT), and dopamine (DA), which are important neurotransmitters closely related to human mental activity, especially emotional activity [6]. Plasma concentrations of neurotransmitters seemed to be closely related to intracerebral concentrations [7],

* Correspondence: guilmeng@iu.edu; 1098127350@qq.com
Department of Neurology, Shanghai Tenth People's Hospital, Tongji University School of Medicine, Shanghai 200072, China

suggesting that plasma concentrations could be used to predict the cerebral concentrations using much less invasive procedures [8]. A hypothesis suggests that immune imbalance is implicated in the pathophysiology of PSD and that IL-6 and TNF-α are key cytokines [9]. Interestingly, nerve growth factor (NGF) [10] and calcitonin gene–related peptide (CGRP) [11] have been reported as relevant factors for depression. Besides, the relationship between the lesion site in the brain and PSD is also controversial [12, 13]. Therefore, a better understanding of biological factors associated with PSD is urgently required.

This retrospective study was conducted on Chinese patients to systematically investigate the correlations of depression development 1 week after ischemic stroke with the following factors: intracerebral neurotransmitters, inflammatory cytokines, NGF, CGRP, and lesion site in the brain.

Methods

Study design

This study was approved by the local ethics committee of Shanghai Tenth People's Hospital. The continuous inpatient electronic medical records at the Department of Neurology, Shanghai Tenth Hospital, were reviewed for an acute cerebral infarction (ACI) between April 2016 and September 2016. After a detailed evaluation with inclusion and exclusion criteria, 83 patients were included in this study (Fig. 1).

Inclusion criteria

Patients who met all of the following inclusion criteria were eligible for the study:

1) Patients who fully understood the purpose of this study, expressed voluntary participation, agreed to sign informed consent, and were willing to bear the relevant risks.
2) Patients who met the criteria proposed at the Fourth Cerebrovascular Disease Conference held by the Chinese Medical Association and were diagnosed with ACI by computed tomography (CT) or magnetic resonance imaging (MRI)
3) Patients who were admitted to hospital within 24 h after stroke onset.

Exclusion criteria

1) Presence of intracranial hemorrhage or subdural hematoma evidenced by cranial CT scan
2) Presence of depression-positive mental disorder within the previous 6 months
3) Presence of disturbance of consciousness or serious cognitive dysfunction
4) Presence of complete aphasia, sensory aphasia, or apraxia
5) Presence of severe infectious diseases such as respiratory system infections, urinary system infections, and gastrointestinal infections; severe heart failure; liver and kidney disease; blood

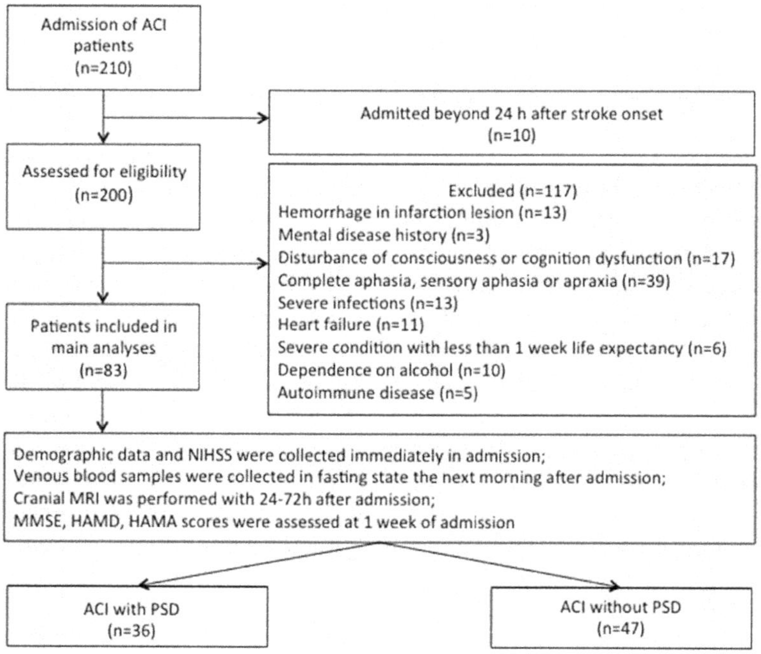

Fig. 1 Flow chart of the study implementation. ACI, Acute cerebral infarction; NIHSS, National Institutes of Health Stroke Scale; MMSE, Mini-Mental State Examination; HAMA, Hamilton Anxiety Scale; HAMD, Hamilton Depression Scale; PSD, post-stroke depression

disorder; immune disease; thyroid disease; epilepsy; or cancer
6) Severe condition with a life expectancy of less than 1 week
7) Pregnant or lactating women
8) Dependence on alcohol, tobacco, or other substances
9) Presence of autoimmune diseases or mental retardation.

At admission, demographic data and history of conventional vascular risk factors were recorded.

Testing indexes of plasma concentrations

Venous blood samples were collected the next morning after admission for basic biochemical tests, fasting and postprandial blood glucose, glycosylated hemoglobin (HbAlc), low-density lipoprotein (LDL), high-density lipoprotein (HDL), and thyroid function. Samples were marked with a unique study number only. Some of the fasting blood was centrifuged, and the serum was stored at −80°C. The concentrations of norepinephrine (NE), 5-HT, dopamine (DA), CGRP, and NGF were detected using enzyme-linked immunosorbent assay.

Detailed assessment and grouping

Stroke severity was assessed using the National Institutes of Health Stroke Scale (NIHSS) [14] at the time of admission. The mental state was assessed using Mini-Mental State Examination (MMSE), Hamilton Depression Scale (HAMD), and Hamilton Anxiety Scale (HAMA) by trained neurologists at 1 week of admission.

CT brain scans were obtained routinely in the emergency room, and it was also possible that the patient was sent to the inpatient Neurology department directly before the cranial CT if the symptoms and signs were quite typical, thus in this situation, cranial CT was performed in Neurology department immediately after admission. Cranial MRI was performed within 24–72 h after admission to assess the site of the brain infarct.

Patients with HAMD scores greater than or equal to 8 were included in the PSD group [15]. Patients with HAMD scores less than 8 were enrolled in the non-PSD group. Finally, the 2 groups included 36 and 47 patients, respectively.

Statistical analysis

The Kolmogorov–Smirnov test was used to determine whether the metrological data followed the normal distribution. Continuous variables, which followed a normal distribution, were expressed as mean ± standard deviation ($x \pm s$). Patients with PSD and without PSD were compared using the independent two-sample *t* test or Mann–Whitney *U* test. The chi-square/Fisher's exact test was used for categorical variables. Variables having a *P* value less than 0.1 in the univariate analysis were selected and evaluated using multivariate logistic regression models with the conditional forward selection method to minimize confounding and examine their independent contributions of what we adjusted for. All statistical assessments were two tailed, and a *P* value less than 0.05 was considered statistically significant. Statistical analyses were performed using SPSS 22.0 statistical software (SPSS Inc., IL, USA).

Results

General patient characteristics

A total of 210 patients presented to the Neurology department at the Shanghai Tenth Hospital for ACI between April 2016 and September 2016. Eighty-three of them were found to fulfill the criteria for further analysis.

The average age was 69.4 years (range 50–86 years); 51.8% were men (Table 1). Fifty-nine patients (71.1%) had a history of hypertension, 38 (45.8%) had diabetes mellitus, and 13 (15.7%) had atrial fibrillation.

Thirty-six (43.4%) of the 83 enrolled patients with ACI were diagnosed as having PSD during their hospitalization. In general, patients with PSD were more likely to present with higher NIHSS scores (median, 3 vs 1), higher HAMD scores (median, 8 vs 0), higher HAMA scores (median, 6.5 vs 0), and lower MMSE scores (median, 25 vs 29) than did patients without PSD (Table 1), indicating that the neurological deficits were more serious in the PSD group. PSD was more likely to occur in patients with frontal lesions (41.7% vs 19.15%) and parietal lesions (16.7% vs 14.9%).

Tests for biochemical indicators

Several laboratory tests were conducted to examine the differences in biochemical indicators between the two groups. As a result, patients with PSD were more likely to present with lower TT3 levels (average 1.1 vs 1.3 μg/L), but no significant difference in thyroid-stimulating hormone (TSH) levels was reported (Table 2).

This study also found that the monoamine neurotransmitters were significantly lower and the levels of IL-6 and TNF-α were significantly higher in the PSD group than in the non-PSD group (Table 2). Moreover, patients with PSD were more likely to present with lower NGF levels (average 6.5 vs 8.1 ng/L); no significant difference in CGRP levels was found (Table 2).

Logistic regression analysis

Univariate logistic regression identified the following demographic and clinical characteristics associated with PSD: frontal lesions [odds ratio (OR) 3.02; $P = 0.028$], NIHSS scores (OR 2.08 per 1-point increase in NIHSS scores; $P < 0.001$), HAMD scores (OR 2.63 per 1-point increase in HAMD scores; $P < 0.001$), HAMA scores

Table 1 Baseline characteristics of patients with ACI and with and without PSD

Characteristics	All Patients ($n = 83$)	PSD ($n = 36$)	Non-PSD ($n = 47$)	*P* value
Age, y, mean (SD)	69.0(9.9)	67.9(9.1)	69.8(10.4)	0.397
Sex				
Male	43(51.8)	22(61.1)	21(44.7)	0.138
Female	40(48.2)	14(38.9)	26(55.3)	
Medical history				
Hypertension	59(71.1)	24(66.7)	35(74.5)	0.437
Diabetes mellitus	38(45.8)	16(44.4)	22(46.8)	0.830
Atrial fibrillation	13(15.7)	4(11.1)	9(19.2)	0.318
Lesion location				
Frontal	24(28.9)	15(41.7)	9(19.2)	0.025*
Temporal	8(9.6)	4(11.1)	4(8.5)	0.982
Parietal	13(15.7)	6(16.7)	7(14.9)	0.049*
Occipital	7(8.4)	3(8.3)	4(8.5)	1.000
Basal ganglia	42(50.6)	19(52.8)	23(48.9)	0.729
Cerebellum	3(3.6)	1(2.8)	2(4.3)	1.000
Brain stem	12(14.2)	4(11.1)	8(17.0)	0.448
Corona radiata	34(41.0)	16(44.4)	18(38.3)	0.573
Neurophysiological test scores, median (IQR)				
NHISS	1(1–2)	3(1–6)	1(0–2)	< 0.001#
HAMD	2(0–6)	9.4(8.5–10.8)	0(0–1)	< 0.001#
HAMA	2(0–7)	6.5(5–9)	0(0–1)	< 0.001#
MMSE	27(25–30)	25(22–27)	29(26–30)	< 0.001#

P values comparing persons with and without PSD. *$P < 0.05$ vs non-PSD group; #$P < 0.001$ vs non-PSD group
Numbers (%) are provided unless otherwise specified
HAMA Hamilton Anxiety Scale, *HAMD* Hamilton Depression Scale *IQR* interquartile range, *MMSE* Mini-Mental State Examination, *NIHSS* National Institutes of Health Stroke Scale, *PSD* post-stroke depression, *SD* standard deviation

(OR 2.10 per 1-point increase in HAMA scores; $P < 0.001$), and MMSE scores (OR 0.77 per 1-point decrease in MMSE scores; $P = 0.001$)]. In multivariable logistic regression, only NIHSS scores (OR 1.84 per 1-point increase in NIHSS scores; $P = 0.023$) and HAMD scores (OR 2.38 per 1-point increase in HAMD scores; $P < 0.001$) were independent demographic and clinical predictors of PSD ($P < 0.05$) (Table 3).

Univariate logistic regression identified the following biochemical indicators associated with PSD: TT3 (OR 0.01; $P < 0.001$), NE (OR 0.99; $P < 0.001$), DA (OR 0.85; $P < 0.001$), 5-HT (OR 0.99; $P < 0.001$), IL-6 (OR 3.23; $P < 0.001$), TNF-α (OR 1.03; $P < 0.001$), and NGF (OR 0.55; $P < 0.001$). In multivariable logistic regression, only DA (OR 0.64; $P = 0.014$), 5-HT (OR 0.99; $P = 0.046$), TNF-α (OR 1.05; $P = 0.044$), and NGF (OR 0.06; $P = 0.022$) were independent biochemical predictors of PSD ($P < 0.05$) (Table 4).

The multivariable logistic regression equation was logit(P) = 1/2(− 6.36 + 0.61 × NIHSS + 0.87 × HAMD + 46.25–0.45 × DA − 0.01 × 5-HT + 0.04 × TNF-α − 2.8 × NGF).

Discussion

This study investigated the risk factors associated with PSD, such as demographic factors, clinical characteristics, and biochemical factors. NIHSS scores, MMSE scores, HAMA scores, HAMD scores, monoamine neurotransmitters, inflammatory cytokines, NGF, and the lesion site in the brain were found to be related to PSD, whereas CGRP was not related to PSD. Importantly, the study found that NIHSS and HAMD scores were demographic and clinical characteristics independently associated with PSD. Moreover, DA, 5-HT, TNF-α, and NGF levels were biochemical indicators independently associated with PSD.

As shown in Tables 1 and 3, significant differences were found in NIHSS, HAMD, HAMA, and MMSE scores between the two groups, indicating that neurological deficits were more serious in the PSD group. Other studies also showed the same results [16, 17]. Further, a significant difference was found in frontal and parietal lesions between the two groups. Likewise, a study showed the involvement of subcutaneous pathway

Table 2 Biochemical indicators of patients with ACI and with and without PSD

Variables, mean(SD)	PSD ($n = 36$)	Non-PSD ($n = 47$)	P value
TT3, μg/L	1.1(0.2)	1.3(0.2)	< 0.001#
TT4, μg/L	79.8(10.6)	81.1(11.0)	0.587
TSH, uIU/mL	1.6(0.9)	1.5(0.7)	0.629
LDL, mmol/L	2.5(0.9)	2.6(0.9)	0.622
HDL, mmol/L	1.2(0.3)	1.2(0.4)	0.549
FBG, mmol/L	6.8(2.2)	6.3(2.0)	0.338
2hPBG, mmol/L	10.2(4.6)	9.6(4.5)	0.548
HbAlc, %	6.1(1.5)	6.2(1.8)	0.793
NE, ng/L	931.8(172.9)	1237.8(296.5)	< 0.001#
DA, ng/L	46.7(10.2)	64.7(8.9)	< 0.001#
5-HT, ng/L	821.7(228.4)	1065.9(144.3)	< 0.001#
IL-6, ng/L	4.6(1.0)	3.4(0.9)	< 0.001#
TNF-α, ng/L	224.4(44.1)	164.9(43.7)	< 0.001#
NGF, ng/L	6.5(1.5)	8.1(1.6)	< 0.001#
CGRP, pg/ml	41.9(6.1)	38.3(13.8)	0.112

P values compare persons with and without PSD. #$P < 0.001$ vs non-PSD group
Data are displayed as mean (standard deviation)
CGRP calcitonin gene-related peptide, *DA* dopamine, *FBG* fasting blood glucose, *5-HT* 5-hydroxytryptamine, *HbA1c* glycosylated hemoglobin, type A1c, *HDL* high-density lipoprotein, *IL-6* interleukin 6, *LDL* low-density lipoprotein, *NE* norepinephrine, *NGF* nerve growth factor, *2hPBG* 2-h postprandial blood glucose, *PSD* post-stroke depression, *SD* standard deviation, *TNF-α* tumor necrosis factor-α, *TSH* thyroid-stimulating hormone, *TT3* total triiodothyronine, *TT4* total thyroxine

in the frontal lobe, especially the caudate nucleus, globus pallidus, internal capsule knee, and left superior hemisphere [12]; however, other studies showed no significant correlation between the lesion site and PSD [13, 18]. Unlike the present study, Vahid-Ansari et al. developed a preclinical model of PSD in mice by inducing a unilateral ischemic lesion in the medial prefrontal cortex after stroke [19]. The results regarding the value of lesion site in predicting disease outcome are still controversial. Therefore, retrospective trials with larger series of patients with PSD are warranted to demonstrate the value of various lesion sites.

Monoamine neurotransmitters include mainly noradrenaline (NE), 5-HT, and DA. The somata of these neurons are located in the brainstem, and the axons reach the frontal cortex through the thalamus and basal ganglia. If any of the aforementioned locations are damaged, the levels of monoamine neurotransmitters decrease, resulting in depression [20]. Likewise, as shown in Table 2, it was found that NE, 5-HT, and DA levels were significantly lower in the PSD group than in the non-PSD group, supporting the hypotheses of monoamine neurotransmitters. Similarly, reduced DA concentrations in ischemic striatum have been demonstrated in a mouse model of chronic PSD [21]. In addition to monoamine neurotransmitters, a low plasma

Table 3 Univariate and multivariable analyses of demographic and clinical predictors of PSD in patients with ACI

	Univariate		Multivariate	
	OR (95% CI)	P value	OR (95% CI)	P value
Age, yrs	0.98(0.94,1.03)	0.392		
Female vs. Male	1.95(0.81,4.71)	0.140		
Hypertension				
Yes vs. no	0.69(0.26,1.78)	0.438		
Diabetes mellitus				
Yes vs. no	0.91(0.38,2.17)	0.830		
Atrial fibrillation				
Yes vs. no	0.53(0.15,1.88)	0.323		
Lesion location				
Frontal				
Yes vs. no	3.02(1.13,8.06)	0.028*		
Temporal				
Yes vs. no	1.34(0.31,5.78)	0.692		
Parietal				
Yes vs. no	1.14(0.35,3.75)	0.826		
Occipital				
Yes vs. no	0.98(0.21,4.67)	0.977		
Basal ganglia				
Yes vs. no	1.17(0.49,2.78)	0.729		
Cerebellum				
Yes vs. no	0.64(0.06,7.38)	0.723		
Brain stem				
Yes vs. no	0.61(0.17,2.21)	0.451		
Corona radiata				
Yes vs. no	1.29(0.53,3.11)	0.573		
Neurophysiological test scores				
NIHSS	2.08(1.42,3.06)	< 0.001#	1.84(1.09,3.12)	0.023*
HAMD	2.63(1.74,3.96)	< 0.001#	2.38(1.61,3.50)	< 0.001#
HAMA	2.10(1.56,2.83)	< 0.001#		
MMSE	0.77(0.65,0.90)	0.001**		

CI confidence interval, *HAMA* Hamilton Anxiety Sale, *HAMD* Hamilton Depression Scale, *MMSE* Mini-Mental State Examination, *NIHSS* National Institutes of Health Stroke Scale, *OR* odds ratio
*$P < 0.05$; #$P < 0.001$

glutamate has also been reported to be associated with early-onset PSD recently [22].

This study found the levels of IL-6 and TNF-α significantly higher in the PSD group than in the non-PSD group. Inflammatory cytokines are implicated in the pathogenesis of PSD. Spalletta et al. [23] believed that increased inflammatory cytokines after stroke induced damage in the marginal zone by activating indoleamine-2,3-dioxygenase, leading to 5-HT depletion in the secondary edge system. Besides, inflammatory cytokines can also affect the protective cytokines and some

Table 4 Univariate and Multivariable Analysis for Biochemical Predictors of PSD in Patients With ACI

	Univariate		Multivariate	
	OR (95% CI)	*P* value	OR (95% CI)	*P* value
TT3, μg/L	0.00(0.000,0.04)	< 0.001#		
TT4, μg/L	0.99(0.95,1.03)	0.582		
TSH, uIU/mL	1.15(0.66,2.03)	0.625		
LDL, mmol/L	0.89(0.56,1.41)	0.618		
HDL, mmol/L	0.66(0.17,2.56)	0.438		
FBG, mmol/L	1.11(0.90,1.36)	0.337		
2hPBG, mmol/L	1.03(0.94,1.13)	0.543		
HbA1c, %	0.97(0.74,1.26)	0.790		
NE, ng/L	0.99(0.99,0.99)	< 0.001#		
DA, ng/L	0.85(0.79,0.90)	< 0.001#	0.64(0.45,0.91)	0.014*
5-HT, ng/L	0.99(0.99,1.00)	< 0.001#	0.99(0.98,1.00)	0.046*
IL-6, ng/L	3.23(1.90,5.48)	< 0.001#		
TNF-α, ng/L	1.03(1.02,1.04)	< 0.001#	1.05(1.00,1.09)	0.044*
NGF, ng/L	0.55(0.41,0.76)	< 0.000#	0.06(0.01,0.67)	0.022*
CGRP, pg/ml	1.03(0.99,1.07)	0.146		

CI confidence interval, *CGRP* calcitonin gene-related peptide, *DA* dopamine, *FBG* fasting blood glucose, *5-HT* 5-hydroxytryptamine, *HbA1c* glycosylated hemoglobin, type A1c, *HDL* high-density lipoprotein, *IL-6* interleukin 6, *LDL* low-density lipoprotein, *NE* norepinephrine, *NGF* nerve growth factor, *OR* odds ratio, *2hPBG* 2-h postprandial blood glucose, *PSD* post-stroke depression, *SD* standard deviation, *TNF-α* tumor necrosis factor-α, *TSH* thyroid-stimulating hormone, *TT3* total triiodothyronine, *TT4* total thyroxine

*$P < 0.05$; #$P < 0.001$

neurotransmitters in the brain, thus indirectly promoting the occurrence of PSD. Moreover, some studies have shown the overexpression of inflammatory cytokines in patients with cerebral ischemic stroke [24, 25]. Similarly, IL-6, IL-10, TNF-α, and interferon-γ levels increased to different degrees in patients with PSD, corresponding well with the result shown in the patients with PSD in the present study [9, 26]. Interestingly, increased serum IL-18 levels were also suggested as a biomarker for PSD [27].

NGF, a secretory protein first found in neurotrophic factors, inhibits apoptosis and promotes survival, growth, and differentiation of neurons [28]. Some studies have suggested increased NGF expression in cerebral ischemia [29, 30]. This study found the serum NGF levels to be significantly lower in the PSD group than in the non-PSD group. Likewise, several studies have found the NGF levels to be significantly lower in the severe depression group than in the normal control group [31, 32]. Other studies showed that elevated serum NGF levels could significantly ameliorate the depression symptoms and improve the quality of life [33, 34]. Unlike the present study, several studies suggested no correlation between depression and NGF [35, 36]. The differences in patient groups and experimental design might account for the difference in results.

Further, CGRP, an active peptide of 37 amino acids widely distributed in the nervous and cardiovascular system, has potent vasodilator and neuroprotective effects [37]. The CGRP synthesis was known to increase when nerve damage or inflammatory responses occurred [38]. The present study found that CGRP levels were higher in the PSD group than in the non-PSD group, but with no statistically significant difference. Unlike the present study, Shao et al. showed that CGRP immunoreactivity (CGRP-ir) concentration in the cerebrospinal fluid and hippocampus increased in rats with PSD and the administration of CGRP into the ischemic rats increased depression-like behaviors in a dose-dependent manner [11]. A study also found that CGRP antagonists could significantly ameliorate the depression symptoms [39]. The difference in sample size might account for the diversity in results.

Only 83 patients were examined in the present study and the stroke severity of sample was not high. Hence, the results must be confirmed by conducting large-sample studies. The reason for this minimally affected sample was the strict inclusion and exclusion criteria. It is common that patients with higher NIHSS always have aphasia with different degrees of severity, and old-age patients have multiple-system and multiple-organ disorders, and cognition dysfunction, which were all part of the exclusion criteria. However, the preliminary risk factor model provided more confidence to take action for individuals with higher stroke severities. Besides, a potential limitation of this study was the inherent differences between the participants in this clinical trial and the general population of stroke survivors. Another limitation was the absence of medical assessment record of the previous mental states before the stroke onset because the depression history was sometimes not objective for depressive patients without illness perception/cognition. Furthermore, the ideal time for testing the levels of plasma parameters in patients with acute stroke still needs further longitudinal studies. Nevertheless, the results were noteworthy because this novel study systematically investigated the correlations of depression after ischemic stroke with the following factors: neurotransmitters, inflammatory cytokines, NGF, CGRP, and lesion site in the brain.

Overall, it is speculated that the inflammatory response can aggravate the injury in ischemic regions and, meanwhile, lead to 5-HT depletion, increase in DA level, and inhibition of NGF expression, thereby promoting the development of PSD. However, the relationship between inflammatory response with PSD and ideal optimum plasma biomarkers still needs further investigation. The findings of this study might be helpful in preventing PSD and ensuring the adequacy of treatment. All stroke survivors should be screened early for depression. It is critical that patients with PSD are provided with appropriate treatment. Also, larger studies with longer follow-up should be conducted in the future.

Conclusions

The risk factors for PSD were identified as higher NIHSS scores, higher HAMD scores, lower DA level, lower 5-HT level, higher tumor necrosis factor-α level, and lower NGF level. These results might be useful for clinicians in recognizing and treating depression in patients after a stroke.

Abbreviations

2hPBG: 2-h postprandial blood glucose; 5-HT: 5-hydroxytryptamine; ACI: Acute cerebral infarction; CGRP: Calcitonin gene–related peptide; CGRP-ir: CGRP immunoreactivity; CI: Confidence interval; CT: Computed tomography; DA: Dopamine; FBG: Fasting blood glucose; HAMA: Hamilton anxiety scale; HAMD: Hamilton depression scale; HbAlc: Glycosylated hemoglobin; HDL: High-density lipoprotein; IL-6: Interleukin 6; IQR: Interquartile range; LDL: Low-density lipoprotein; MMSE: Mini-mental state examination; MRI: Magnetic resonance imaging; NE: Noradrenaline; NGF: Nerve growth factor; NIHSS: National institutes of health stroke scale; OR: Odds ratio; PSD: Post-stroke depression; SD: Standard deviation; TNF-α: Tumor necrosis factor-α; TSH: Thyroid-stimulating hormone; TT3: Total triiodothyronine; TT4: Total thyroxine

Acknowledgments

The authors thank the patients for their commitment to this research and Professor Kyle Stuart for the English improvement.

Funding

This study was supported by the International Exchange Program for Graduate Students, Tongji University (No. 2016020033), and the National Natural Science Foundation of China (81771131).

Authors' contributions

GM and YZ conceived and designed the study. YT and XL performed the experiments. LL and XL analyzed and prepared the manuscript. XM and GM analyzed the data and wrote the manuscript. All authors read and approved the final manuscript.

Competing interests

The authors declare that they have no competing interests.

References

1. Hackett ML, Pickles K. Part I: frequency of depression after stroke: an updated systematic review and meta-analysis of observational studies. Int J Stroke. 2014;9(8):1017–25.
2. Stern-Nezer S, Eyngorn I, Mlynash M, Snider RW, Venkatsubramanian C, Wijman CAC, Buckwalter MS. Depression one year after hemorrhagic stroke is associated with late worsening of outcomes. NeuroRehabilitation. 2017;41(1):179–87.
3. Arauz A, Rodriguez-Agudelo Y, Sosa AL, Chavez M, Paz F, Gonzalez M, Coral J, Diaz-Olavarrieta C, Roman GC. Vascular cognitive disorders and depression after first-ever stroke: the Fogarty-Mexico stroke cohort. Cerebrovasc Dis. 2014;38(4):284–9.
4. Zhang Y, He JR, Liang HB, Lu WJ, Yang GY, Liu JR, Zeng LL. Diabetes mellitus is associated with late-onset post-stroke depression. J Affect Disord. 2017;221:222–6.
5. Liu R, Yue Y, Jiang H, Lu J, Wu A, Geng D, Wang J, Lu J, Li S, Tang H, et al. A risk prediction model for post-stroke depression in Chinese stroke survivors based on clinical and socio-psychological features. Oncotarget. 2017;8(38):62891–9.
6. Parker G, Brotchie H. Mood effects of the amino acids tryptophan and tyrosine: 'Food for Thought' III. Acta Psychiatr Scand. 2011;124(6):417–26.
7. Gao HQ, Zhu HY, Zhang YQ, Wang LX. Reduction of cerebrospinal fluid and plasma serotonin in patients with post-stroke depression: a preliminary report. Clin Invest Med. 2008;31(6):E351–6.
8. Lang D, Ude C, Wurglics M, Schubert-Zsilavecz M, Klein J. Brain permeability of bilobalide as probed by microdialysis before and after middle cerebral artery occlusion in mice. J Pharm Pharm Sci. 2010;13(4):607–14.
9. Su JA, Chou SY, Tsai CS, Hung TH. Cytokine changes in the pathophysiology of poststroke depression. Gen Hosp Psychiatry. 2012;34(1):35–9.
10. Xiong P, Zeng Y, Wan J, Xiaohan DH, Tan D, Lu J, Xu F, Li HY, Zhu Z, Ma M. The role of NGF and IL-2 serum level in assisting the diagnosis in first episode schizophrenia. Psychiatry Res. 2011;189(1):72–6.
11. Shao B, Zhou YL, Wang H, Lin YS. The role of calcitonin gene-related peptide in post-stroke depression in chronic mild stress-treated ischemic rats. Physiol Behav. 2015;139:224–30.
12. Vataja R, Pohjasvaara T, Leppävuori A, Mäntylä R, Aronen HJ, Salonen O, Kaste M, Erkinjuntti T. Magnetic resonance imaging correlates of depression after ischemic stroke. Arch Gen Psychiatry. 2001;58(10):925–31.
13. Karakus K, Kunt R, Memis CO, Kunt DA, Dogan B, Ozdemiroglu F, Sevincok L. The factors related to early-onset depression after first stroke. Psychogeriatrics. 2017; doi: 10.1111/psyg.12266.
14. Lyden P, Brott T, Tilley B, Welch KM, Mascha EJ, Levine S, Haley EC, Grotta J, Marler J. Improved reliability of the NIH stroke scale using video training. NINDS TPA Stroke Study Group. Stroke. 1994;25(11):2220–6.
15. Hamilton M. A rating scale for depression. J Neurol Neurosurg Psychiatry. 1960;23:56–62.
16. Yang S, Hua P, Shang X, Cui Z, Zhong S, Gong G, Humphreys GW. A significant risk factor for poststroke depression: the depression-related subnetwork. J Psychiatry Neurosci. 2015;40(4):259–68.
17. Zhang L, Sui R, Zhang L, Zhang Z. Morphological and metabolic alteration of cerebellum in patients with post-stroke depression. Cell Physiol Biochem. 2016;40(3–4):420–30.
18. Berg A, Palomaki H, Lehtihalmes M, Lonnqvist J, Kaste M. Poststroke depression: an 18-month follow-up. Stroke. 2003;34(1):138–43.
19. Vahid-Ansari F, Lagace DC, Albert PR. Persistent post-stroke depression in mice following unilateral medial prefrontal cortical stroke. Transl Psychiatry. 2016;6(8):e863.
20. Santos M, Gold G, Kovari E, Herrmann FR, Hof PR, Bouras C, Giannakopoulos P. Neuropathological analysis of lacunes and microvascular lesions in late-onset depression. Neuropathol Appl Neurobiol. 2010;36(7):661–72.
21. Kronenberg G, Balkaya M, Prinz V, Gertz K, Ji S, Kirste I, Heuser I, Kampmann B, Hellmann-Regen J, Gass P, et al. Exofocal dopaminergic degeneration as antidepressant target in mouse model of poststroke depression. Biol Psychiatry. 2012;72(4):273–81.
22. Geng LY, Qian FY, Qian JF, Zhang ZJ. The combination of plasma glutamate and physical impairment after acute stroke as a potential indicator for the early-onset post-stroke depression. J Psychosom Res. 2017;96:35–41.
23. Spalletta G, Bossu P, Ciaramella A, Bria P, Caltagirone C, Robinson RG. The etiology of poststroke depression: a review of the literature and a new hypothesis involving inflammatory cytokines. Mol Psychiatry. 2006;11(11):984–91.
24. Li F, Pendy JT Jr, Ding JN, Peng C, Li X, Shen J, Wang S, Geng X. Exercise rehabilitation immediately following ischemic stroke exacerbates inflammatory injury. Neurol Res. 2017;39(6):530–537.

25. Yang B, Hamilton JA, Valenzuela KS, Bogaerts A, Xi X, Aronowski J, Mays RW, Savitz SI. Multipotent adult progenitor cells enhance recovery after stroke by modulating the immune response from the spleen. Stem Cells. 2017; 35(5):1290–1302.
26. Spalletta G, Cravello L, Imperiale F, Salani F, Bossu P, Picchetto L, Cao M, Rasura M, Pazzelli F, Orzi F, et al. Neuropsychiatric symptoms and interleukin-6 serum levels in acute stroke. J Neuropsychiatry Clin Neurosci. 2013;25(4):255–63.
27. Yang L, Zhang Z, Sun D, Xu Z, Zhang X, Li L. The serum interleukin-18 is a potential marker for development of post-stroke depression. Neurol Res. 2010;32(4):340–6.
28. Ducassou S, Prouzet-Mauleon V, Deau MC. Brunet de la grange P, Cardinaud B, Soueidan H, Quelen C, Brousset P, Pasquet JM, Moreau-Gaudry F et al: MYB-GATA1 fusion promotes basophilic leukaemia: involvement of IL33 and nerve growth factor receptors. J Pathol. 2017;242(3):347–57.
29. Chen C, Zhang W, Lou BD, Pan J, Cao Y, Zhong F, Zhou WJ, Wu J. Effect of Electroacupuncture stimulation of acupoints of the pericardium meridian on serum NGF and Nogo-a contents and cerebral NGF and Nogo-a expression in cerebral ischemia rats. Zhen Ci Yan Jiu. 2015;40(2):94–8.
30. Dmitrieva VG, Stavchansky VV, Povarova OV, Skvortsova VI, Limborska SA. Dergunova LV: [effects of ischemia on the expression of neurotrophins and their receptors in rat brain structures outside the lesion site, including on the opposite hemisphere]. Mol Biol. 2016;50(5):775–84.
31. Wiener CD, de Mello FS, Pedrotti Moreira F, Bittencourt G, de Oliveira JF, Lopez Molina M, Jansen K, de Mattos Souza LD, Rizzato Lara D, Portela LV, et al. Serum levels of nerve growth factor (NGF) in patients with major depression disorder and suicide risk. J Affect Disord. 2015;184:245–8.
32. Oglodek EA, Just MJ, Szromek AR, Araszkiewicz A. Melatonin and neurotrophins NT-3, BDNF, NGF in patients with varying levels of depression severity. Pharmacological Rep. 2016;68(5):945–51.
33. Filho CB, Jesse CR, Donato F, Giacomeli R, Del Fabbro L, da Silva AM, de Gomes MG, Goes AT, Boeira SP, Prigol M, et al. Chronic unpredictable mild stress decreases BDNF and NGF levels and Na(+),K(+)-ATPase activity in the hippocampus and prefrontal cortex of mice: antidepressant effect of chrysin. Neuroscience. 2015;289:367–80.
34. Kaihola H, Olivier J, Poromaa IS, Akerud H. The effect of antenatal depression and selective serotonin reuptake inhibitor treatment on nerve growth factor signaling in human placenta. PLoS One. 2015;10(1):e0116459.
35. Kheirouri S, Noorazar SG, Alizadeh M, Dana-Alamdari L. Elevated brain-derived Neurotrophic factor correlates negatively with severity and duration of major depressive episodes. Cogn Behav Neurol. 2016;29(1):24–31.
36. Cirulli F, Alleva E. The NGF saga: from animal models of psychosocial stress to stress-related psychopathology. Front Neuroendocrinol. 2009;30(3):379–95.
37. Hind WH, Tufarelli C, Neophytou M, Anderson SI, England TJ, O'Sullivan SE. Endocannabinoids modulate human blood-brain barrier permeability in vitro. Br J Pharmacol. 2015;172(12):3015–27.
38. Muzzi M, Buonvicino D, De Cesaris F, Chiarugi A. Acute and chronic triptan exposure neither alters rodent cerebral blood flow nor worsens ischemic brain injury. Neuroscience. 2017;340:1–7.
39. Jiao J, Opal MD, Dulawa SC. Gestational environment programs adult depression-like behavior through methylation of the calcitonin gene-related peptide gene. Mol Psychiatry. 2013;18(12):1273–80.

10

The intracerebral hemorrhage acutely decreasing arterial pressure trial II (ICH ADAPT II) protocol

Laura Gioia[1], Ana Klahr[1], Mahesh Kate[1], Brian Buck[1], Dariush Dowlatshahi[2], Thomas Jeerakathil[1], Derek Emery[3] and Kenneth Butcher[1*]

Abstract

Background: Aggressively lowering blood pressure (BP) in acute intracerebral hemorrhage (ICH) may improve outcome. Although there is no evidence that BP reduction changes cerebral blood flow, retrospective magnetic resonance imaging (MRI) studies have demonstrated sub-acute ischemic lesions in ICH patients. The primary aim of this study is to assess ischemic lesion development in patients randomized to two different BP treatment strategies. We hypothesize aggressive BP reduction is not associated with ischemic injury after ICH.

Methods: The Intracerebral Hemorrhage Acutely Decreasing Blood Pressure Trial II (ICH ADAPT II) is a phase II multi-centre randomized open-label, blinded-endpoint trial. Acute ICH patients (N = 270) are randomized to a systolic blood pressure (SBP) target of <140 or <180 mmHg. Acute ICH patients within 6 h of onset and two SBP measurements ≥140 mmHg recorded >2 mins apart qualify. SBP is managed with a pre-defined treatment protocol. Patients undergo MRI at 48 h, Days 7 and 30, with clinical assessment at Day 30 and 90. The primary outcome is diffusion weighted imaging (DWI) lesion frequency at 48 h. Secondary outcomes include cumulative DWI lesion rate frequency within 30 days, absolute hematoma growth, prediction of DWI lesion incidence, 30-day mortality rates, day 90 functional outcome, and cognitive status.

Discussion: This trial will assess the impact of hypertensive therapies on physiological markers of ischemic injury. The findings of this study will provide evidence for the link, or lack thereof, between BP reduction and ischemic injury in ICH patients.

Keywords: Blood Pressure, Intracerebral Hemorrhage, DWI, MRI, Stroke, Clinical Trial

Background

Acute management of elevated blood pressure (BP) in acute intracerebral hemorrhage (ICH) remains an area of clinical equipoise. Phase III studies have failed to demonstrate marked improvements in clinical outcome when BP is lowered aggressively [1, 2]. The most recent trial demonstrated a trend to worse outcomes in patients in whom BP was lowered to 120–140 mmHg [2]. Although aggressive BP reduction has not been associated with lower cerebral perfusion [3], magnetic resonance imaging (MRI) studies have reported acute and subacute ischemic lesions in 14–41% of ICH patients [4–9]. These lesions have been associated with aggressive BP treatment as well as unfavorable clinical outcomes but these data are all retrospective [4, 5, 9]. Therefore, we designed a prospective randomized study to definitively determine whether acute BP reduction is associated with an elevated risk of ischemic injury, detected with diffusion-weighted imaging (DWI).

* Correspondence: ken.butcher@ualberta.ca
[1]Division of Neurology, University of Alberta, 7th Floor Clinical Sciences Building, 11350-83rd Avenue, Edmonton, AB T6G 2B7, Canada
Full list of author information is available at the end of the article

Methods

Study design

The Intracerebral Hemorrhage Acutely Decreasing Arterial Pressure Trial II (ICH ADAPT II) is a phase II multi-center prospective, randomized, open-label study with blinded-evaluation (PROBE). Eligible ICH patients are randomized 1:1 to systolic BP (SBP) targets of <140 or <180 mmHg (Fig. 1). This study is registered with clinicaltrials.gov (NCT02281838). The primary study aim is to assess DWI lesion frequency in patients randomized to aggressive versus conservative BP targets.

Patient population

Inclusion criteria

- Patients ≥18 years with spontaneous ICH ≤6 h from onset
- Two SBP measurements ≥140 mmHg recorded >2 min apart
- Hematoma volume on CT <90 mL, as estimated using the ABC/2 method [10]
- Onset ≤6 h prior to randomization
- Glasgow Coma Scale (GCS) ≥5 prior to randomization

Exclusion criteria

- Definite contraindication to BP reduction (i.e. severe arterial stenosis, MoyaMoya disease)
- Definite indication for BP reduction (i.e. hypertensive encephalopathy or aortic dissection)
- Contraindication to MRI (i.e. cardiac pacemaker)
- Suspected secondary cause of ICH
- Ischemic stroke <90 days
- Planned hematoma resection
- Pre-morbid modified Rankin score (mRS) ≥3
- Life expectancy <6 months
- Early implementation of palliative care

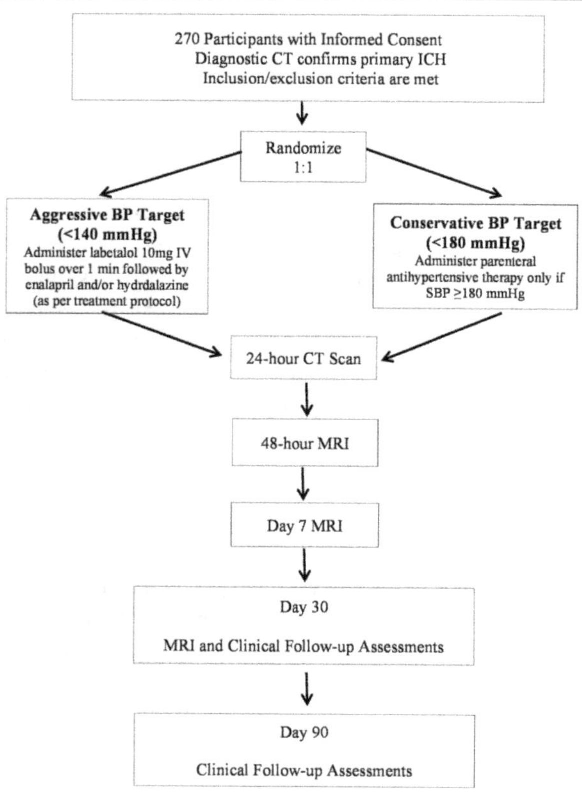

Fig. 1 Study Schema

Randomization

All patients undergo standard screening assessments including BP, GCS, and National Institutes of Health Stroke Scale (NIHSS) scores prior to randomization (Table 1). A centralized web-based randomization process is used to assign BP treatment target.

Interventions

BP Management

The assigned BP target is achieved and maintained using an intravenous antihypertensive drug bolus protocol (Table 2). Patients in the aggressive BP target (SBP <140 mmHg) group immediately receive a 10 mg intravenous (IV) bolus of labetalol, followed by repeated boluses designed to lower systolic BP to <140 mmHg within 60 min of randomization. The protocol utilizes IV enalapril and hydralazine boluses as well.

Patients randomized to the conservative arm (SBP <180 mmHg group) are treated with antihypertensive agents only if SBP ≥180 mmHg. BP and heart rate (HR) are continuously monitored non-invasively for the first 24 h.

Imaging Procedures

Baseline: Diagnostic non-contrast computed tomography (CT) scan. This consists of 5 mm slices, no gap (120 kvp, 300 mA per slice) through the entire brain (18–20 slices with a 512 × 512 matrix).

24-h: Repeat CT scan at 24 ± 3 h to assess for hematoma expansion and peri-hematoma edema volume.

48-h: MRI at 48 ± 12 h, including a T1-weighted sagittal localizer, T2-weighted images, DWI (the primary endpoint), Fluid-attenuated Inverse Recovery (FLAIR), Susceptibility Weighted Imaging (SWI), and pulse Arterial Spin Labeling (ASL; optional sequence). DWI sequences are combined to form isotropic (trace) diffusion images and Apparent Diffusion Coefficient (ADC) maps are generated from these raw data. ADC maps are used to ensure all lesions represent true diffusion restriction and not T2 shine through effects. FLAIR sequences are also utilized to assess chronic small vessel ischemic changes. SWI sequences are used to assess the burden (number, total volume and topography) of cerebral microbleeds. Pulse ASL data is used to generate blood flow maps to determine if DWI lesions are correlated with hypoperfusion. All image analyses are completed centrally by raters blinded to BP treatment group allocation.

Table 1 Summary of trial procedures

	Screening/Randomization	24 ± 3 h	48 ± 12 h	Day 7 ± 2	Day 30 ± 5	Day 90 ± 30
Eligibility Criteria	□					
Signed Informed Consent	□					
Past Medical History	□					
Vital Signs (BP, HR) Monitoring	□	□	□	□	□	□
Medications	□			□	□	□
CT scan	□	□				
MRI scan			□	□	□	
NIHSS	□	□	□	□	□	□
Glasgow Coma Scale	□	□	□	□	□	□
Modified Rankin Scale	□			□	□	□
Montreal Cognitive Assessment	□			□	□	□
Barthel Index, EuroQOL					□	□
AE/SAE Reporting		□	□	□	□	□
End of Study Report						□

Days 7 and 30: MRI repeat at Days 7 ± 2 and 30 ± 5 to assess for new DWI lesion development and evolution of those previously identified.

Clinical assessments

In-hospital clinical assessments (24 h, 48 h, day 7 and hospital discharge) of neurological deterioration are performed using GCS and NIHSS. Discharge mRS scores is obtained to assess disability and Montreal Cognitive Assessment (MoCA) to determine cognitive changes. This latter assessment is relevant as development of DWI lesions may impair cognition in ICH patients. All neurological, disability, and cognitive assessments are repeated at days 30 and 90.

Primary outcome

The primary endpoint is DWI lesion frequency on the 48-h MRI, which is the time point DWI lesions have most commonly been observed after ICH [4–9]. This is also the time point most relevant to acute BP reduction.

Secondary outcomes

- Hematoma growth at 24 h
  - *Hypothesis*: The mean hematoma growth will be smaller in the SBP <140 mmHg group.
- Cumulative DWI lesion rate frequency within 30 days
  - *Hypothesis:* The rate of DWI lesion development will be higher in the SBP <140 mmHg group.
- Day 30 mortality rates
  - *Hypothesis:* DWI lesion development will predict mortality, which should be independent of BP randomization.
- Day 90 mRS scores
  - *Hypothesis:* Median mRS will be positively correlated with number of DWI lesions.
- Day 90 MoCA
  - *Hypothesis:* MoCA scores will be lower in patients with DWI lesions.

Data safety monitoring body (DSMB)

The DSMB (Additional file 1) reviews the proportion of patients with neurological deterioration within 48 h (defined as an increase in NIHSS ≥4 points), 90-day mortality and all serious adverse events (SAE) after 33% and 67% of patients are enrolled. The committee may modify or stop the trial at any point.

Sample size estimates

The sample size is based on an observed DWI lesion frequency of 26% in the <180 mmHg target group [4–9]. The odds ratio for DWI lesion occurrence is 1.03 per decrease in mmHg of mean arterial pressure (MAP) between baseline and the MRI scan [5]. In ICH ADAPT I, MAP in the aggressive treatment group decreased by an average of 28 mmHg at the time of the primary endpoint assessment. Assuming a similar treatment effect in ICH ADAPT II, the predicted effect of SBP reduction <140 mmHg is an odds ratio of DWI lesion incidence of 1.84. The trial has been powered to detect a 0.84 (relative) increase in the frequency of DWI lesions in the <140 mmHg target group. The predicted absolute increase in the proportion of patients with DWI lesions is 22%.

Hypotheses:

H_0: The proportion of patients with DWI lesions in the < 140 mmHg treatment arm will be ≤ 0.48.

Table 2 Acute BP treatment protocols

A. <140 mmHg Target Group	
	Target SBP <140 mmHg within 30 min of randomization
Monitoring	• Record BP/HR q[a]5 min during active treatment; q15 min × 1 h, q30 min × 5 h and q1h × 18 h
Labetalol (IV)	• Labetalol test dose: 10 mg bolus over 1 min • If SBP ≥140 mmHg and HR >55 BPM, repeat 10 mg bolus in 5 min. • 10–20 mg IV push q5 min until SBP <140 mmHg or HR <55 BPM • Maximum labetalol dose: 300 mg/24 h
And Enalapril (IV) (If available)	• Enalapril 1.25 mg bolus
And/or Hydralazine (IV)	If BP persistently >140 mmHg: • Hydralazine test dose: 5 mg IV bolus over 1 min • If SBP ≥140 mmHg, repeat 5 mg IV bolus in 5 min • 10–20 mg IV bolus q5 min until SBP <140 mmHg • Maximum hydralazine dose = 240 mg/24 h
Continuous IV Infusions (ICU admission)	If BP persistently >140 mmHg: • Labetalol infusion 2–8 mg/min (maximum 300 mg/24 h) and/or hydralazine infusion 50–150 µg/min
Maintenance Therapy	
Maintain SBP <140 mmHg × 24 h minimum	
IV treatment prn[b]	If SBP >140 mmHg at any point: • Labetalol (10–20 mg) / hydralazine (10–20 mg) boluses. Record BP/HR 5 and 15 min later • Enalapril 1.25 mg q6 h if SBP >140 mmHg • If SBP ≤135 mmHg or HR <55 BPM, hold maintenance dose
B. <180 mmHg Target Group	
	Protocol to be used <u>only</u> if SBP ≥180 mmHg
Monitoring	• as listed above
Labetalol (IV)	• Labetalol test dose: 10 mg bolus over 1 min • If SBP ≥180 mmHg and HR >55 BPM, repeat 10 mg bolus in 5 min. • 10–20 mg IV push q5 min until SBP <180 mmHg or HR <55 BPM • Maximum labetalol dose: 300 mg/24 h
Hydralazine (IV)	If BP persistently >180 mmHg: • Hydralazine test dose: 5 mg IV bolus over 1 min • If SBP ≥180 mmHg, repeat 5 mg IV bolus in 5 min • 10–20 mg IV bolus q5 min until SBP <180 mmHg • Maximum hydralazine dose = 240 mg/24 h
Maintenance Therapy	
IV treatment prn	If SBP >180 mmHg at any point during 24 h: • Labetalol (10–20 mg) / hydralazine (10–20 mg) boluses. Record BP/HR 5 and 15 min later

[a]q = every, [b]prn = when necessary

H_A: The proportion of patients with DWI lesions in the < 140 mmHg treatment arm will be > 0.48.

The primary analysis will be a one-sided test of proportions at the alpha = 0.025 level. A sample size of 180 evaluable patients will be required to reject the null hypothesis with 80% power (alpha = 0.025). To account for withdrawal of consent and missing data related to early death and MRI contraindications, the sample size has been increased to 270 patients.

Statistical analyses

The primary endpoint will be tested using Fisher's Exact test. There will be no interim analyses for efficacy or futility.

Discussion

Elevated BP has been associated with hematoma growth, mortality, and disability after ICH [11]. However, the most recent clinical trial data have revived concerns about the safety of very aggressive BP reduction [2]. It is unknown if this trend to worse outcome is related to cerebral ischemic changes, but it is one possible mechanism [12]. There are mixed data regarding the development of ischemic lesions after ICH and its association with BP. Retrospective studies have suggested that there is a negative, positive, and even no correlation between the two [5, 8, 13, 14].

The current trial utilizes a physiological endpoint that is more sensitive to ischemic injury to determine whether aggressive BP reduction in ICH patients exacerbates DWI lesion development, in individual patients. We have previously conducted a trial, ICH ADAPT I, in which ICH patients were randomized to aggressive (SBP <150 mmHg) versus conservative (SBP <180 mmHg) BP management strategies [3]. We did not find a difference in peri-hematoma cerebral blood flow (CBF) in these two groups. Most importantly, the magnitude of BP change was not related to regional CBF [3]. In contrast, several studies indicate that delayed cerebral ischemia, evident on MRI scan only, is common within the first week after ICH [4–9]. Although the majority of peri-hematoma DWI hyperintensities result from plasma derived edema,[15] true diffusion restriction representing bioenergetic compromise in this region and topographically remote areas are also present in some patients [4–9]. These DWI lesions tend to be small but are still a subject of concern as longitudinal studies indicate the probability of death/dependence at one year is increased between five and six-fold in these patients [13, 16].

Canadian Stroke Best Practices recommendations for hyperacute stroke care recognize the safety of aggressively reducing SBP [17]. Furthermore, current American Heart Association/American Stroke Association guidelines advise lowering SBP <140 mmHg given its potential to improve patient prognosis in ICH patients, but more aggressive treatment is not encouraged [18]. These recommendations are based primarily on the results of two phase III studies which have failed to demonstrate an increase in the proportion of patients with good clinical outcomes when BP is lowered aggressively [1, 2]. In the Intensive Blood Pressure Reduction in Acute Cerebral Hemorrhage Trial (INTERACT II), 2839 ICH patients were randomized within 6 h of symptom onset to a SBP target of <140 or <180 mmHg. The rate of death/disability was similar in the <140 mmHg target group (52%) and the <180 mmHg target group (55.3%; odds ratio with intensive treatment, 0.87; 95% CI, 0.75 to 1.01; $p = 0.06$) [1]. In the Antihypertensive Treatment of Acute Cerebral Hemorrhage II (ATACH II), patients were randomized earlier (4.5 rather than 6 h after symptom onset) to the aggressive and conservative BP strategies [2]. This trial recruited 1000 ICH patients, in which the primary outcome of death and disability (GCS >5) was observed in 38.7% vs. 37.7% in the aggressive vs. conservative treatment, respectively. The investigators concluded that aggressive antihypertensive therapy did not improve outcome.

At this point the optimal BP treatment strategy remains unknown. It has been hypothesized that an earlier intervention (e.g., in the prehospital setting) may be needed to improve patient prognosis, and small clinical trials have demonstrated the feasibility and safety of hyperacute BP management in stroke patients [19, 20]. However, it may be that in some patients aggressive BP reduction precipitate and/or exacerbate ischemic lesion development. This can only be addressed with a randomized controlled trial specifically addressing this endpoint.

In conclusion, ICH ADAPT II will provide evidence for the link, or lack thereof, between BP reduction and ischemic injury. This will add support for the safety of early systolic BP reduction to <140 mmHg, or alternatively a more nuanced approach to acute hypertension management in ICH patients.

Abbreviations

ADC: Apparent diffusion coefficient; ASL: Arterial spin labeling; ATACH II: Antihypertensive treatment of acute cerebral hemorrhage II; BP: Blood pressure; CBF: Cerebral blood flow; CT: Computed tomography; DSMB: Data safety monitoring body; DWI: Diffusion-weighted imaging; FLAIR: Fluid-attenuated inverse recovery; GCS: Glasgow coma scale; ICH ADAPT II: Intracerebral Hemorrhage Acutely Decreasing Blood Pressure Trial II; ICH: Intracerebral hemorrhage; INTERACT II: Intensive blood pressure reduction in acute cerebral hemorrhage II; MAP: Mean arterial pressure; MoCA: Montreal cognitive assessment; MRI: Magnetic resonance imaging; mRS: Modified Rankin scale; NIHSS: National Institutes of Health Stroke Scale; PROBE: Prospective, randomized, open-label study with blinded-evaluation; SAE: Serious adverse events; SBP: Systolic blood pressure; SWI: Susceptibility Weighted Imaging

Acknowledgements
Not applicable.

Funding
The trial is funded by the Heart and Stroke Foundation of Canada (GIA G-14-0006004).

Authors' contributions
LG, AK, and KB drafted the manuscript. AK and KB will be involved in the main data analysis. LG, MK, BB, DD, TJ, DE, and KB are involved in data collection. KB designed the trial and wrote the protocol. All authors read and approved the final manuscript.

Competing interests
The authors declare that they have no competing interests.

Author details
[1]Division of Neurology, University of Alberta, 7th Floor Clinical Sciences Building, 11350-83rd Avenue, Edmonton, AB T6G 2B7, Canada. [2]Division of Neurology, University of Ottawa, Ottawa, ON, Canada. [3]Department of Diagnostic Imaging, University of Alberta, Edmonton, AB, Canada.

References
1. Anderson CS, Heeley E, Huang Y, Wang J, Stapf C, Delcourt C, et al. Rapid blood-pressure lowering in patients with acute intracerebral hemorrhage. N Engl J Med. 2013;368:2355–65.
2. Qureshi AI, Palesch YY, Barsan WG, Hanley DF, Hsu CY, Martin RL, et al. Intensive Blood-Pressure Lowering in Patients with Acute Cerebral Hemorrhage. N Engl J Med. 2016;375(11):1033–43.
3. Butcher KS, Jeerakathil T, Hill M, Demchuk AM, Dowlatshahi D, Coutts SB, et al. The intracerebral hemorrhage acutely decreasing arterial pressure trial. Stroke. 2013;44(3):620–6.
4. Prabhakaran S, Gupta R, Ouyang B, John S, Temes RE, Mohammad Y, et al. Acute brain infarcts after spontaneous intracerebral hemorrhage: a diffusion-weighted imaging study. Stroke. 2010;41:89–94.
5. Menon RS, Burgess RE, Wing JJ, Gibbons MC, Shara NM, Fernandez S, et al. Predictors of highly prevalent brain ischemia in intracerebral hemorrhage. Ann Neurol. 2012;71:199–205.
6. Kang DW, Han MK, Kim HJ, Yun SC, Jeon SB, Bae HJ, et al. New ischemic lesions coexisting with acute intracerebral hemorrhage. Neurology. 2012;79:848–55.
7. Gregoire SM, Charidimou A, Gadapa N, Dolan E, Antoun N, Peeters A, et al. Acute ischaemic brain lesions in intracerebral haemorrhage: multicentre cross-sectional magnetic resonance imaging study. Brain. 2011;134:2376–86.
8. Kimberly WT, Gilson A, Rost NS, Rosand J, Viswanathan A, Smith EE, et al. Silent ischemic infarcts are associated with hemorrhage burden in cerebral amyloid angiopathy. Neurology. 2009;72:1230–5.
9. Garg RK, Liebling SM, Maas MB, Nemeth AJ, Russell EJ, Naidech AM. Blood pressure reduction, decreased diffusion on MRI, and outcomes after intracerebral hemorrhage. Stroke. 2012;43:67–71.
10. Kothari RU, Brott T, Broderick JP, Barsan WG, Sauerbeck LR, Zuccarello M, et al. The ABCs of measuring intracerebral hemorrhage volumes. Stroke. 1996; 27(8):1304–5.
11. Butcher K, Laidlaw J. Current intracerebral haemorrhage management. J Clin Neurosci. 2003;10(2):158–67.
12. Prabhakaran S, Naidech AM. Ischemic brain injury after intracerebral hemorrhage: a critical review. Stroke. 2012;43(8):2258–63.
13. Singer OC, Kurre W, Humpich MC, Lorenz MW, Kastrup A, Liebeskind DS, et al. Risk assessment of symptomatic intracerebral hemorrhage after thrombolysis using DWI-Aspects. Stroke. 2009;40(8):2743–8.
14. Brazzelli M, Sandercock Peter AG, Chappell Francesca M, Celani Maria G, Righetti E, Arestis N, et al. Magnetic resonance imaging versus computed tomography for detection of acute vascular lesions in patients presenting with stroke symptoms. Cochrane Database Syst Rev. 2009; doi:10.1002/14651858.CD007424.pub2.

15. Butcher KS, Baird T, MacGregor L, Desmond P, Tress B, Davis S. Perihematomal edema in primary intracerebral hemorrhage is plasma derived. Stroke. 2004;35(8):1879–85.
16. Murat Arsava E, Kayim-Yildiz O, Oguz KK, Akpinar E, Topcuoglu MA. Elevated Admission Blood Pressure and Acute Ischemic Lesions in Spontaneous Intracerebral Hemorrhage. J Stroke Cerebrovasc Dis. 2013;22(3):250–4.
17. Casaubon LK, Boulanger J, Blacquiere D, Boucher S, Brown K, Goddard T, et al. Canadian stroke best practice recommendations: hyperacute stroke care guidelines, update 2015. Int J Stroke. 2015;10(6):924–40.
18. Hemphill JC, Greenberg SM, Anderson CS, Becker K, Bendok BR, Cushman M, et al. Guidelines for the management of spontaneous intracerebral hemorrhage. Stroke. 2015;46(7):2032–60.
19. Shaw L, Price C, Mclure S, Howel D, Mccoll E, Younger P, et al. Paramedic Initiated Lisinopril For Acute Stroke Treatment (PIL-FAST): results from the pilot randomised controlled trial. Emerg Med J. 2014;31(12)994–9.
20. Right T, Ankolekar S, Fuller M, Cross I, Renton C, Cox P, et al. Feasibility of an ambulance-based stroke trial, and safety of glyceryl trinitrate in ultra-acute stroke: the rapid intervention with glyceryl trinitrate in hypertensive stroke trial (RIGHT, ISRCTN66434824). Stroke. 2013;44:3120–8.

11

Development and validation of a score for evaluating comprehensive stroke care capabilities: J-ASPECT Study

Akiko Kada[1*], Kunihiro Nishimura[2], Jyoji Nakagawara[3], Kuniaki Ogasawara[4], Junichi Ono[5], Yoshiaki Shiokawa[6], Toru Aruga[7], Shigeru Miyachi[8], Izumi Nagata[9], Kazunori Toyoda[10], Shinya Matsuda[11], Akifumi Suzuki[12], Hiroharu Kataoka[13], Fumiaki Nakamura[2], Satoru Kamitani[14], Koji Iihara[15] and the J-ASPECT Study Collaborators

Abstract

Background: Although the Brain Attack Coalition recommended establishing centers of comprehensive care for stroke and cerebrovascular disease patients, a scoring system for such centers was lacking. We created and validated a comprehensive stroke center (CSC) score, adapted to Japanese circumstances.

Methods: Of the selected 1369 certified training institutions in Japan, 749 completed an acute stroke care capabilities survey. Hospital performance was determined using a 25-item score, evaluating 5 subcategories: personnel, diagnostic techniques, specific expertise, infrastructure, and education. Consistency and validity were examined using correlation coefficients and factorial analysis.

Results: The CSC score (median, 14; interquartile range, 11–18) varied according to hospital volume. The five subcategories showed moderate consistency (Cronbach's $\alpha = 0.765$). A strong correlation existed between types of available personnel and specific expertise. Using the 2011 Japanese Diagnosis Procedure Combination database for patients hospitalized with stroke, four constructs were identified by factorial analysis (neurovascular surgery and intervention, vascular neurology, diagnostic neuroradiology, and neurocritical care and rehabilitation) that affected in-hospital mortality from ischemic stroke, intracerebral hemorrhage, and subarachnoid hemorrhage. The total CSC score was related to in-hospital mortality from ischemic stroke (odds ratio [OR], 0.973; 95% confidence interval [CI], 0.958–0.989), intracerebral hemorrhage (OR, 0.970; 95% CI, 0.950–0.990), and subarachnoid hemorrhage (OR, 0.951; 95% CI, 0.925–0.977), with varying contributions from the four constructs.

Conclusions: The CSC score is a valid measure for assessing CSC capabilities, based on the availability of neurovascular surgery and intervention, vascular neurology, diagnostic neuroradiology, and critical care and rehabilitation services.

Keywords: Ischemia, Stroke, Hemorrhage, Cerebrovascular circulation, Risk factors

Background

Stroke is the fourth leading cause of mortality and the most common cause of permanent morbidity in Japan, causing an enormous socioeconomic burden. The public health implications of stroke care globally, including in Japan, are profound. Despite accelerating progress in stroke therapy, implementation of appropriate acute treatment remains essential for decreasing the associated mortality and permanent morbidity. In 2000, the Brain Attack Coalition discussed the concept of primary stroke centers and later proposed the design of comprehensive stroke centers (CSCs) [1, 2]. Most stroke patients can be adequately treated at a primary stroke center (PSC), and the Joint Commission established programs for the certification and performance measurement of PSCs [3]. The concept and recommended key components of a CSC enable intensive patient care and the use of specialized techniques that are not available at most PSCs [1, 4]. To continuously monitor the efficiency of care, reliable

* Correspondence: akiko.kada@nnh.go.jp
[1]Department of Clinical Trials and Research, Clinical Research Center, National Hospital Organization Nagoya Medical Center, 4-1-1 Sannomaru, Naka-ku, Nagoya, Aichi 460-0001, Japan
Full list of author information is available at the end of the article

measures of hospital capabilities and performance are needed. Although the Joint Commission and several US states have started certification processes for PSCs and CSCs [5–8], an established, simple scoring system does not exist to evaluate the comprehensive acute stroke care capabilities of CSCs. To this end, a simple tool for assessing CSC capabilities would be useful for monitoring service quality and enabling its improvement [4]. In 2010, we started the J-ASPECT study (Nationwide survey of Acute Stroke care capacity for Proper dEsignation of Comprehensive stroke cenTer in Japan) to establish optimal nationwide implementation of stroke centers to improve acute stroke outcomes. We modified the above recommendations to reflect the specific circumstances in Japan and developed a CSC score; this tool was validated using the nationwide Diagnosis Combination Procedure (DPC) database, created during the first year of this study.

Methods

Content validity

In the first step of the J-ASPECT study, we investigated the current conditions of stroke hospitals in Japan. We created a 49-item questionnaire examining various aspects of stroke care, including medical systems, emergency systems, stroke rehabilitation, education, and medical performance. Some recommended items, such as ventriculostomy availability, were excluded from our questionnaire for the sake of simplicity and to increase the survey response rate since the items seemed identical to the recommendations of board-certified (BC) neurosurgeons in Japan. Other items, such as availability of transesophageal echocardiography, were excluded because of their very low expected usage, which would make an evaluation of their impact on mortality rates difficult. In February 2011, the questionnaire was mailed to 1369 certified training institutions belonging to the Japan Neurosurgical Society, the Japanese Society of Neurology, and the Japan Stroke Society. Based on this questionnaire, the overall organizational and staffing levels of the hospitals, in terms of CSC capacity, were scored following the Brain Attack Coalition recommendations, after reviewing the literature describing CSCs and conducting a thorough discussion with an expert panel [9]. Advanced acute stroke care capabilities were assessed based on 25 items divided into 5 subcategories (listed in Table 1). One point was assigned for each recommended item that the hospital met, resulting in a maximum total score of 25; subcategory scores were also calculated.

Table 1 The availability of comprehensive stroke center score components

Components	Items	Item No	Number	Percent
Personnel	Neurologists	1	358	47.8
	Neurosurgeons	2	694	92.7
	Endovascular physicians	3	272	36.3
	Critical care medicine	4	162	21.6
	Physical medicine and rehabilitation	5	113	15.1
	Rehabilitation therapy	6	742	99.1
	Stroke rehabilitation nurses	7	102	13.6
Diagnostics (24/7)	CT[a]	8	742	99.1
	MRI[b] with diffusion	9	647	86.4
	Digital cerebral angiography	10	602	80.4
	CT angiography	11	627	83.7
	Carotid duplex ultrasound	12	257	34.3
	TCD[c]	13	121	16.2
Specific expertise	Carotid endarterectomy	14	603	80.5
	Clipping of intracranial aneurysm	15	685	91.5
	Hematoma removal/draining	16	689	92.0
	Coiling of intracranial aneurysm	17	360	48.1
	Intra-arterial reperfusion therapy	18	498	66.5
Infrastructure	Stroke unit	19	132	17.6
	Intensive care unit	20	445	59.4
	Operating room staffed 24/7	21	451	60.2
	Interventional services coverage 24/7	22	279	37.2
	Stroke registry	23	235	31.4
Education	Community education	24	369	49.3
	Professional education	25	436	58.2

[a]computed tomography; [b]magnetic resonance imaging; [c]transcranial Doppler

Consistency

Cronbach's α was calculated to evaluate the consistency between the 5 CSC score subcategories used for assessing CSC capabilities. To determine the influence of each subcategory, α-values were also calculated for all combinations of the four subcategories. Correlations between the 25 CSC score items were determined using tetrachoric correlation coefficients to evaluate individual items measured with different constructs.

Construct validity

Factorial analysis, based on tetrachoric correlation coefficients [10], was performed using principal factor analysis to explore possible potential groupings of the 25 items into a more limited number of components. The selection of the number of components was based on the Eigen values. To understand the meaning of the components, promax rotation was used.

Predictive validity

Using the Japanese DPC database for patients hospitalized with strokes during the 2011 fiscal year, we examined the differential effects of the items on mortality and poor outcomes (modified Rankin Scale: 3–6, at discharge) associated with ischemic stroke (IS), intracerebral hemorrhage (ICH), and subarachnoid hemorrhage (SAH). This cross-sectional survey used the DPC discharge database for the institutions participating in the J-ASPECT study. The DPC database is a mixed-case classification system that is linked with the lump-sum payment system, launched in 2002 by the Ministry of Health, Labor and Welfare of Japan [11]. In 2010, approximately 1388 acute care hospitals, representing about 50% of the total hospital beds, had adopted the DPC data system. Data regarding practices were obtained from the DPC database; the attending physician is responsible for each patient's clinical data entry. The details of this database have been described elsewhere [12].

Of the 749 hospitals that responded to the institutional survey of advanced stroke care capabilities, 256 agreed to participate in the DPC discharge database study. Consecutive patients, hospitalized between April 1, 2010 and March 31, 2011, were identified in the annual discharge database using the International Classification of Diseases (ICD)-10 diagnosis codes related to IS (I63.0-9), nontraumatic ICH (I61.0-9, I62.0-1, I62.9), and SAH (I60.0-9). Patients with scheduled admissions were excluded from analysis. This research was approved by the Institutional Review Board of the National Cerebral and Cardiovascular Center and, if required, by the participating hospitals.

We used hierarchical logistic regression models to determine relationships between hospital CSC scores, reflecting the capacities they were equipped with, and mortality. Each model had two levels of hierarchy (hospital and patient), and considered the random effects of hospital variables as well as the fixed effects of CSC scores, patient age and sex, and Japan Coma Scale (JCS) scores. Interactions such as those between the JCS and CSC scores were not included in the model. The analyses were performed using SAS, version 9.3 (SAS Institute, Cary, NC, USA), and R, version 3.2.0 (R Core Team, R Foundation for Statistical Computing, Vienna, Austria).

Results

Of the selected 1369 certified training institutions, 749 (55%) responded to the acute stroke care capability survey. Among the surveyed hospitals, 62% had more than 300 beds, and 51% had more than 200 acute patients (Table 2). Clipping of intracranial aneurysms (IAs) was performed more frequently than any other procedure (median/hospital, 15), followed by craniotomy removal of ICH (6), intravenous infusion of recombinant tissue plasminogen activator (5), and coiling of IAs (3). The availability of each item is shown in Table 1. Even within the same component, the availability of each item varied. Low availability values were noted for IA coiling (48.1%) in the specific expertise component and for stroke units (17.6%) in the infrastructure component.

Table 2 Hospital characteristics

Beds per hospital, n (%)	
20–49	16 (2.1)
50–99	30 (4.0)
100–299	232 (31.0)
300–499	260 (34.7)
> 500	207 (27.6)
Unknown	4 (0.5)
Acute stroke patients per hospital, n (%)	
≤ 49	51 (6.8)
50–99	78 (10.4)
100–199	199 (26.6)
200–299	155 (20.7)
> 300	228 (30.4)
Unknown	38 (5.1)
Treated patients per hospital, median (IQR[a])	
Tissue plasminogen activator	5 (2–10)
Intra-arterial thrombolysis/percutaneous angioplasty	0 (0–2)
Carotid endarterectomy	1 (0–4)
Carotid stenting	1 (0–7)
Extracranial-intracranial bypass surgery	1 (0–5)
Clipping of intracranial aneurysm	15 (6–27)
Coiling of intracranial aneurysm	3 (0–11)
Craniotomy hematoma removal	6 (2–12)
Stereotactic hematoma removal	0 (0–3)
Endoscopic hematoma removal	0 (0–0)

[a]interquartile range

The distribution of CSC score components, by hospital, is shown in Table 3. The median CSC score was 14 (interquartile range, 11–18). These components showed moderate consistency (Cronbach's $\alpha = 0.765$, for the total score). Removal of any one component resulted in Cronbach's α falling in the range of 0.668–0.776, indicating the absence of substantial influence of individual components. High correlations between the survey components pertaining to personnel and specific expertise were observed (Table 4). For example, there were high correlations between neurosurgeon availability and carotid endarterectomy ($r = 0.821$; items 2 and 14), clipping of IAs ($r = 0.936$; items 2 and 15), and hematoma removal/drainage ($r = 0.949$; items 2 and 16). Similarly, endovascular physician availability was strongly correlated with

Table 3 The distribution of comprehensive stroke center score components and their consistency

Components	Mean	SD	Median	IQR[a]	Cronbach's α
Personnel	3.26	1.25	3	2–4	0.724
Diagnostic	4.00	1.28	4	4–5	0.741
Specific expertise	3.79	1.48	4	3–5	0.668
Infrastructure	2.06	1.43	2	1–3	0.674
Education	1.07	0.83	1	0–2	0.776
Total Score	14.18	4.57	14	11–18	0.765

[a]interquartile range

coiling of IAs (r = 0.932; items 3 and 17) and intra-arterial reperfusion therapy (r = 0.842; items 3 and 18). Other relationships regarding diagnostics, infrastructure, and education did not stand out.

Factorial analysis, based on promax rotation, revealed four constructs (Table 5). The first pattern contained items pertaining to neurovascular surgery and intervention, such as endovascular physician availability, coiling of IAs, intra-arterial reperfusion therapy, 24/7 interventional services coverage, carotid endarterectomy, hematoma removal/drainage, clipping of IAs, neurosurgeon availability, rehabilitation therapy, 24/7 operating room staffing, and stroke rehabilitation nurse availability. The first pattern had the largest explained variance (43% of total variance). The second pattern included imaging modalities mainly associated with diagnostic neuroradiology (e.g., computed tomography, computed tomography angiography, digital cerebral angiography, and diffusion-weighted magnetic resonance imaging) and intensive care units. The third pattern contained items related to vascular neurology: transcranial Doppler, carotid duplex ultrasound, professional education, community education, stroke registry, and available stroke units. The fourth pattern represented neurocritical care and rehabilitation, and included the availability of neurologists, physical medicine and rehabilitation, and critical care medicine.

A total of 53,170 patients in the cohort were analyzed; the in-hospital mortality was 7.8% for IS, 16.8% for ICH, and 28.1% for SAH (Table 6). Table 7 shows the impact of hospital capacity for each of the 25 items on mortality. Among the four constructs obtained using factorial analysis, the availability of neurologists in neurocritical care and rehabilitation was significantly associated with reduced mortality of patients with IS ($P < 0.05$). The 24/7 availability of interventional service coverage in neurovascular surgery and intervention ($P < 0.05$), availability of intensive care units in diagnostic neurology, and physical medicine and rehabilitation in neurocritical care and rehabilitation ($P < 0.05$) were related to SAH mortality. The total CSC score was related to the mortality associated with IS (OR, 0.973; 95% CI, 0.958–0.989), ICH (OR, 0.970; 95% CI, 0.950–0.990), and SAH (OR, 0.951; 95% CI, 0.925–0.977).

The proportions of poor outcomes (modified Rankin Scale, 3–6) were 49.2% for IS, 65.3% for ICH, and 56.4% for SAH (Table 6). In contrast to mortality, the total CSC score was not significantly associated with poor outcomes in patients having any type of stroke (Table 8). The impact of hospital capacity for each of the 25 items on poor outcomes differed from that for mortality in some aspects. For example, among patients with IS, stroke unit availability were significantly associated with a reduced proportion of poor outcomes ($P < 0.05$). Among patients with ICH and SAH, no significant association was observed between the availability of any item and poor outcomes.

Discussion

We evaluated the consistency and validity of the CSC score; based on the Cronbach's α value of 0.765, the five components were moderately consistent [13]. The validity of the score was evaluated using factorial analysis, which revealed four major constructs. Although the four constructs were determined by the five components: personnel, diagnostic techniques, specific expertise, infrastructure, and education, this study showed a high correlation between the survey components pertaining to personnel and specific expertise. The unique fact that BC neurosurgeons comprise more than 95% of BC endovascular physicians, in Japan, may explain why personnel, specific expertise, and infrastructure components closely related to these different treatment aspects were grouped into the same construct (neurovascular surgery and intervention). Considering their influence on the variance of the CSC scores, temporal trends and geographical disparities focused on this construct may provide critical information for proper accreditation and implementation of CSCs.

With regard to the predictive validity of the CSC score, the four constructs had different effects on mortality and poor outcomes in patients with IS, ICH, and SAH. The availability of neurologists involved in neurocritical care and rehabilitation was significantly associated with reduced in-hospital morality in patients with IS. Recently, the treatment paradigm for acute IS has been changing rapidly, such that the critical role of endovascular intervention following tissue plasminogen activator infusion, for acute IS, has been established by several recent randomized controlled trials (MR Clean, ESCAPE, EXTEND-IA) [14–16]. Of note, however, the acute stroke care survey used in this study and the DPC database were both implemented before these evidences were published in 2015. The availability of BC neurosurgeons at more than 90% of the participating hospitals suggests the importance of multidisciplinary acute stroke care [17].

Table 4 Correlation coefficients between the 25 survey items

Item No[a]	1	2	3	4	5	6	7	8	9	10	11	12	13	14	15	16	17	18	19	20	21	22	23	24	25
1	1.000																								
2	-0.071	1.000																							
3	0.201	0.671	1.000																						
4	0.282	0.243	0.244	1.000																					
5	0.520	0.063	0.259	0.476	1.000																				
6	0.334	0.282	0.239	-0.190	0.140	1.000																			
7	0.171	0.072	0.248	0.054	0.117	0.125	1.000																		
8	0.300	0.451	0.265	0.202	0.037	0.392	0.007	1.000																	
9	-0.018	0.500	0.325	0.054	-0.025	0.043	0.047	0.636	1.000																
10	-0.027	0.827	0.490	0.255	0.058	0.132	-0.005	0.616	0.594	1.000															
11	-0.132	0.701	0.264	0.201	-0.050	0.017	0.055	0.632	0.614	0.830	1.000														
12	0.120	0.215	0.118	0.198	0.016	-0.196	0.158	0.306	0.357	0.332	0.295	1.000													
13	0.155	0.435	0.361	0.156	0.036	-0.142	0.102	0.194	0.287	0.492	0.372	0.713	1.000												
14	0.095	0.821	0.639	0.238	0.155	0.234	0.138	0.281	0.363	0.694	0.492	0.196	0.305	1.000											
15	0.029	0.936	0.669	0.208	0.073	0.253	0.123	0.414	0.405	0.840	0.675	0.253	0.521	0.885	1.000										
16	0.010	0.949	0.709	0.227	0.053	0.263	0.105	0.431	0.429	0.831	0.663	0.256	0.512	0.865	0.987	1.000									
17	0.215	0.648	0.932	0.283	0.270	0.228	0.373	0.262	0.288	0.486	0.243	0.220	0.386	0.648	0.695	0.729	1.000								
18	0.092	0.784	0.842	0.209	0.226	0.215	0.289	0.234	0.407	0.646	0.391	0.247	0.418	0.754	0.793	0.821	0.874	1.000							
19	0.185	0.378	0.277	0.109	0.045	0.049	0.373	0.197	0.333	0.340	0.193	0.206	0.260	0.345	0.408	0.395	0.307	0.357	1.000						
20	0.154	0.358	0.256	0.237	0.086	-0.230	0.012	0.451	0.197	0.416	0.374	0.187	0.229	0.325	0.403	0.416	0.265	0.243	0.291	1.000					
21	0.291	0.599	0.603	0.205	0.155	0.314	0.180	0.484	0.287	0.583	0.429	0.193	0.386	0.714	0.756	0.718	0.564	0.515	0.443	0.382	1.000				
22	0.273	0.515	0.912	0.226	0.218	0.229	0.376	0.347	0.277	0.464	0.224	0.217	0.400	0.538	0.594	0.626	0.895	0.762	0.321	0.283	0.697	1.000			
23	0.203	0.314	0.360	0.145	0.210	0.014	0.213	0.059	0.342	0.357	0.253	0.287	0.406	0.373	0.425	0.451	0.385	0.405	0.381	0.165	0.369	0.362	1.000		
24	0.193	0.346	0.298	0.080	0.134	0.188	0.104	0.179	0.219	0.234	0.079	0.249	0.414	0.266	0.337	0.334	0.293	0.314	0.408	0.174	0.303	0.344	0.315	1.000	
25	0.038	0.425	0.230	0.025	0.073	-0.114	0.055	0.012	0.312	0.292	0.260	0.193	0.289	0.373	0.422	0.395	0.267	0.359	0.417	0.101	0.282	0.221	0.311	0.576	1.000

[a]Item No in Table 1

Table 5 Factor analysis

		Factor 1	Factor 2	Factor 3	Factor 4
		Neurovascular surgery and intervention	Diagnostic neuroradiology	Vascular neurology	Neurocritical care and rehabilitation
	Proportion explained	0.43	0.25	0.19	0.14
Item No	Items	Standardized loadings (pattern matrix)			
3	Endovascular physicians	***0.91***[d]	-0.07	-0.04	0.12
17	Coiling of intracranial aneurysm	***0.89***	-0.11	0.04	0.15
18	Intra-arterial reperfusion therapy	***0.88***	0.00	0.10	-0.05
22	Interventional services coverage 24/7	***0.80***	-0.09	0.05	0.23
14	Carotid endarterectomy	***0.76***	0.24	-0.01	-0.10
16	Hematoma removal/draining	***0.75***	**0.37**	0.06	-0.16
15	Clipping of intracranial aneurysm	***0.73***	**0.37**	0.08	-0.16
2	Neurosurgeons	***0.69***	**0.43**	0.02	-0.22
6	Rehabilitation therapy	***0.59***	0.07	-0.63	0.18
21	Operating room staffed 24/7	***0.59***	0.28	0.00	0.18
7	Stroke rehabilitation nurses	***0.34***	-0.36	0.21	0.20
8	CT[a]	-0.03	***0.89***	-0.21	**0.34**
11	CT angiography	0.08	***0.84***	0.06	-0.17
10	Digital cerebral angiography	**0.36**	***0.70***	0.08	-0.10
9	MRI[b] with diffusion	0.03	***0.59***	0.23	-0.06
20	Intensive care unit	-0.06	***0.50***	0.17	0.22
13	TCD[c]	0.02	0.15	***0.71***	0.04
12	Carotid duplex ultrasound	-0.31	0.26	***0.72***	0.16
25	Professional education	0.23	-0.15	***0.63***	-0.23
24	Community education	0.21	-0.17	***0.56***	0.07
23	Stroke registry	0.24	-0.08	***0.52***	0.10
19	Stroke unit	0.23	-0.05	***0.49***	0.06
1	Neurologists	-0.02	-0.02	0.02	***0.85***
5	Physical medicine and rehabilitation	0.10	-0.09	0.00	***0.72***
4	Critical care medicine	-0.09	0.25	0.14	***0.55***

[a]computed tomography; [b]magnetic resonance imaging; [c]transcranial Doppler; [d]values > 0.300 are shown in bold font

The association between the availability of a stroke care unit and the increased proportion of favorable outcomes after IS, observed in this study, is consistent with a 2009 Cochrane review conducted by the Stroke Unit Trialists' Collaboration that showed the benefits of stroke unit care in terms of reducing death, dependency, and institutional care [18].

The SAH-associated mortality was higher than that associated with IS or ICH, and the condition of the patients with SAH was also more severe and required more urgent intervention. Accordingly, the availability of items representing SAH treatment, such as 24/7 interventional service coverage, intensive care unit, and BC physical medicine and rehabilitation, showed the greatest effects on mortality. The critical role of endovascular coil embolization for ruptured IAs was previously established by the International Subarachnoid Aneurysms Trial [19]. Using Nationwide Inpatient Survey data, Qureshi et al. reported a significant increase in endovascular treatment as well as a decrease in in-hospital mortality (2000–2002, 27%; 2004–2006, 24%) in patients with SAH after publication of the International Subarachnoid Trial (ISAT) in 2002 [20]. However, whether the ISAT results can be generalized to all patients with SAH is questionable because most of the patients enrolled in the study were patients with good clinical grades, having small, anterior circulation aneurysms.

The second common cause of SAH-related death and poor functional outcome is rebleeding [21], and early treatment of the ruptured aneurysm is known to lower the incidence of rebleeding. Intensive care unit and 24/7

Table 6 Demographics of the patient cohort at diagnosis, mortality, and severe disability at discharge

	Total		IS[a]		ICH[b]		SAH[c]	
	(*n* = 53170)		(*n* = 32671)		(*n* = 15699)		(*n* = 4934)	
	N	%	N	%	N	%	N	%
Male	29353	55.2	18816	57.6	9030	57.5	1584	32.1
Age (years)								
18–50	3515	6.6	1328	4.1	1271	8.1	927	18.8
51–60	5824	11.0	2742	8.4	2171	13.8	934	18.9
61–70	11744	22.1	6894	21.1	3640	23.2	1242	25.2
71–80	15825	29.8	10342	31.7	4466	28.4	1048	21.2
81–106	16262	30.6	11365	34.8	4151	26.4	783	15.9
Hypertension	39918	75.1	22531	69.0	13281	84.6	4229	85.7
Diabetes mellitus	13725	25.8	9318	28.5	3278	20.9	1174	23.8
Hyperlipidemia	15015	28.2	11104	34.0	2529	16.1	1412	28.6
Smoking (n = 44842)	12761	24.0	8188	25.1	3540	22.5	1074	21.8
Japan Coma Scale								
0	19635	36.9	15027	46.0	3620	23.1	1024	20.8
1-digit code	19371	36.4	12375	37.9	5934	37.8	1117	22.6
2-digit code	6937	13.0	3396	10.4	2705	17.2	852	17.3
3 digit code	7227	13.6	1873	5.7	3440	21.9	1941	39.3
Emergency admission by ambulance	31995	60.2	17336	53.1	10909	69.5	3830	77.6
Mortality	6522	12.3	2535	7.8	2630	16.8	1384	28.1
Poor outcome (modified Rankin Scale 3–6) at discharge. (*N* = 51719)	28238	54.6	15566	49.2	10044	65.3	2721	56.4

[a]ischemic stroke; [b]intracerebral hemorrhage; [c]subarachnoid hemorrhage

interventional coverage availability were significant factors associated with decreasing in-hospital mortality after SAH. These findings are explained by the importance of early obliteration of ruptured aneurysms for preventing rebleeding and by the early detection and appropriate treatment of vasospasms, another important cause of morbidity and mortality in patients with SAH. The study provided additional evidence that the availability of endovascular treatment and surgical clipping may reduce in-hospital mortality in patients with SAH [22]. Another recent study also showed that an early mobilization program for patients with aneurysmal SAH is feasible and safe [23]. In addition, appropriate nutritional care from the acute stage is reported to be essential for improving functional outcomes and reducing post-SAH mortality [24]. Taken together, the significant association between the availability of BC physical medicine and rehabilitation and reduced mortality observed in our study reinforces the importance of comprehensive care capabilities, including early rehabilitation and nutritional care for patients with SAH, to prevent complications. Further investigation is required to understand the role of BC physical medicine and rehabilitation in reducing SAH-associated mortality.

Finally, the total CSC score correlated with reduced mortality for all types of stroke, supporting the usefulness of this score as a comprehensive measure of acute stroke care capabilities. Another study showed that hemorrhagic stroke patients admitted to CSCs were more likely to receive neurosurgical and endovascular treatments and to be alive at 90 days than patients admitted to other hospitals. The authors used certification by the New Jersey Department of Health and Senior Services to identify CSCs. The impacts of CSCs on mortality determined in that study are similar to the results obtained using our simple scoring system [25].

In contrast to its impact on in-hospital mortality, the total CSC score did not show a significant impact on poor functional outcomes in patients with any type of stroke. Similarly, no specific item had a significant impact on poor outcomes in patients with hemorrhagic stroke. In patients with IS, the significant role of the presence of a stroke unit in reducing poor outcomes, observed in the present study, was consistent with the results of a previous report [26]. A validation study investigating functional outcomes using the DPC database may be necessary to explain the disparities between the total CSC scores (and specific items) on mortality and poor functional outcomes.

Table 7 The effect of items on mortality

Item No	Items	IS[a] (n = 32671)			ICH[b] (n = 15699)			SAH[c] (n = 4934)		
		OR[d]	95% CI[e]		OR	95% CI		OR	95% CI	
3	Endovascular physicians	0.832	0.653	1.060	0.896	0.671	1.198	1.309	0.906	1.891
17	Coiling of intracranial aneurysm	1.062	0.832	1.355	1.075	0.797	1.451	0.982	0.667	1.444
18	Intra-arterial reperfusion therapy	1.155	0.931	1.434	0.919	0.706	1.194	0.854	0.608	1.201
22	Interventional services coverage 24/7	1.071	0.831	1.379	1.145	0.844	1.555	0.674[j]	0.458	0.992
14	Carotid endarterectomy	0.945	0.708	1.262	0.833	0.595	1.165	0.789	0.503	1.237
15 and 16	Clipping of intracranial aneurysm and hematoma removal/draining	0.798	0.465	1.368	0.537	0.266	1.088	0.359	0.082	1.564
2	Neurosurgeons	0.905	0.530	1.546	1.513	0.744	3.077	0.840	0.230	3.071
6	Rehabilitation therapy	1.000			1.000			1.000		
21	Operating room staffed 24/7	0.986	0.826	1.176	0.956	0.769	1.187	1.217	0.921	1.610
7	Stroke rehabilitation nurses	1.021	0.831	1.253	1.019	0.803	1.293	1.074	0.803	1.436
8	CT[f]	0.963	0.208	4.462	0.515	0.035	7.590	1.000		
11	CT angiography	1.127	0.877	1.449	0.820	0.608	1.107	0.978	0.662	1.446
10	Digital cerebral angiography	0.840	0.652	1.082	1.243	0.917	1.684	1.068	0.722	1.580
9	MRI[g] with diffusion	1.117	0.849	1.471	0.844	0.605	1.176	0.897	0.581	1.383
20	Intensive care unit	1.032	0.897	1.188	0.964	0.813	1.144	0.795[j]	0.640	0.988
13	TCD[h]	0.852	0.699	1.038	0.879	0.700	1.105	1.222	0.930	
12	Carotid duplex ultrasound	1.039	0.889	1.215	1.021	0.849	1.228	1.119	0.891	1.406
25	Professional education	0.907	0.765	1.076	1.061	0.868	1.296	0.954	0.751	1.212
24	Community education	0.948	0.810	1.109	0.908	0.753	1.094	0.800	0.636	1.006
23	Stroke registry	0.895	0.781	1.026	0.861	0.732	1.013	0.915	0.749	1.118
19	Stroke unit	0.993	0.838	1.177	0.887	0.724	1.086	0.871	0.679	1.118
1	Neurologists	0.854[j]	0.742	0.982	1.043	0.881	1.234	1.110	0.901	1.367
5	Physical medicine and rehabilitation	1.025	0.844	1.245	0.976	0.777	1.225	0.746[j]	0.562	0.991
4	Critical care medicine	0.967	0.825	1.134	0.993	0.823	1.200	0.895	0.712	1.126
	Total CSC[i] score	0.973[j]	0.958	0.989	0.970[j]	0.950	0.990	0.951[j]	0.925	0.977

[a]ischemic stroke; [b]intracerebral hemorrhage; [c]subarachnoid hemorrhage; [d]*OR* odds ratio adjusted by hierarchical logistic model including patient age, sex, Japan Coma Scale scores, and hospital variables; [e]*CI* confidence interval; [f]computed tomography; [g]magnetic resonance imaging; [h]transcranial Doppler; [i]comprehensive stroke center; [j]$P < 0.05$ (hierarchical logistic model)

Strengths and limitations of the present study

First, this study is limited by a possible selection bias because hospitals actively working to improve stroke care were more likely to respond to the questionnaire. However, the coverage of the J-ASPECT Study group, which collaborates with the Japan Neurosurgical Society and the Japanese Congress of Neurological Surgeons, was broad enough to provide a reliable study sample. Second, information bias might have existed (self-reporting, recall, and nonresponse). Third, the CSC score mainly evaluated structural measures and did not consider their utilization, supported with real data. To assess clinical practice quality, the use of process measures is preferred [27], but process measures, such as electrocardiogram monitoring and pulse oximetry, were not considered in this scoring system [4, 28]. However, strong correlations between survey components pertaining to personnel and specific expertise (e.g., availability of neurosurgeons and carotid endarterectomy) were observed in this study, suggesting that these items may not be considered as purely structural, but may have characteristics of both structural and process measures. We are planning to develop a new registry system in the J-ASPECT Study to include key metrics required for certification of CSCs in the US, in addition to the DPC database, to study and monitor the association of such quality metrics on mortality and morbidity of acute stroke patients, in Japan. Fourth, in-hospital mortality was selected as an outcome measure to test the validity of the CSC score. A recent systematic review showed that hospital mortality does not necessarily reflect the quality of clinical practice because mortality is affected

Table 8 The effect of items on poor outcome (modified Rankin Scale 3–6)

Item		IS[a]			ICH[b]			SAH[c]		
No	Items	(n = 31640)			(n = 15391)			(n = 4821)		
		OR[d]	95% CI[e]		OR	95% CI		OR	95% CI	
3	Endovascular physicians	1.180	0.890	1.563	0.896	0.671	1.198	1.267	0.856	1.875
17	Coiling of intracranial aneurysm	0.838	0.634	1.106	1.075	0.797	1.451	0.933	0.618	1.407
18	Intra-arterial reperfusion therapy	0.990	0.777	1.261	0.919	0.706	1.194	0.704	0.487	1.017
22	Interventional services coverage 24/7	0.969	0.725	1.295	1.145	0.844	1.555	0.928	0.615	1.400
14	Carotid endarterectomy	1.293	0.946	1.768	0.833	0.595	1.165	0.838	0.511	1.376
15 and 16	Clipping of intracranial aneurysm and hematoma removal/draining	0.763	0.427	1.364	0.537	0.266	1.088	0.553	0.065	4.693
2	Neurosurgeons	1.026	0.582	1.807	1.513	0.744	3.077	4.449	0.987	20.041
6	Rehabilitation therapy	1.000	.	.	1.000	.	.	1.000	.	.
21	Operating room staffed 24/7	0.883	0.723	1.078	0.956	0.769	1.187	0.959	0.712	1.290
7	Stroke rehabilitation nurses	0.874	0.693	1.101	1.019	0.803	1.293	0.877	0.641	1.200
8	CT[f]	1.328	0.296	5.956	0.515	0.035	7.590	1.000	.	.
11	CT angiography	1.227	0.931	1.617	0.820	0.608	1.107	0.877	0.579	1.329
10	Digital cerebral angiography	0.912	0.685	1.213	1.243	0.917	1.684	1.274	0.842	1.928
9	MRI[g] with diffusion	0.940	0.706	1.252	0.844	0.605	1.176	0.793	0.490	1.284
20	Intensive care unit	0.987	0.842	1.156	0.964	0.813	1.144	1.000	0.795	1.259
13	TCD[h]	0.966	0.773	1.208	0.879	0.700	1.105	1.152	0.858	1.547
12	Carotid duplex ultrasound	1.183	0.988	1.415	1.021	0.849	1.228	1.206	0.945	1.538
25	Professional education	0.892	0.737	1.079	1.061	0.868	1.296	1.015	0.782	1.317
24	Community education	1.144	0.957	1.368	0.908	0.753	1.094	0.871	0.680	1.116
23	Stroke registry	0.981	0.840	1.146	0.861	0.732	1.013	0.860	0.695	1.065
19	Stroke unit	0.783[j]	0.645	0.952	0.887	0.724	1.086	0.878	0.676	1.141
1	Neurologists	1.137	0.969	1.335	1.043	0.881	1.234	1.096	0.877	1.370
5	Physical medicine and rehabilitation	1.163	0.934	1.449	0.976	0.777	1.225	0.979	0.725	1.322
4	Critical care medicine	1.113	0.929	1.334	0.993	0.823	1.200	1.062	0.830	1.360
	Total CSC[i] score	0.995	0.977	1.014	1.007	0.984	1.030	0.978	0.950	1.008

[a]ischemic stroke; [b]intracerebral hemorrhage; [c]subarachnoid hemorrhage; [d]OR odds ratio adjusted by hierarchical logistic model including patient age, sex, Japan Coma Scale scores, and hospital variables; [e]CI: confidence interval; [f]computed tomography; [g]magnetic resonance imaging; [h]transcranial Doppler; [i]comprehensive stroke center; [j]$P < 0.05$ (hierarchical logistic model)

to a greater extent by the patients' condition rather than by the quality of practice [29]. Possible correlations between specific items and mortality in patients with IS may have been missed because of the relatively low in-hospital mortality associated with these patients; a larger study is necessary to resolve this issue. Fifth, the DPC-based payment system contains limited information regarding patient condition severity beyond post-discharge data and the National Institute of Health Stroke (NIHSS) Scale, Glasgow Coma Scale (GCS), ICH-, or Hunt-Hess severity scores, upon admission. Nevertheless, the JCS is a useful tool for evaluating stroke severity. Notably, the importance of the JCS, published in 1974, for predicting stroke outcomes has been recently reconfirmed [9, 30]. Further study is necessary to validate the results of the present study with other patient-level measurements, such as the NIHSS, GCS, etc. Despite the above limitations, clear correlations were revealed between the CSC score and in-hospital mortality in patients with all types of strokes. In future work, the score's components should be weighted according to stroke type, based on their influence on patient outcomes.

Conclusions

The CSC score is a valid measure for assessing the capabilities of CSCs with regard to the availability of neurovascular surgery and intervention, vascular neurology, diagnostic neuroradiology, and neurocritical care and rehabilitation. The total CSC score was associated with mortality in patients with IS, ICH, and SAH, with varying contributions from the four abovementioned constructs.

Abbreviations

BC: Board-certified; CI: Confidence interval; CSC: Comprehensive stroke center; DPC: Diagnosis combination procedure; GCS: Glasgow coma scale; IA: Intracranial aneurysm; ICH: Intracerebral hemorrhage; IS: Ischemic stroke; ISAT: International subarachnoid trial; JCS: Japan coma scale; NIHSS: National institute of health stroke; OR: Odds ratio; PSC: Primary stroke center; SAH: Subarachnoid hemorrhage

Acknowledgements

We thank Drs. Manabu Hasegawa, Tomoatsu Tsuji, and Yasuhiro Nishijima for their helpful discussions, Profs. Takamasa Kayama and Nobuo Hashimoto for their supervision of the Japan Neurosurgical Society collaboration, and Ms. Arisa Ishitoko for her secretarial assistance.

Funding

This work was supported by Grants-in-Aid from the Ministry of Health, Labor and Welfare of Japan and JSPS KAKENHI Grant Number 25293314 (principal investigator: KI). This research was partially supported by the Practical Research Project for Life-Style related Diseases, including Cardiovascular Diseases and Diabetes Mellitus, from the Japan Agency for Medical Research and Development.

Authors' contributions

KI initiated the collaborative project. AK, KN, SK, and KI designed the study, drafted and revised the article. AK, KN, SK monitored data collection and analyzed the data. JN, KO, JO, YS, TA, SM, IN, KT, SM, AS, HK, FN designed the study, and validated the survey questions from the views of physicians and experts. All authors read and approved the final manuscript.

Competing interests

KI has received grants from Nihon Medi-Physics, AstraZeneca, and Otsuka Pharmaceutical. JN has received an unrestricted research grant from Nihon Medi-Physics. IN has received lecture honoraria from Otsuka Pharmaceutical and Sanofi.

Author details

[1]Department of Clinical Trials and Research, Clinical Research Center, National Hospital Organization Nagoya Medical Center, 4-1-1 Sannomaru, Naka-ku, Nagoya, Aichi 460-0001, Japan. [2]Center for Cardiovascular Disease Information, National Cerebral and Cardiovascular Center, Suita, Japan. [3]Integrative Stroke Imaging Center, National Cerebral and Cardiovascular Center, Suita, Japan. [4]Department of Neurosurgery, Iwate Medical University, Morioka, Japan. [5]Chiba Cardiovascular Center, Ichihara, Japan. [6]Department of Neurosurgery, Kyorin University, Mitaka, Japan. [7]Showa University, Tokyo, Japan. [8]Department of Neurosurgery, Osaka Medical College, Takatsuki, Japan. [9]Kokura Memorial Hospital, Fukuoka, Japan. [10]Departments of Cerebrovascular Medicine, National Cerebral and Cardiovascular Center, Suita, Japan. [11]Department of Preventive Medicine and Community Health, University of Occupational and Environmental Health, Kita-Kyushu, Japan. [12]Akita Prefectural Hospital Organization Research Institute for Brain and Blood Vessels, Akita, Japan. [13]Department of Neurosurgery, National Cerebral and Cardiovascular Center, Suita, Japan. [14]Department of Public Health, Graduate School of Medicine, The University of Tokyo, Tokyo, Japan. [15]Department of Neurosurgery, Graduate School of Medical Sciences, Kyushu University, Fukuoka, Japan.

References

1. Alberts MJ, Hademenos G, Latchaw RE, Jagoda A, Marler JR, Mayberg MR, et al. Recommendations for the establishment of primary stroke centers. Brain Attack Coalition. JAMA. 2000;283:3102–9.
2. Alberts MJ, Latchaw RE, Selman WR, Shephard T, Hadley MN, Brass LM, et al. Recommendations for comprehensive stroke centers: a consensus statement from the Brain Attack Coalition. Stroke. 2005;36:1597–616.
3. Reeves MJ, Parker C, Fonarow GC, Smith EE, Schwamm LH. Development of stroke performance measures: definitions, methods, and current measures. Stroke. 2010;41:1573–8.
4. Leifer D, Bravata DM, Connors 3rd JJ, Hinchey JA, Jauch EC, Johnston SC, et al. Metrics for measuring quality of care in comprehensive stroke centers: detailed follow-up to Brain Attack Coalition comprehensive stroke center recommendations: a statement for healthcare professionals from the American Heart Association/American Stroke Association. Stroke. 2011;42:849–77.
5. Markovchick VJ, Moore EE. Optimal trauma outcome: trauma system design and the trauma team. Emerg Med Clin North Am. 2007;25:643–54.
6. Joint Commission on Accreditation of Healthcare Organizations. Updated Primary Stroke Center Certification appendix for the disease-specific care manual. Jt Comm Perspect. 2005;25:3–6.
7. Gropen TI, Gagliano PJ, Blake CA, Sacco RL, Kwiatkowski T, Richmond NJ, et al. Quality improvement in acute stroke: the New York State Stroke Center Designation Project. Neurology. 2006;67:88–93.
8. Stradling D, Yu W, Langdorf ML, Tsai F, Kostanian V, Hasso AN, et al. Stroke care delivery before vs after JCAHO stroke center certification. Neurology. 2007;68:469–70.
9. Iihara K, Nishimura K, Kada A, Nakagawara J, Toyoda K, Ogasawara K, et al. The impact of comprehensive stroke care capacity on the hospital volume of stroke interventions: a nationwide study in Japan: J-ASPECT Study. J Stroke Cerebrovasc Dis. 2014;23:1001–18.
10. Kubinger KD. On artificial results due to using factor analysis for dichotomous variables. Psychol Sci. 2003;45:106–10.
11. Yasunaga H, Ide H, Imamura T, Ohe K. Impact of the Japanese Diagnosis Procedure Combination-based Payment System on cardiovascular medicine-related costs. Int Heart J. 2005;46:855–66.
12. Iihara K, Nishimura K, Kada A, Nakagawara J, Ogasawara K, Ono J, et al. Effects of comprehensive stroke care capabilities on in-hospital mortality of patients with ischemic and hemorrhagic stroke: J-ASPECT Study. PLoS ONE. 2014;9:e96819.
13. Terwee CB, Bot SD, de Boer MR, van der Windt DA, Knol DL, Dekker J, et al. Quality criteria were proposed for measurement properties of health status questionnaire. J Clin Epidemiol. 2007;60:34–42.
14. Berkhemer OA, Fransen PS, Beumer D, van den Berg LA, Lingsma HF, Yoo AJ, et al. A randomized trial of intraarterial treatment for acute ischemic stroke. N Engl J Med. 2015;372:11–20.
15. Goyal M, Demchuk AM, Menon BK, Eesa M, Rempel JL, Thornton J, et al. Randomized assessment of rapid endovascular treatment of ischemic stroke. N Engl J Med. 2015;372:1019–30.
16. Campbell BC, Mitchell PJ, Kleinig TJ, Dewey HM, Churilov L, Yassi N, et al. Endovascular therapy for ischemic stroke with perfusion-imaging selection. N Engl J Med. 2015;372:1009–18.
17. Decker C, Chhatriwalla E, Gialde E, Garavalia B, Summers D, Quinlan ME, et al. Patient-centered decision support in acute ischemic stroke: Qualitative study of patients' and providers' perspectives. Circ Cardiovasc Qual Outcomes. 2015;8 Suppl 3:S109–16.
18. Sun Y, Paulus D, Eyssen M, Maervoet J, Saka O. A systematic review and meta-analysis of acute stroke unit care: what's beyond the statistical significance? BMC Med Res Methodol. 2013;13:132.
19. Molyneux AJ, Kerr RS, Yu LM, Clarke M, Sneade M, Yarnold JA, et al. International subarachnoid aneurysm trial (ISAT) of neurosurgical clipping versus endovascular coiling in 2143 patients with ruptured intracranial aneurysms: a randomized comparison of effect on survival, dependency, seizures, rebleeding, subgroups, and aneurysm occlusion. Lancet. 2005; 366:809–17.
20. Qureshi AI, Vazquez G, Tariq N, Suri MF, Lakshminarayan K, Lanzino G. Impact of International Subarachnoid Aneurysm Trial results on treatment of ruptured intracranial aneurysms in the United States. Clinical article. J Neurosurg. 2011;114:834–41.

21. Broderick JP, Brott TG, Duldner JE, Tomsick T, Leach A. Initial and recurrent bleeding are the major causes of death following subarachnoid hemorrhage. Stroke. 1994;25:1342–7.
22. Spetzler RF, McDougall CG, Albuquerque FC, Zabramski JM, Hills NK, Partovi S, et al. The Barrow Ruptured Aneurysm Trial: 3-year results. J Neurosurg. 2013;119:146–57.
23. Olkowski BF, Devine MA, Slotnick LE, Veznedaroglu E, Liebman KM, Arcaro ML, et al. Safety and feasibility of an early mobilization program for patients with aneurysmal subarachnoid hemorrhage. Phys Ther. 2013;93:208–15.
24. Nagano A, Yamada Y, Miyake H, Domen K, Koyama T. Increased resting energy expenditure after endovascular coiling for subarachnoid hemorrhage. J Stroke Cerebrovasc Dis. 2016;25:813–8.
25. McKinney JS, Cheng JQ, Rybinnik I, Kostis JB, for the Myocardical Infarction Data Acquisition System Study Group. Comprehensive stroke centers may be associated with improved survival in hemorrhagic stroke. J Am Heart Assoc. 2015;4:e001448.
26. Minematsu K, Uehara T, Yasui N, Hata T, Ueda T, Okada Y, et al. Effects of stroke unit on patient outcome: a prospective multicenter study in Japan. Jpn J Stroke. 2007;29:59–64.
27. Lilford RJ, Brown CA, Nicholl J. Use of process measures to monitor the quality of clinical practice. BMJ. 2007;335:648–50.
28. Uehara T, Yasui N, Okada Y, Hasegawa Y, Nagatsuka K, Minematsu K. Which should be the essential components of stroke centers in Japan? A survey by questionnaires sent to the directors of facilities certified by the Japan Stroke Society. Cerebrovasc Dis. 2014;37:409–16.
29. Pitches DW, Mohammed AM, Lilford RJ. What is the empirical evidence that hospitals with higher-risk adjusted mortality rates provide poorer quality care? A systematic review of the literature. BMC Health Serv Res. 2007;7:91.
30. Shigematsu K, Nakano H, Watanabe Y. The eye response test alone is sufficient to predict stroke outcome–reintroduction of Japan Coma Scale: A cohort study. BMJ Open. 2013;3:e002736.

12

CDKN2BAS gene polymorphisms and the risk of intracranial aneurysm in the Chinese population

Yunchang Chen[1], Gancheng Li[1], Haiyan Fan[1], Shenquan Guo[1], Ran Li[1], Jian Yin[1], Xin Zhang[1], Xifeng Li[1], Xuying He[1] and Chuanzhi Duan[1,2*]

Abstract

Background: CDKN2BAS gene polymorphisms has been shown to correlation with intracranial aneurysm(IA) in the study of foreign people. The study, the author selected the Chinese people as the research object to explore whether CDKN2BAS gene polymorphisms associated with Chinese patients with IA.

Methods: We selected 200 patients(52.69 ± 11.50) with sporadic IA as experimental group, 200 participants(49.99 ± 13.00) over the same period to the hospital without cerebrovascular diseases as control group. Extraction of peripheral blood DNA, applying polymerase chain reaction(PCR)-ligase detection reaction (LDR) identified CDKN2BAS Single nucleotide polymorphism(SNP) locus genotype: rs6475606, rs1333040, rs10757272, rs3217992, rs974336, rs3217986, rs1063192. The differences in allelic and genotype frequencies between the patient and control groups were evaluated by the chi-square test or Fisher's exact tests.

Results: The genotype of rs1333040 and rs6475606 shown association with sporadic IA($X^2 = 8.545$, $P = 0.014$; $X^2 = 10.961$, $P = 0.004$; respectively);the C allele of rs6475606 showed reduction the occurrence of IA; the rs1333040 and rs6475606 associated with hemorrhage, the C allele of rs1333040 could lower the risk of hemorrhage, and rs6475606 will not, rs1333040 also associated with aneurysm size.

Conclusion: Our research shows that variant rs1333040 and rs6475606 of CDKN2BAS related to the Chinese han population of sporadic IAs occurs. This study confirms the association between CDKN2BAS and IAs.

Keywords: CDKN2BAS gene, Polymorphisms, Intracranial aneurysms

Background

IA is a complex disease affecting human health, it is the primary cause of subarachnoid hemorrhage. According to statistics, in the event of rupture of IA, patients' mortality and morbidity is 30 and 25%, respectively. It is generally accepted that IA influenced both by genetic and environmental risk factors. Environmental factors including smoking, drinking, hypertension, diabetes and so on. Genetic factors, there are a number of human genes associated with the occurrence and development of IA [1, 2, 22]. Genome-wide association study(GWAS) as a kind of method research on diseases, which applied to study of IA has found associated with these chromosomes:4q(EDNRA),5q31.3,6q24.2,8q12.1(SOX17), 9p21.3 (CDKN2A/CDKN2B/CDKN2BAS),10q24.32(CNNM2), 12q22,13q13.1(KL/STARD13), 18q11.2(RBBP8), 20p2.1 [3, 7, 9, 10, 17, 20, 21].

CDKN2BAS located in chromosome 9p21, a 3.8 kb long non-coding RNA(lncRNA) expressed in the opposite direction from INK4A-ARF-INK4B gene cluster, it is associated with a variety of human diseases, such as prostate cancer, stomach cancer, pancreatic cancer, leukemia, glioma, colorectal cancer, lung cancer, diabetes and aneurysm [4, 5, 14, 16]. There has been a lot of scholar studies supported CDKN2BAS gene multiple SNPs loci associated with IA. Hashikata confirmed

* Correspondence: doctor_duanZJ@163.com
[1]Department of Neurosurgery, The National Key Clinic Specialty, The Neurosurgery Institute of Guangdong Province, Guangdong Provincial Key Laboratory on Brain Function Repair and Regeneration, Zhujiang Hospital, Southern Medical University, Guangzhou 510282, China
[2]Department of Neurosurgery, Southern Medical University, Zhujiang Hospital, 253# industry road, Guangzhou, Guangdong 510282, China

rs1333040 associated with familial and sporadic IA in Japanese [8]. Foroud and his colleagues study United States population also confirmed CDKN2BAS SNP loci could lead to susceptibility of IA on the basis of predecessors' research results, and believe rs6475606 have significant effect on IA [6]; another research on Japanese found that rs10757272 is a new susceptibility locus of IA, and confirmed rs10757278 associated with IA [13]; other chromosome gene polymorphism loci showed association with intracranial aneurysm, such as rs6841581(4q), rs12411886(10q), rs6538595(12q), rs9315204(13q), but the CDKN2BAS SNP loci were replicated successfully the most time in later studies [12, 21]. Due to the limitation of the study sample size, these studies credibility is not so high, the relationship between CDKN2BAS SNP loci and IA needs more study.

Whether CDKN2BAS SNP loci associated with China IAs patients has not been reported. Taking into account the same gene mutation rates is differ greatly in different populations and the genetic heterogeneity between races of people, so we use the database to find the minor allele frequency(MAF ≥ 0.05) of CDKN2BAS SNP loci at an $r^2 > 0.8$ threshold in Chinese population, including rs3217992, rs974336, rs3217986, rs1063192, explore CDKN2BAS SNP effect on IAs, hope to provide new strategies for prevention and treatment of IAs.

Methods

The research object

This study was supported by Zhujiang Hospital of Southern Medical University ethics com- mittee, all the participants reported themselves to be of Han residents, have signed informed consent. Zhujiang Hospital is located in developed areas of China—Guangzhou, where the people from other provinces of China accounts for a large part of city population, and popul- ation flow is also very frequent, so the subjects of this study are representative. All particip- ants exclude genetic history, family history and history of malignancy, controlling the age between 18 and 80 years.

Within 14 months, this study recruited 200 patients with sporadic IAs, the median age was 52.69 ± 11.50 years. Patients with IAs diagnosed by computed tomography angiography(CTA), magnetic resonance angiography(MRA) or digital subtraction angiography(DSA) has at least one aneurysm. For the diagnosis of hemorrhage caused by aneurysms, especially ruptured IAs, not only combined with clinical symptoms, but also confirmed by the DSA results eventually. All cases with confirmed IAs based on DSA were retrospectively reviewed by 2 independent doctors, a neuroradiologist and a neurosurgeon, they are all experienced in the diagnosis of aneurysms. All patients in the study underwent either craniotomy or interventional therapy to confirm the correct diagnosis of IAs again.

During the same period, 200 blood donors form a control group for the study, with a median age of 49.99 ± 13.00. Considering the prevalence of IAs vary between 0.2 and 9% of the population, this study does not recruit volunteers from the outside, control participants were patients(such as cerebral hemorrhage, cerebral trauma, epilepsy) from the Department of Neurosurgery of Zhujiang Hospital, as most of them have imaging data(computed tomography(CT), magnetic resonance imaging(MRI), MRA) and clinical information excluded the presence of aneurysms. Controls were eliminate diseases not only including polycystic kidney disease, Malaysia's syndrome, systemic lupus erythematosus (SLE), etc., but also severity of neurological diseases.

The subjects fully considered the balance and comparable of the baseline data during collection process, genomic DNA was extracted from Peripheral whole blood use kit, using agarose gel electrophoresis to detect the DNA integrity, ensure the follow-up test smoothly.

Genotyping and SNP selection of CDKN2BAS

Through foreign research literatures found the highest positive sites correlation with IAs, they are rs1333040, rs6475606, rs10757272; and using genetic database Hapmap (http://hapmap.org), Haploview (http://www.broad.mit.edu/mpg/haploview) found the tagSNP loci of CDKN2BAS in Chinese population, including rs3217992, rs974336, rs3217986, rs1063192; so the seven sites as this research objects, SNP genotyping by PCR-LDR in Shanghai Biowing Applied Biotechnology Co., Ltd. The seven SNPs primer sequences and PCR length are given in Table 1; these SNPs probe sequences and LDR length are read in Table 2. PCR and LDR manipulated as previous describe [18], Firstly, PCR amplification of SNP sites in 20ul master mix, containing 2ul 1 × buffer, 0.6ul Mg++, 2ul dNTPs, 0.2ul Taq polymerase, 4ul 1 × Q-solution, 0.4ul primer mix and 9.8ul ddH^2O, after thoroughly incorporated, take 19ul partial shipments in PCR reaction tube and add 1ul genomic DNA of samples, set the following program on Gene Amp PCR system (model 9600, Perkin Elmer): denaturing at 95 °C for 15 min; then denaturing at 94 °C for 30 s, annealing at 56 °C for 1 min, extension at 72 °C for 1 min, repeat 35 cycles; also need to extend 7 min under 72 °C temperature. Secondly, LDR performed to further amplification in 10ul volume of Multiplex LDR mixture, before operation LDR add the same as volume ddH^2O to PCR amplification product, the LDR mixture containing resultant PCR product of 1ul, 1ul probe mix, 0.05ul Taq DNA ligase, and 6.95ul ddH^2O, after thoroughly incorporated, take 9ul partial shipments in PCR reaction tube and add 1ul PCR amplification product, set LDR conditions: initial denaturing at 95 °C for 2 min, followed by

Table 1 Primer sequences and PCR length

Primer name	sequence(5-3) up	low	PCR length
rs1333040	TAATGGGATGGAGTGCAGGG	AACCTCCATGAGAACTGGCT	193
rs3217986	CTCCACCAGATAGCAGAGGG	CCACCACCTCATCCTGTGTA	176
rs10757272	CCTGAGGAGAAGAGAAGGGC	TGGGGCACATGATTCCAAAA	180
rs6475606	AAAGGAAGAACATGGCACCC	TTGTAGAACACAACAACCCC	87
rs1063192	GTGTAATATAGTACTGTGGG	CTTGTGGAATCTTTCCTAAT	85
rs974336	CAGACATCAGAGACCTGAAC	GCAGGTGGAGCCATTTAAAG	78
rs3217992	GGAATTAATTTTTACATGGC	TGGGTATCAATTACCACCTG	67

35 cycles of denaturing at 94 °C for 30 s, and annealing at 50 °C for 2 min, mix 1ul of LDR product with 0.6ul ROX(ABI.GS-500), after denaturing at 95 °C for 2 min, in the ice cold snap, following capillary electrophoresis, meanwhile applying Genemapper(ABI, Inc.) for data analysis and genotyping.

Statistical analysis

Hardy-Weinberg equilibrium tested by chi-square in control, allelic and genotype frequencies are evaluated by chi-square test or Fisher's exact tests, all data analysis using SPSS 20.0, considering statistical differences when *P* value is less than 0.05.

Results

Clinical background of patients

The clinical information of the study participants was summarized in Table 3. Female patients with IAs accounted for 61.5%, is 1.60 times of male patients, and consistent with other related reports [18, 23]. The baseline data balanced between the experimental group and the control group, including gender, smoking, drinking, hypertension and diabetes. Patients with IAs also make specific statistic about aneurysm number and position. There were 90 patients with IAs located in the posterior communicating artery and internal carotid artery, 41 patients in the anterior cerebral artery and 32 patients in posterior cerebral artery. The numbers of patients with

Table 2 Probe sequences and LDR length

Probename	sequence(5-3)	LDR length
rs1333040_modify	P-CATTCTTACCTCTGACCCTCTTTTTTTTTTTTTTTTTT-FAM	
rs1333040_C	TTTTTTTTTTTTTTTTCTTCCTCTCTGTCCCAGCGGTAG	77
rs1333040_T	TTTTTTTTTTTTTTTTTTCTTCCTCTCTGTCCCAGCGGTAA	79
rs3217986_modify	P-CCTCTCTTACCCCTCTGCTATTTTTTTTTTTTTTTTTTTTT-FAM	
rs3217986_A	TTTTTTTTTTTTTTTTTTAGCATCTGTCGTCGCTTGCACAT	82
rs3217986_C	TTTTTTTTTTTTTTTTTTTTAGCATCTGTCGTCGCTTGCACAG	84
rs10757272_modify	P-CTTCTTACGACCTTTCATAATTTTTTTTTTTTTTTTTTTTTTTT-FAM	
rs10757272_C	TTTTTTTTTTTTTTTTTTTTATAATAAAACATTGCAACATTCG	87
rs10757272_T	TTTTTTTTTTTTTTTTTTTTTTATAATAAAACATTGCAACATTCA	89
rs6475606_modify	P-CTTTCACTGAGTGTCCATTATTTTTTTTTTTTTTTTTTTTTTTTTTT-FAM	
rs6475606_C	TTTTTTTTTTTTTTTTTTTTTTCCAAAAATGATGATGATAGCCAG	92
rs6475606_T	TTTTTTTTTTTTTTTTTTTTTTTTCCAAAAATGATGATGATAGCCAA	94
rs1063192_modify	P-GTTGTCATTAGGAAAGATTCTTTTTTTTTTTTTTTTTTTTTTTTTTTTTT-FAM	
rs1063192_C	TTTTTTTTTTTTTTTTTTTTTTTTTCTTTAGTTTCCCTTAATATCAG	97
rs1063192_T	TTTTTTTTTTTTTTTTTTTTTTTTTTTCTTTAGTTTCCCTTAATATCAA	99
rs974336_modify	P-AAAGTTTTCACCCAGTGCAGTTTTTTTTTTTTTTTTTTTTTTTTTTTTTTTTT-FAM	
rs974336_A	TTTTTTTTTTTTTTTTTTTTTTTTTTCATTTAAAGAAACACCTAATTGT	102
rs974336_G	TTTTTTTTTTTTTTTTTTTTTTTTTTTTCATTTAAAGAAACACCTAATTGC	104
rs3217992_modify	P-AATACAACCAGGTGGTAATTTTTTTTTTTTTTTTTTTTTTTTTTTTTTTTTTTTTTTTTT-FAM	
rs3217992_A	TTTTTTTTTTTTTTTTTTTTTTTTTTTTTGGCATTGATAAGTTACTATTTT	107
rs3217992_G	TTTTTTTTTTTTTTTTTTTTTTTTTTTTTTTGGCATTGATAAGTTACTATTTC	109

Table 3 Characteristics of patients with IAs vs. controls

	Aneurysms group	Controls group	X^2 value	*P* value
Number	200	200		
Male	77(38.5)	78(39.0)		
Female	123(61.5)	122(61.0)	0.011	0.918
Age	52.69 ± 11.50	49.99 ± 13.00	1.639	0.201
Smoking	43(21.5)	40(20.0)		
Non-smoking	157(78.5)	160(80.0)	0.137	0.711
Drinking	44(22.0)	42(21.0)		
Non-drinker	156(78.0)	158(79.0)	0.059	0.808
Hypertension	59(29.5)	54(27.0)		
Non-hypertension	141(70.5)	146(73.0)	0.308	0.579
Diabetes	24(12.0)	22(11.0)		
Non-diabetes	176(88.0)	178(89.0)	0.098	0.754
Site of aneurysm(%)				
ACA	41(20.5)			
PCA	32(16.0)			
ACoA	16(8.0)			
ICA,PCoA	90(45.0)			
MCA	10(5.0)			
other	11(5.5)			
Number of aneurysm(319)				
One	130(65.0)			
Two	35(17.5)			
Three	21(10.5)			
> three	14(7.0)			

ACA anterior cerebral artery, *ACoA* anterior communicating artery, *ICA* internal carotid artery, *MCA* middle cerebral artery, *PCA* posterior cerebral artery, *PCoA* posterior communicating artery

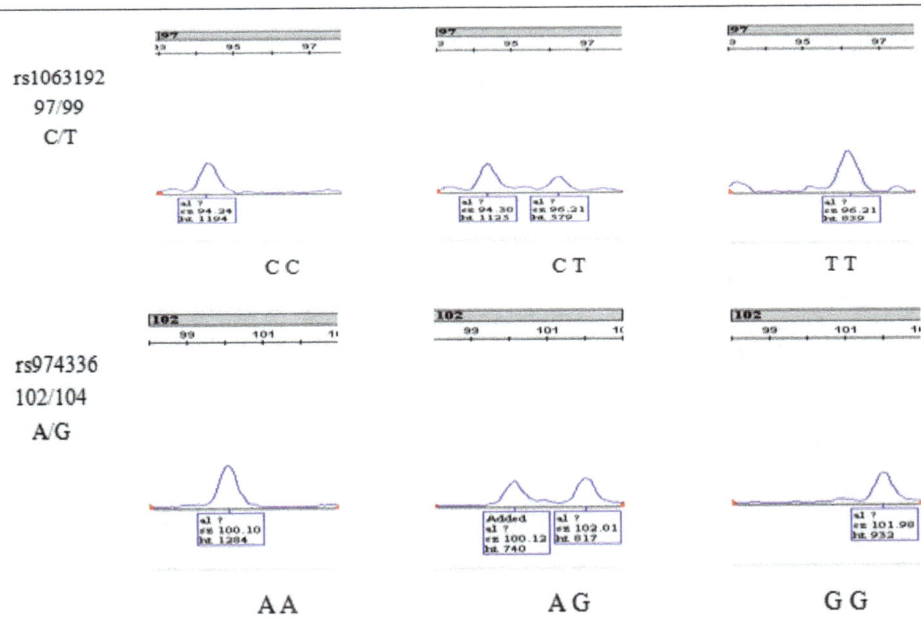

Fig. 1 Two loci of the gene-picture

one aneurysm, two aneurysms, three aneurysms, more than 3 aneurysms are 130, 35, 21, 14 respectively.

Allelic association study with SNPs of CDKN2BAS

We randomly selected two loci of the Genemapper as shown in Fig. 1. The genotype and allele frequency of cases and controls was presented in Table 4. The control group completely accorded with Hardy-Weinberg equilibrium and objects included in the study could represent the crowd finely. The difference in seven sites of genotype and allele frequency was compared with chi-square or Fisher's exact tests. The genotype frequency of rs6475606 show significant difference between cases and controls($X^2 = 10.961$, $P = 0.004$), There also existed difference among groups when compared frequency of TT with CC and CT genotypes combined ($X^2 = 9.008$, OR 1.831 [95% confidence interval 1.232—2.723], $P = 0.003$), the C allele showed reduction the risk of IAs($X^2 = 4.784$, OR 0.710 [95% confidence interval 0.522—0.966], $P = 0.029$). The distribution of the variants rs1333040 was significantly different in genotype frequency among cases and controls($X^2 = 8.545$, $P = 0.014$), and compared frequency of TT with CC and CT genotypes combined, the results were significant($X^2 = 7.295$, OR 1.722 [95% confidence interval 1.159—2.558], $P = 0.007$).

Genotype is related to clinical manifestation

The study aimed to assess the correlation between CDKN2BAS SNP genotypes and clinical presentation(such as hemorrhage, epilepsy, aneurysm location and size) of

Table 4 genotype and allele frequencies of patients with IAs vs. controls

		Aneurysms	Controls	X^2 value	*P* value	OR(95%CI)
rs1333040	CC	19(9.5)	18(9)	8.545	0.014	
	CT	65(32.5)	92(46)			
	TT	116(58)	90(45)			
	CC + CT	84(42)	111(55.5)	7.295	0.007	1.722(1.159—2.558)
C allele		103/297(25.75)	128/272(32)	3.804	0.051	0.737(0.542—1.002)
rs3217986	AA	166(83)	157(78.5)	1.597	0.445	
	AC	32(16)	39(19.5)			
	CC	2(1)	4(2)			
	AC + CC	34(17)	43(21.5)	1.303	0.254	0.748(0.454—1.233)
rs10757272	CC	21(10.5)	22(11)	0.497	0.780	
	CT	97(48.5)	90(45)			
	TT	82(41)	88(44)			
	CC + CT	112(56)	111(55.5)	0.368	0.544	1.131(0.760—1.681)
rs6475606	CC	19(9.5)	17(8.5)	10.961	0.004	
	CT	63(31.5)	95(47.5)			
	TT	118(59)	88(44)			
	CC + CT	82(41)	112(56)	9.008	0.003	1.831(1.232—2.723)
C allele		101/299(25.25)	129/271(32.25)	4.784	0.029	0.710(0.522—0.966)
rs1063192	CC	6(3)	5(2.5)	0.783	0.676	
	CT	56(28)	49(24.5)			
	TT	138(69)	146(73)			
	CC + CT	62(31)	54(27)	0.777	0.378	1.215(0.788—1.872)
rs974336	AA	9(4.5)	3(1.5)	3.983	0.137	
	AG	63(31.5)	74(37)			
	GG	128(64)	123(61.5)			
	AA + AG	72(36)	77(38.5)	0.267	0.605	0.899(0.599—1.348)
rs3217992	AA	61(30.5)	60(30)	1.021	0.600	
	AG	101(50.5)	94(47)			
	GG	38(19)	46(23)			
	AG + GG	139(69.5)	140(70)	0.012	0.913	0.977(0.637—1.496)

OR odds ratio, *CI* confidence intervals, *P* value was considered significant at a level of <0.05

aneurysms(Table 5). Statistical analysis indicated that both of rs1333040 and rs6475606 were associated with hemorrhage. The C allele of rs1333040 reduced the incidence of hemorrhage. The C allele of rs6475606 was over-represented in controls which controversial with it was the risk of hemorrhage($X^2 = 9.626$, OR 2.002 [95% confidence interval 1.286—3.119], $P = 0.002$); and rs13330 40 also related to aneurysm size($P < 0.000$), the C allele was the risk factor of IAs with size < 3 cm($X^2 = 7.358$, OR 2.020 [95% confidence interval 1.207—3.380], $P = 0.007$). The study did not find that CDKN2BAS SNP genotypes was associated with epilepsy and aneurysm location.

Discussion

In this study, we aim to explore CDKN2BAS genetic relationship with Chinese han nationality of IAs. We provided evidence that the variants rs1333040 and rs6475606 were associated with IAs, in agreement with the results of Hashikata et al. and Foroud et al., respectively. Hashikata et al. based on previous results of Genome-wide association studies(GWAS) confirmed rs1333040 association with familial and sporadic IAs in Japanese patients, their study included 419 sporadic IA cases and 408 control subjects; Foroud et al. utilized the similar approach to investigate the role of rs6475606 in 1095 IA cases and 1286 controls, as the size of the sample, our results with theirs differ markedly.

Rs3217992, rs974336, rs3217986, rs1063192 are the highest mutation rate locus of CDKN2BAS gene in Chinese population. We can learn from the Table 4 that the four sites genotype frequency and allele frequency were close in the experimental group and the control group. Statistical results show that these loci loss correlation with sporadic IAs of China(all P values > 0.05), rs6475606, rs1333040 and rs10757272 are the highest positive sites correlation with IAs in overseas study,reflect the Japan and the United States population, rs1333040 and rs6475606 were also replicated, but no association of the variant rs10757272 with sporadic IAs was found in our study, the conflicting results mainly root in genetic heterogeneity in different ethnic populations, additionally, the presence of genetic heterogeneity may be relevant in a bias caused by variation in the prevalence of a positive family history between populations, because familial IAs have a higher risk than sporadic IAs, negative results for this SNP do not exclude CDKN2BAS SNP plays an important role in aneurysms. The other four loci selected in this study which is the highest mutation rates in Chinese population were unrelated to aneurysms, among previous studies, a research thinks disease-causing mutations may be located in MAF < 0.05, and influence the formation of IAs. We also detected statistically significant correlations between CDKN2BAS SNPs and hemorrhage and aneurysm size, rs1333040_C did not work in aneurysm formation, but it could reduce the occurrence of hemorrhage and it was the risk factor of IAs with size < 3 cm; the rs6475606_C could reduce the occurrence of IAs, but the impact of it on hemorrhage and size was not clear, the reason may be related to the research errors.

Table 5 Analysis of genotype and clinical presentation

		Hemorrhage (136 patients)	No Hemorrhage (64 patients)	X^2 value	P value	OR(95%CI)
rs1333040	CC	14(10.29)	5(7.80)			
	CT	31(22.79)	34(53.13)	18.421	0.000*	
	TT	91(66.92)	25(39.07)			
C allele		59/272(21.69)	44/128(34.38)	4.182	0.041	0.631(0.405—0.983)
rs6475606	CC	13(9.56)	6(9.38)			
	CT	26(19.12)	37(57.81)	31.628	0.000*	
	TT	97 (71.32)	21(32.81)			
C allele		52/272(22.43)	49/128(31.25)	9.626	0.002	2.002(1.286—3.119)
		Size(≥3 cm) (72 patients)	Size(<3 cm) (128 patients)	X^2 value	P value	
rs1333040	CC	8(11.11)	11(8.59)			
	CT	6 (8.33)	57(44.53)	28.355	0.000*	
	TT	58(80.56)	60(46.88)			
C allele		22/144(15.28)	79/256(30.86)	7.358	0.007	2.020(1.207—3.380)
rs6475606	CC	7(9.72)	12(9.37)			
	CT	23(31.94)	40(31.25)	0.021	0.989	
	TT	42(58.33)	76(59.38)			

*$P < 0.000$

The sequence of CDKN2BAS gene is so long that it will be very difficult to find the exact loci associated with IA. Rs6475604, rs1333040, rs10757272 associated with IA come from GWAS mostly, these loci are not for more research, and lack of functional studies. IA is a complex genetic disease, the interaction between genes and genes as racial differences will affect the results of our study. CDKN2BAS belongs to long noncoding RNA(lncRNA) and affects the surrounding gene expression indirectly play a role in the disease, Bai Y research results show that CDKN2BAS can regulate the expression of CARD8 level, which affects the progress of atherosclerosis, compare the RNA in aneurysm tissue and normal cerebrovascular, hundreds of lncRNA exists differences, we can't help but question: would CDKN2BAS cause IA formation? Or CDKN2BAS associated with IA could be caused by other lncRNA [2, 15, 19].

The current generally accepted IA is the result of the dual role of genetic and environmental factors, screening finds a large number of genes associated with IA, but these genes effect on IA is too low, thus known that the influence of environmental factors on the disease may be greater, CDKN2BAS gene polymorphism correlated with IA in other population, but has nothing to do with the Chinese people, there is a hypothesis: the environment makes IA more susceptible to CDKN2BAS in other population, although rs3217992, rs974336, rs3217986 and rs1063192 are the highest mutation rate loci of CDKN2BAS gene in Chinese population, influenced by environmental factors, they without associated with IA [11].

In addition to the above mentioned several assumptions, our study associated with the degree and distribution of linkage disequilibrium [1]. Research work in susceptibility genes of IA did not make substantive progress, scholars have been staying at the screening level, but many of genes repeatability is poor, the author considers not all IA are related to gene mutation, genetic, environmental and perhaps many other factors involved in the IA progress, it needs us to further research.

Conclusions

Our study showed that CDKN2BAS polymorphism might be associated with intracranial aneurysms in Chinese population. Additional studies are needed to confirm our finding.

Abbreviations

ACA: Anterior cerebral artery; ACoA: Anterior communicating artery; CI: Confidence intervals; CTA: Computed tomography angiography; DSA: Digital subtraction angiography; GWAS: Genome-wide association study; IA: Intracranial aneurysm; ICA: Internal carotid artery; LDR: Ligase detection reaction; lncRNA: long noncoding RNA; MAF: Minor allele frequency; MCA: Middle cerebral artery; MRA: Magnetic resonance angiography; MRI: Magnetic resonance imaging; OR: Odds ratio; PCA: Posterior cerebral artery; PCoA: Posterior communicating artery; PCR: Polymerase chain reaction; SNP: Single nucleotide polymorphism

Acknowledgments

We thank the DNA donors and the supporting medical staff for making this study possible.

Funding

The authors report no conflict of interest concerning the materials or methods used in this study or the findings specified in this paper. This study was supported by the National Natural Science Foundation of China (Grants No.81271315), National Key Research Development Program (Grants No.2016YFC1300804,2016YFC1300800), Specialized Research Fund for the Doctoral Program of Higher Education (Grants No.20124433110014). The funders had no role in study design, data collection and analysis, decision to publish, or preparation of the manuscript.

Authors' contributions

Author contributions to the study and manuscript preparation include the following. Conception and design: YCC. Acquisition of data: YCC, SQG. Drafting the article: YCC, XZ, HYF. Critically revising the article: all authors. Reviewed submitted version of manuscript: all authors. Statistical analysis: YCC, CZD. Study supervision: CZD, YCC. Approved the final version of the manuscript on behalf of all authors.

Competing interests

The authors declare that they have no competing interests.

References

1. Adeyemo A, Rotimi C. Genetic variants associated with complex human diseases show wide variation across multiple populations. Public Health Genomics. 2010;13(2):72–9. doi:10.1159/000218711.
2. Bai Y, Nie S, Jiang G, Zhou Y, Zhou M, Zhao Y, et al. Regulation of CARD8 expression by ANRIL and association of CARD8 single nucleotide polymorphism rs2043211 (p.C10X) with ischemic stroke. Stroke. 2014;45(2): 383–8. doi:10.1161/STROKEAHA.113.003393.
3. Bilguvar K, Yasuno K, Niemelä M, Ruigrok YM, von Und Zu Fraunberg M, van Duijn CM, et al. Susceptibility loci for intracranial aneurysm in European and Japanese populations. Nat Genet. 2008;40(12):1472–7. doi:10.1038/ng.240.
4. Bochenek G, Hasler R, El Mokhtari NE, Konig IR, Loos BG, Jepsen S, et al. The large non-coding RNA ANRIL, which is associated with atherosclerosis, periodontitis and several forms of cancer, regulates ADIPOR1, VAMP3 and C11ORF10. Hum Mol Genet. 2013;22(22):4516–27. doi:10.1093/hmg/ddt299.
5. Broadbent HM, Peden JF, Lorkowski S. Susceptibility to coronary artery disease and diabetes is encoded by distinct, tightly linked SNPs in the ANRI locus on chromosome 9p. Hum Mol Genet. 2008;17(6):806–14.
6. Foroud T, Koller DL, Lai D, Sauerbeck L, Anderson C, Ko N, et al. Genome-wide association study of intracranial aneurysms confirms role of Anril and SOX17 in disease risk. Stroke. 2012;43(11):2846–52. doi:10.1161/STROKEAHA.112.656397.
7. Foroud T, Lai D, Koller D, Van't Hof F, Kurki MI, Anderson CS, et al. Genome-wide association study of intracranial aneurysm identifies a new association on chromosome 7. Stroke. 2014;45(11):3194–9. doi:10.1161/STROKEAHA.114.006096.
8. Hashikata H, Liu W, Inoue K, Mineharu Y, Yamada S, Nanayakkara S, et al. Confirmation of an Association of Single-Nucleotide Polymorphism rs1333040 on 9p21 with familial and sporadic intracranial aneurysms in Japanese patients. Stroke. 2010;41(6):1138–44. doi:10.1161/STROKEAHA.109.576694.
9. Helgadottir A, Thorleifsson G, Magnusson KP, Grétarsdottir S, Steinthorsdottir V, Manolescu A, et al. The same sequence variant on 9p21 associates with myocardial infarction, abdominal aortic aneurysm and intracranial aneurysm. Nat Genet. 2008;40(2):217–24.
10. Holdt LM, Teupser D. Recent studies of the human chromosome 9p21 locus, which is associated with atherosclerosis in human populations. Arterioscler Thromb Vasc Biol. 2012;32(2):196–206. doi:10.1161/ATVBAHA.111.232678.

11. Hunter DJ. Gene–environment interactions in human diseases. Nat Rev Genet. 2005;6(2):287–98.
12. Koichi Akiyama ANHN, Atsushi Tajima BKKY. Genome-wide association study to identify genetic variants present in Japanese patients harboring intracranial aneurysms. J Hum Genet. 2010;55(10):656–61. doi:10.1038/jhg.2010.82.
13. Low SK, Takahashi A, Cha PC, Zembutsu H, Kamatani N, Kubo M, et al. Genome-wide association study for intracranial aneurysm in the Japanese population identifies three candidate susceptible loci and a functional genetic variant at EDNRA. Hum Mol Genet. 2012;21(9):2102–10. doi:10.1093/hmg/dds020.
14. Nie FQ, Sun M, Yang JS, Xie M, Xu TP, Xia R, et al. Long noncoding RNA ANRIL promotes non-small cell lung cancer cell proliferation and inhibits apoptosis by silencing KLF2 and P21 expression. Mol Cancer Ther. 2015; 14(1):268–77. doi:10.1158/1535-7163.MCT-14-0492.
15. Pan W, Liu L, Wei J, Ge Y, Zhang J, Chen H, et al. A functional lncRNA HOTAIR genetic variant contributes to gastric cancer susceptibility. Mol Carcinog. 2016;55(1):90–6. doi:10.1002/mc.22261.
16. Pasmant E, Sabbagh A, Vidaud M, Bieche I. ANRIL, a long, noncoding RNA, is an unexpected major hotspot in GWAS. FASEB J. 2011;25(2):444–8. doi:10.1096/fj.10-172452.
17. Ruigrok YM, Rinkel GJ. From GWAS to the clinic: risk factors for intracranial aneurysms. Genome Med. 2010;2(9):61. doi:10.1186/gm182.
18. Suo M, Lin Y, Yu H, Song W, Sun K, Song Y, et al. Association of Kallikrein gene polymorphisms with sporadic intracranial aneurysms in the Chinese population. J Neurosurg. 2014;120(6):1397–401. doi:10.3171/2013.11.JNS131036.
19. Wu SC, Kallin EM, Zhang Y. Role of H3K27 methylation in the regulation of lncRNA expression. Cell Res. 2010;20(10):1109–16. doi:10.1038/cr.2010.114.
20. Yasuno K, Bakircioglu M, Low SK, Bilguvar K, Gaal E, Ruigrok YM, et al. Common variant near the endothelin receptor type a (EDNRA) gene is associated with intracranial aneurysm risk. Proc Natl Acad Sci. 2011;108(49): 19707–12. doi:10.1073/pnas.1117137108.
21. Yasuno K, Bilguvar K, Bijlenga P, Low S, Krischek B, Auburger G, et al. Genome-wide association study of intracranial aneurysm identifies three new risk loci. Nat Genet. 2010;42(5):420–5. doi:10.1038/ng.563.
22. Ynte M, Ruigrok GJER. Genetics of intracranial aneurysms. Lancet Neurol. 2005;4(1):179–87.
23. Zhu Y, Li W, Ge M, Xu S, Zhao G, Wang H, et al. Polymorphism rs42524 of COL1A2 and sporadic intracranial aneurysms in the Chinese population. J Neurosurg. 2008;109(6):1060–4. doi:10.3171/JNS.2008.109.12.1060.

13

Paroxysmal freezing of gait in a patient with mesial frontal transient ischemic attacks

Hee Won Hwang, Seung Ha Lee, Chul Hyoung Lyoo and Myung Sik Lee*

Abstract

Background: Rare patients have been reported who developed a mixture of gait disturbances following a focal lesion in the frontal lobe. Thus, the exact location of frontal lesion responsible for a specific gait disturbance is not well defined.

Case presentation: We describe a 47-year-old man who experienced two episodes of paroxysmal freezing of gait of the right leg. During the attacks, he had no motor weakness, sensory change, or disequilibrium. He had past history of panic attacks. Recently, he had been under severe emotional stress. T2 and diffusion brain magnetic resonance imaging scans were normal. So far, the most likely clinical diagnosis might be functional freezing of gait. However, magnetic resonance angiography showed atherosclerosis in the proximal left anterior cerebral artery. Perfusion scans showed a delayed mean transit time in the left mesial frontal lobe. He developed two more attacks during the four months of follow up.

Conclusions: The presented case illustrates that the mesial frontal lobe may be important in the pathophysiology of freezing of gait. We speculate that the supplementary motor area may generate a neuronal command for the initiation of locomotion that in our case may have been inhibited by a transient ischemia.

Keywords: Mesial frontal lobe, Transient ischemic attack, Freezingof gait, Locomotor block

Background

Freezing of gait (FOG) is defined as episodic brief absence or marked reduction of forward progression of the feet despite the intention to walk [1]. Patients with frontal gait disorder may have FOG. However, they frequently have widespread cerebrovascular lesions and present various combinations of additional gait disturbances including start and turn hesitation, short steps, shuffling, and postural instability. Thus, in patients with frontal gait disorder, exact location of brain lesion responsible for FOG is difficult to decipher [2].

Rare patients have been reported who developed FOG following a focal lesion involving the dorsal midbrain tegmentum, suggestive of important role of mesencephalic locomotor region in the locomotor initiation [3–5]. However, frontal lobe, especially the supplementary motor area, plays also a prominent role in the initiation and control of human locomotion [1]. Here, we describe a patient who developed paroxysmal FOG of the right leg associated with left mesial frontal transient ischemic attacks (TIAs).

Case presentation

A 47-year-old man visited the emergency room due to two incidents of transient locomotor blocks. He had a past history of panic attacks. Recently, he had been under severe emotional stress. When he attempted to walk at the pedestrian crossing on the green light, his right foot was glued to the ground. He sat down and massaged his right leg with both hands. Several seconds later, he could walk normally again. Two hours later, when he attempted to run while walking, his right foot was again stuck to the ground for several seconds. During the attacks, there were no knee trembling of the frozen leg. He denied any motor weakness, sensory change, or dyskinesia of the arms or legs. On

* Correspondence: mslee@yuhs.ac
Department of Neurology, Gangnam Severance Hospital, Yonsei University College of Medicine, Eonjuro 211, Gangnam-gu, Seoul, South Korea

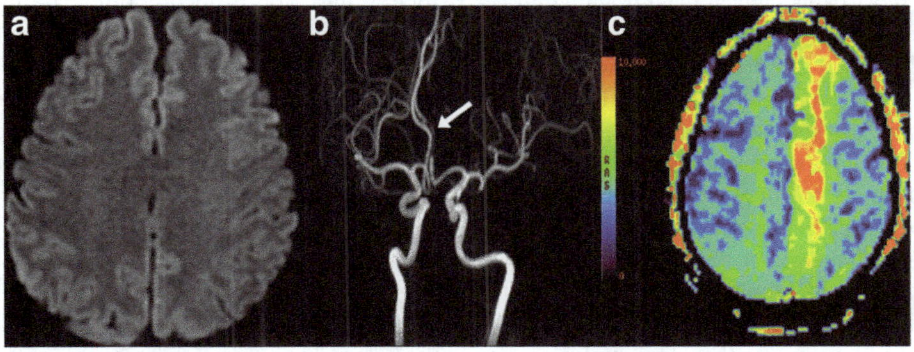

Fig. 1 **a** Diffusion axial brain MRI scan shows no abnormalities. **b** Cerebral MR angiography shows atherosclerotic narrowing in the left anterior cerebral artery (*arrow*). **c** Perfusion axial brain MRI scan shows delayed mean transit time in the left mesial frontal lobe

neurological examination, he had no motor, sensory, or cerebellar dysfunctions. T2 and diffusion brain magnetic resonance imaging (MRI) scans were normal (Fig. 1a). However, magnetic resonance (MR) angiography showed atherosclerosis in the proximal left anterior cerebral artery (Fig. 1b). Perfusion scans showed a delayed mean transit time in the left mesial frontal lobe, including the supplementary motor area and cingulate cortex (Fig. 1c). Routine laboratory tests were all normal, including CBC, liver function tests, renal function tests, urine analysis, electrocardiography, and chest x-ray studies. There was no hyperlipidemia. Screening tests for autoimmune disease (e.g. ANA, Ani-dsDNA antibodies, P-ANCA, C-ANCA, Anti-Cardiolipin antibodies Ig M andIg G) were all negative. Transthoracic echocardiography study showed no abnormalities. Interictal electroencephalography (EEG) studies revealed no abnormalities. During four months of follow up period, he had been treated with low dose aspirin, but he developed two more attacks when he attempted walking.

Conclusion and discussion

The presented case developed paroxysmal locomotor blocks. There were no motor weakness, sensory changes, or cerebellar ataxia. The attacks were induced by sudden movements of the leg as in paroxysmal kinesigenic dyskinesia, but there was no dyskinesia. Unlike the typical FOG observed in patients with degenerative parkinsonism, the present patient developed FOG in open spaces and there was no hastening or alternating knee trembling-like leg movements. Besides, he did not have any parkinsonian features [1]. T2 and diffusion weighted brain MRI studies showed no lesions (Fig. 1a). He had past history of panic attacks and recently had been under severe emotional

Table 1 Reported patients with gait disturbances or postural instabilities following a lesion confined to the frontal lobe

Reference	Lesion sites	Gait disturbances & postural instabilities	Other neurologic deficits	Characters of lesion
Sakakibara et al. [14]	bilateral medial frontal	shuffling gait	tinnitus, deafness, hallucination, versive seizure, disorientation, inattention	MRI: neurosarcoidosis
Chung et al. [19]	Lt. medial frontal	gait initiation disturbance	severe bilateral lower extremity bradykinesia	MRI: ischemic stroke
Nadeau et al. [20]	Bilateral parasaggital white matter	gait ignition difficulty	bilateral paratonia, retropulsion in sitting position	MRI: Primary CNS lymphoma
Ducruet et al. [15]	Rt. medial frontal	ataxic gait	Lt. hemiparesis	CT: hemorrhage
Wada et al. [16]	Rt. SMA	astasia		MRI: infarction
Robbins et al. [18]	Rt. Parasagittal frontal	freezing of gait	speech impairment, axial bradykinesia, balance disturbance	MRI: cortical vein thrombosis
Frassanito et al. [17]	Rt. basal frontal	gait instability		MRI: tumor excision
Della et al. [21]	Bilateral frontal	gait apraxia	spastic paraplegia, disequilibrium, loss of postural reflexes	MRI: infarction
Present case	Lt. mesial frontal	freezing of gait of the right leg		MRI: ischemia

CT computerized tomography, *MRI* magnetic resonance imaging, *SMA* supplementary motor area

stress. So far, the most likely clinical diagnosis might be a functional FOG [6].

However, cerebral MR angiography showed atherosclerosis in the left anterior cerebral artery (Fig. 1b) and perfusion MR scans showed ischemia in the left mesial frontal lobe (Fig. 1c). The presented case did not develop sensory dysfunctions or motor weakness during the attacks, probably because the lesion was remote from the sensory pathways and unilateral proximal limb receives motor inputs from the bilateral supplementary motor areas [7]. Indeed, about 20% of patients with anterior cerebral infarctions develop neither leg weakness nor sensory changes [8].

FOG occurs rarely as a form of bilateral akinetic seizure. Such FOG is precipitated by standing up, gait initiation, turning, stumbling, or startle induced by unexpected auditory or tactile stimuli [9]. Because mesial frontal epileptic discharge can hardly be detected by conventional EEG studies, epileptic origin of FOG can not be excluded in the presented case [10]. However, increased neuronal excitability in TIA causes dyskinesia (so call 'shaking TIA') rather than epileptic motor arrest [11]. FOG has been reported in patents who had widespread cerebral and bilateral basal ganglia lesions associated with hypoxia, carbon monoxide poisoning, wasp sting allergy, orpantothenate kinase associated neurodegeneration, as well as primary degenerative parkinsonism [12]. A recent neuronal network mapping study attributed FOG to the dorsal medial cerebellum [13]. FOG may also occur in patients with a focal brain lesion. The most often reported focal lesion is in the unilateral or bilateral dorsal midbrain tegmentum [3–5]. However, some patients had progressive worsening of gait disturbances and extensive subcortical white matter changes that obscured the causal relationship between the midbrain lesion and FOG [3].

We reviewed the literature and identified eight patients who developed gait disturbances or postural instabilities following a focal lesion in the frontal lobe. As the present case, seven of the eight patients had lesions in the mesial frontal lobe (Table 1) [14–21]. They developed various gait disturbances, inducing ataxic gait, shuffling gait, astasia, or FOG. At least four patients have been reported who developed FOG following a mesial frontal lesion associated with cortical vein thrombosis, lymphoma, or infarction [18–21]. However, they had additional neurological deficits that may disturb locomotor initiation (e.g. short steps, severe leg bradykinesia, spastic paraplegia, paratonia, retropulsion, loss of postural reflexes, and balance disturbance).

The presented patient developed isolated paroxysmal FOG associated with mesial frontal TIAs. This finding indicates that the mesialfrontal lobe, probably the supplementary motor area, generates a neuronal command for the initiation of locomotion. The mesial frontal lobe lesion seemed to disrupt transmission of a locomotor initiation command from the mesial frontal cortex to the locomotor pattern generators in the subcortical (e.g. nucleus accumbens and ventral pallidum), brainstem (e.g. pedunculopontine nucleus, cuneiform nucleus, and subcuneiform nucleus),and spinal cord [1, 22].

Abbreviations

ANA: Anti-nuclear antibodies; Anti-dsDNA: Anti-double stranded DNA antibodies; C-ANCA: Cytoplasmic anti-neutrophil cytoplasmic antibodies; CBC: Complete blood counts; FOG: Freezing of gait; MR: Magnetic resonance; MRI: Magnetic resonance imaging; P-ANCA: Perinuclear anti-neutrophil cytoplasmic antibodies

Acknowledgements

Not applicable.

Funding

We received no funding support.

Authors' contributions

HWH collected data, analyzed and wrote the manuscript. SHL analyzed the data and revised the manuscript. CHL analyzed the data and revised the manuscript. MSL designed the study, analyzed the data and revised the manuscript. All authors read and approved the final manuscript.

Competing interests

The authors declare that they have no competing interests.

References

1. Nutt JG, Bloem BR, Giladi N, Hallett M, Horak FB, Nieuwboer A. Freezing of gait: moving forward on a mysterious clinical phenomenon. Lancet Neurol. 2011;10:734–44.
2. Nutt J, Marsden CD, Thompson PD. Human walking and higher-level gait disorders, particularly in the elderly. Neurology. 1993;44:268–79.
3. Kuo SH, Kenney C, Jankovic J. Bilateral pedunculopontine nuclei strokes presenting as freezing of gait. Mov Disord. 2008;23:616–9.
4. Hathout GM, Bhidayasiri R. Midbrain ataxia: an introduction to the mesencephalic locomotor region and the pedunculopontine nucleus. Am J Roentgenol. 2005;184:953–6.
5. Ishihara S, Kano O, Ikeda K, Shimokawa R, Kawabe K, Iwasaki Y. Clinicoradiological changes of brain NK/T cell lymphoma manifesting pure akinesia: a case report. BMC Neurol. 2011;11:137. doi:10.1186/1471-2377-11-137.
6. Shill H, Gerber P. Evaluation of clinical diagnostic criteria for psychogenic movement disorders. Mov Disord. 2006;21:1163–8.
7. Schneider R, Gautier JC. Leg weakness due to stroke. Site of lesions, weakness patterns and causes. Brain. 1994;117:347–54.
8. de Freitas GR, Devuyst G, van Melle G, Bogousslavsky J. Motor strokes sparing the leg. Arch Neurol. 2000;51:513–8.
9. Toledano R, García-Morales I, Kurtis MM, Pérez-Sempere A, Ciordia R, Gil-Nagel A. Bilateral akinetic seizures: a clinical and electroencephalographic description. Epilepsia. 2010;51:2108–15.
10. Norman S. Mesial frontal epilepsy. Epilepsia. 1998;39:S49–61.
11. Lee MS, Kim WJ, Lyoo CH, Kim SJ, Suh GI. Giant somatosensory evoked potential in a patient with shaking TIA. Mov Disord. 2009;24:2301–4.

12. Lyoo CH, Prokisch H, Meitinger T, Lee SY, Kim DH, Lee MS. Anticholinergic-responsive gait freezing in a patient with pantothenate kinase-associatedneurodegeneration. Mov Disord. 2008;23:283–4.
13. Fasano A, Laganiere SE, Lam S, Fox MD. Lesions causing freezing of gait localize to a cerebellar functional network. Ann Neurol. 2017;81:129–41.
14. Sakakibara R, Hattori T, Uchiyama T, Yamanishi T. Micturitional disturbance in a patient with neurosarcoidosis. Neurourol Urodyn. 2000;19:273–7.
15. Ducruet AF, Kellner CP, Connolly ES, Meyers PM. Endovascular occlusion of a ruptured transitional aneurysm associated with a developmental venous anomaly. Neurosurg Focus. 2009;26:E8. doi:10.3171/2009.1.FOCUS08291.
16. Wada Y, Nishimura Y. Isolated astasia in acute infarction of the supplementary-motor area. BMJ Case Rep. 2010; doi:10.1136/bcr.01.2010.2618.
17. Frassanito P, D'Angelo L, Massimi L, Lauriola L, Novello M, Di Rocco C, et al. Sudden paraplegia in a case of apparently isolated frontal embryonaltumour with abundant neuropil and true rosettes. Br J Neurosurg. 2012;26:284–6.
18. Robbins MS, Verghese J, Antoniello D. Isolated gait apraxia from an acute unilateral parasagittal lesion. Clin Neurol Neurosurg. 2011;113:782–4.
19. Chung SJ, Im JH, Lee JH, Lee MC. Stuttering and gait disturbance after supplementary motor area seizure. Mov Disord. 2004;19:1106–9.
20. Nadeau SE. Gait apraxia: further clues to localization. Eur Neurol. 2007;58:142–5.
21. Della SS, Francescani A, Spinnier H. Gait apraxia after bilateral supplementary motor area lesion. J Neurol Neurosurg Psychiatry. 2002;72:77–85.
22. Lee MS, Rinne JO, Marsden CD. The pedunculopontine nucleus: its role in the genesis of movement disorders. Yonsei Med J. 2000;41:167–84.

Stroke unit care in germany: the german stroke registers study group (ADSR)

Steffi Hillmann[1*], Silke Wiedmann[1,2], Viktoria Rücker[1], Klaus Berger[3], Darius Nabavi[4], Ingo Bruder[5], Hans-Christian Koennecke[6], Günter Seidel[7], Björn Misselwitz[8], Alfred Janssen[9], Christoph Burmeister[10], Christine Matthis[11], Otto Busse[12], Peter Hermanek[13], Peter Ulrich Heuschmann[1,2,14], on behalf of the German Stroke Register Study Group (ADSR)

Abstract

Background: Factors influencing access to stroke unit (SU) care and data on quality of SU care in Germany are scarce. We investigated characteristics of patients directly admitted to a SU as well as patient-related and structural factors influencing adherence to predefined indicators of quality of acute stroke care across hospitals providing SU care.

Methods: Data were derived from the German Stroke Registers Study Group (ADSR), a voluntary network of 9 regional registers for monitoring quality of acute stroke care in Germany. Multivariable logistic regression analyses were performed to investigate characteristics influencing direct admission to SU. Generalized Linear Mixed Models (GLMM) were used to estimate the influence of structural hospital characteristics (percentage of patients admitted to SU, year of SU-certification, and number of stroke and TIA patients treated per year) on adherence to predefined quality indicators.

Results: In 2012 180,887 patients were treated in 255 hospitals providing certified SU care participating within the ADSR were included in the analysis; of those 82.4% were directly admitted to a SU. Ischemic stroke patients without disturbances of consciousness ($p < .0001$), an interval onset to admission time ≤3 h ($p < .0001$), and weekend admission ($p < .0001$) were more likely to be directly admitted to a SU. A higher proportion of quality indicators within predefined target ranges were achieved in hospitals with a higher proportion of SU admission ($p = 0.0002$). Quality of stroke care could be maintained even if certification was several years ago.

Conclusions: Differences in demographical and clinical characteristics regarding the probability of SU admission were observed. The influence of structural characteristics on adherence to evidence-based quality indicators was low.

Keywords: Stroke unit care, Quality of health care, Quality indicators, Stroke register

Background

Overwhelming evidence from RCTs showed efficacy of stroke unit (SU) care [1] with data from RCTs being replicated in routine care in different countries and different SU settings [2–5]. In German SUs, specific focus is given to management and treatment of patients in the hyper acute phase, including multimodal monitoring of vital functions, rapid diagnosis, and early initiation of secondary prevention [6]. Independent certification of SUs is performed mainly by the German Stroke Society (DSG) and the German Stroke Foundation (SDSH) [7]. Furthermore, stroke units are certified according to regional criteria of the federal states [8]. However, not all patients treated at hospitals providing SU care were admitted to SU. Available data on SU care in Germany are mainly based on routine data [9, 10] estimating for example that about 56.9% of all ischemic stroke (IS) patients in 2012 were admitted to a hospital with a specialized SU care in Germany [9]. However, routine data do not include detailed clinical relevant information such as stroke severity and comorbidities. Thus, it is currently unclear, if the demographic and clinical

* Correspondence: steffi.hillmann@uni-wuerzburg.de
[1]Institute of Clinical Epidemiology and Biometry (ICE-B) Würzburg, Josef-Schneider-Str. 2 / D7, 97080 Würzburg, Germany
Full list of author information is available at the end of the article

characteristics influence direct access of stroke patients to a SU. Furthermore, previous studies did not investigate variations in quality of stroke care by SU structures in Germany. Thus, it is unclear to what extent structural characteristics of the respective hospitals, such as certification procedures or percentage of stroke patients admitted to a SU, might influence quality of care provided. Therefore, we investigated the influence of demographic and clinical characteristics of patients on direct admission to a SU as well as the influence of the structural characteristics on adherence to evidence-based quality indicators among hospitals providing SU care in Germany.

Methods

The german stroke registers study group (ADSR)

Data were derived from the German Stroke Registers Study Group (ADSR), a voluntary network of 9 regional registers (Bavaria, Baden-Württemberg, Berlin, Hamburg, Hesse, North Rhine, Northwest Germany, Rhineland-Palatinate, and Schleswig-Holstein), which was founded in 1999 for monitoring quality of acute stroke care in Germany [11]. Data are collected mainly electronically, with predefined completeness and plausibility checks, by the respective quality assurance projects [12]. For example: date of ever treatment must be after the date of admission. Only plausible datasets were evaluated and sent to the data-pooling center. Each regional stroke register sends the complete data set in regular intervals to the data-pooling center (University of Würzburg, 2011-2015) [11]. Participation within a regional register of the ADSR is mandatory for all SUs in Germany certified according to the criteria of the DSG and the SDSH (see below) as well as for all hospitals in several regions [12].

Stroke unit definition

SUs were certified according to criteria of the German Stroke Society (DSG) and the German Stroke Foundation (SDSH) [13] and supported by the LGA InterCert [8]. SUs certified according to these criteria are distinguished into regional SUs and supra-regional SUs, depending on equipment and expertise [6]. Regional SUs have to treat at least 250 patients per year in at least 4 beds [14]. Supra-regional SUs have further demands on structural and procedural requirements [13, 14]. For example, interventional neuroradiology and neurosurgery and all relevant therapeutic and diagnostic facilities for stroke diagnosis, treatment, and management have to be available [6]. Additionally, a minimum of 450 patients per year treated in at least 6 monitoring beds are essential for certification of supra-regional SUs [14]. The minimum number of stroke patients per year was increased up to at least 500 in 2012 [13]. Beside these criteria, certification procedures by the local government of some federal states are also applied (i.e. Baden-Württemberg).

Hospital characteristics

Analyses were restricted to hospitals with a certified SU, according to criteria of the DSG, the SDSH or to regional criteria by the federal states that provided complete information regarding the admitting department. Investigated structural characterisis of participating hospitals providing SU care included: percentage of patients directly admitted to a SU (SU/general ward/intensive care unit/other), percentage of patients admitted directly to a SU (<60%, 60-80%, >80%), year of first certification of the respective SU (2000-2002, 2003-2005, 2006-2008, 2009-2012), and number of stroke and Transient Ischemic Attack (TIA) patients treated per year (<250, 250-500, >500-750, >750).

Quality Indicators

A set of evidence based patient-oriented quality indicators was defined to measure quality of acute stroke care in participating hospitals. A standardized process was initiated for developing a set of evidence based quality indicators between 2003 and 2006 [11]. The process contained a systematic literature review, external independent validation and the conduction of a prospective pilot study [11]. The quality indicator set is updated on a regular basis every 2-3 years [15]. Target values of quality indicators were defined to indicate good quality of stroke care based on distribution within the data, national recommendations and expert consensus by the working group [15]. For the present analysis, the following set of 11 patient-oriented QIs with defined target values were used with definitions published previously [12]: early antithrombotic therapy; antithrombotic therapy – secondary prevention; anticoagulant therapy; brain imaging in patients with suspected strokes; vascular imaging in IS and TIA; screening for dysphagia; early rehabilitation – physiotherapy/occupational therapy; early rehabilitation – speech therapy; early mobilization; patients who arrived at the hospital within two hours from symptom onset and received brain imaging within one hour; early systemic thrombolytic therapy in eligible patients.

Achievement of quality indicators

Achievement of QIs was defined by reaching previously defined target values [12]. The proportion of achieved QIs was calculated by the number of QIs fulfilled in patients divided by the number of QIs that a patient could have fulfilled, according to the defined eligibility criteria of the respective QI.

Statistical analysis

The following regional stroke audits were included in the present analyses: Hesse, Bavaria, Northwest Germany, Baden-Württemberg, North Rhine and the Berlin Stroke Register. Three regional stroke audits (Hamburg, Rhineland-Palatinate, and Schleswig-Holstein) were excluded because of missing or not comparable information on SU admission. Detailed descriptive and univariate analyses were performed to describe the demographic and clinical characteristics of the patients. Multivariable logistic regression analyses were performed to estimate the characteristics of ischemic stroke patients being admitted to a SU including: age (age group: ≤64y, ≥65y and ≤74y, ≥75y and ≤84y, ≥85y); sex; comorbidities (atrial fibrillation, diabetes mellitus, hypertension, previous stroke, hyperlipidemia); time from onset to admission (≤2h, >2-3h, >3-6h, >6-24h, >24h-48h, >48h, unknown); NIHSS (≤3, >4-15, ≥15) [16]; and day of admission (weekday, weekend). Analyses were adjusted for regional audits. The association between hospital characteristics and the achievement of given target values to a defined set of evidence based quality indicators was assessed by Generalized Linear Mixed Models (GLMM). GLMM was used to estimate the p-values and regression coefficients for the differences in the percentage of fulfilled quality indicators regarding the structure of the hospital (percentage of patients being admitted to a SU, year of certification of the respective SU, and the number of stroke and TIA patients treated per year) and individual characteristics (age [categories], sex, stroke classification [ischemic stroke (IS), intracerebral hemorrhage (ICH), Transient Ischemic Attack (TIA), other], day of admission [weekday/weekend], and NIHSS on admission [categories]). The variable hospital was added as a random effect to model the correlations within the hospitals. Analyses were restricted to patients without missing values in the respective variables. The number of missing values ranged from 0.1% in age to 3.8% in NIHSS. Regarding the variables "interval onset to admission" and "day of admission", no comparable information was provided in one regional stroke register. Therefore, we performed a sensitivity analysis for the multivariable logistic regression analysis including all patients with missing information as own category. Statistical significance was determined at an alpha level of 0.05. Statistical analyses were performed using the SAS 9.3 Software Package, SAS Institute Inc., Cary, NC, USA.

Ethics

The data pooling was approved by the ethics committee of the Charité-Universitätsmedizin Berlin (EA4/043/10) and is registered by the University of Würzburg (214/11). The identity of the individual patients was completely anonymous. Therefore, no specific informed consent was obtained by patients. The investigators who performed the data analyzes were blinded to hospital identities. These identities are only known by the coordinating center of the respective regional stroke registers [11].

Results

In 2012,180,887 patients were included in the analysis from 255 hospitals providing certified SU care: of those, 149,001 patients have been directly admitted to SUs (82.4%) The range of SU admission between the regional stroke audits was 77.9% - 84.6%. Median age of all patients was 74 years (IQR 64-82), 49.1% were women. 66.4% had an (IS), 6.3% had an intracerebral hemorrhage (ICH), 25.9% had a transient ischemic attack (TIA), and 1.4% of strokes were undefined or subarachnoid hemorrhage. Demographical and clinical characteristics of all patients treated in hospitals with a certified SU by direct SU admission are provided in Table 1. The proportion of patients receiving thrombolysis therapy without admission on a SU was relatively high (10.9%). This was due to the high number of thrombolysis therapy at Intensive Care Units (data not shown).

IS patients admitted on weekends ($p < .0001$), with an interval-onset-admission time less than 3 h ($p < .0001$), with hypertension ($p < .0001$), and hyperlipidemia ($p < .0001$) are more likely, and patients with a previous stroke (0.0055) were less likely to be admitted directly to a SU. Contrary, patients with a severe stroke (NIHSS >15) had a lower probability of being admitted to a SU ($p < .0001$) (Table 2). Results remained stable in a sensitivity analysis including all stroke subtypes, except for age. Patients younger than 85 years were more likely to be admitted on a SU ($p = 0.0031$). An additional sensitivity analysis based on all data including missing information as separate categories showed no substantial differences (data not shown).

Quality indicators

Results of achieved QIs by structural and individual factors are presented in Table 3. In hospitals with a SU, overall a mean of 93.7% (SD 13.3) of the QIs were within the predefined target ranges. The proportion of patients admitted to SUs ($p = 0.0002$) had a significant impact on the achievement of quality indicators, whereas year of certification ($p = 0.3014$) and number of treated patients ($p = 0.7238$) showed no significant impact. Results remained stable in a sensitivity analysis stratifying by admission on a SU (Additional file 1: Table S1).

Discussion

Demographic and clinical factors influencing admission to a SU were identified in a large sample of hospitals across Germany. Results of our study show that patients admitted to SUs have milder strokes, suffer more from high blood pressure or hyperlipidemia, and are admitted earlier after stroke onset. A higher proportion of quality

Table 1 Demographic and clinical characteristics of the patients

	Hospital with certified SU	Admission on a SU		*P*-value
		Yes	No	
No of centers	255			
No of patients, n	180,887	149,001	31,886	
Age, y				<.0001
Mean (SD)	72.0 (13.4)	72.1 (13.3)	71.6 (14.0)	
Median (IQR)	74 (64 – 82)	74 (64 – 82)	74 (63 – 82)	
Age categories, y, %				<.0001
< 65	25.8	25.4	27.3	
65-74	24.6	24.8	23.9	
75-84	32.6	32.8	31.5	
≥ 85	17.0	16.9	17.3	
Stroke subtype, %				<.0001
IS	66.4	67.5	61.5	
ICH	6.3	4.9	13.0	
TIA	25.9	26.7	22.2	
other (unclassified, SAH)	1.4	0.9	3.3	
Women, %	49.1	48.9	50.4	<.0001
Comorbidities, %				
Atrial fibrillation	25.8	26.0	24.7	<.0001
Diabetes mellitus	26.5	26.8	25.2	<.0001
Hypertension	82.6	83.2	79.5	<.0001
Previous stroke	24.6	24.9	23.1	<.0001
Hyperlipidemia	51.1	52.8	43.4	<.0001
Thrombolysis after IS, %	14.6	15.3	10.9	<.0001
Interval onset admission, hours, %[a]				<.0001
< =2	20.7	21.7	15.9	
> 2-3	9.2	9.7	6.9	
> 3-6	15.3	16.0	11.9	
> 6-24	16.2	17.1	12.2	
> 24-48	5.7	5.7	5.6	
> 48	9.2	7.0	19.8	
unknown	23.8	22.9	27.7	
Neurological signs within 24h after admission, %				
Paresis	55.3	55.9	52.2	<.0001
Aphasia	27.5	27.4	28.2	0.0065
Dysarthria	34.6	35.2	31.5	<.0001
Disturbed level of consciousness	9.0	6.9	18.6	<.0001
NIHSS on admission,				
Median (IQR)	3 (1-7)	3 (1-7)	3 (1-10)	<.0001
NIHSS on admission, %				<.0001
< 4	55.5	55.6	55.1	
4-15	35.0	36.4	27.9	
> 15	9.5	8.0	17.0	

Table 1 Demographic and clinical characteristics of the patients *(Continued)*

Day of admission				<.0001
Weekday	73.7	73.1	76.3	
Weekend	26.3	26.9	23.7	
Length of stay, days				<.0001
Mean (SD)	8.8 (7.3)	8.7 (6.9)	9.5 (9.0)	
Median (IQR)	7 (4-11)	7 (4-11)	7 (4-12)	

[a]information not available in 1 regional stroke audit

Table 2 Probability for admission of patients with ischemic stroke on a Stroke Unit (demographical and clinical characteristics)

	OR (95% CI) $n = 88,316$	*P*-values
Age categories		0.0664
< 65	1	
65-74	1.03 (0.97 - 1.08)	
75-84	1.00 (0.95 - 1.05)	
≥ 85	0.95 (0.89 - 1.01)	
Sex		
Men	1	0.3088
Women	0.98 (0.94 - 1.02)	
Comorbidities		
Atrial fibrillation	1.02 (0.98 - 1.07)	0.2998
Diabetes mellitus	0.99 (0.95 - 1.03)	0.4659
Hypertension	1.13 (1.08 - 1.19)	<.0001
Previous stroke	0.94 (0.90 - 0.98)	0.0055
Hyperlipidemia	1.26 (1.21 - 1.31)	<.0001
Interval onset admission, hours[a]		
< =2	1	<.0001
> 2-3	0.94 (0.87 - 1.02)	
> 3-6	0.88 (0.83 - 0.94)	
> 6-24	0.90 (0.85 - 0.96)	
> 24-48	0.61 (0.56 - 0.66)	
> 48	0.19 (0.18 - 0.20)	
unknown	0.43 (0.41 - 0.46)	
NIHSS admission		
≤ 3	1	<.0001
≥ 4- ≤ 15	1.30 (1.25 - 1.36)	
> 15	0.55 (0.52 - 0.59)	
Day of admission[a]		
weekday	1	<.0001
weekend	1.12 (1.08 - 1.17)	

[a]no information in one regional stroke register

indicators were fulfilled in hospitals with a higher proportion of patients being directly admitted to a SU.

Our findings are comparable with previous studies showing that patients treated on a SU tends to be younger on average, had a higher prevalence of comorbidities, especially atrial fibrillation, and hypertension, and were more conscious [3, 17]. Older patients might be more likely to be admitted to a geriatric or general ward, especially older patients with multiple pathologies and greater degrees of frailty [18]. We found a slightly higher probability for patients directly admitted to SUs on weekends. This might be explained by certification requirements of SUs resulting in better staffing of SUs compared to other wards on weekends which could lead to a preferred admission to a SU. Data on quality of care on weekends are heterogeneous. Most studies demonstrate a poorer quality of care, and negative effects for patients being admitted on weekends [18–21], whereas others do not confirm these findings [22–24].

Adherence to given target values of evidence-based QIs was significantly associated with the proportion of patients admitted to a SU. That means, more patients receive guideline-recommended therapy if they are treated on a SU. This implies that ischemic stroke patients should be treated on a SU. But, not all quality indicators are relevant for patients not being treated on a SU – e.g. patients with intracerebral hemorrhage treated on an Intensive Care Unit. This higher quality of stroke care might be the result of a more specific training of the medical staff of SU (doctors, nurses, and therapists) in acute stroke management. A higher proportion of quality standards met in patients admitted to a SU was also reported by Rudd et al [18]. We found no association between proportion of fulfilled QIs and year of first certification, or the annual number of stroke patients treated. We assume that the quality of stroke care could be maintained even if certification was several years ago. This finding is in contrast to other studies reporting a higher level of quality of care and better outcomes for patients in higher volume SUs [25–27]. Our results suggest that certification requirements of the DSG and the SDSH might ensure quality of SU care independently from the number of patients treated on a local SU per

Table 3 Achieved QIs by structural factors in hospitals with certified SUs[a]

	Hospitals with certified Stroke Units		Regression coefficient in % (95%-CI)[b]	*P*-values
	No of hospitals	Mean (SD) % achieved QIs		
Overall/Intercept	255	93.7 (13.3)	86.8 (79.4 – 94.3)	
SU admission within hospitals with SU, %				
< 60	16	87.6 (18.5)	0	0.0002
60-80	63	92.7 (14.3)	4.4 (1.2 – 7.5)	
> 80	176	94.4 (12.4)	5.7 (2.7 – 8.6)	
Year of certification[c]				
2000-2002	31	94.2 (12.5)	0	0.3014
2003-2005	42	93.3 (13.3)	-0.9 (-2.6 – 0.7)	
2006-2008	32	93.8 (14.2)	0.7 (-1.3 – 2.9)	
2009-2012	81	93.6 (13.3)	-0.6 (-2.1 – 0.9)	
No of patients				
< 250	11	94.4 (12.9)	0	0.7238
250-500	62	92.4 (15.1)	1.8 (-4.9 – 8.4)	
> 500-750	80	94.0 (13.1)	2.4 (-4.1 – 8.9)	
> 750	102	93.7 (13.0)	1.8 (-4.7 – 8.3)	

[a]11 quality indicators; [b]analysis adjusted for individual level factors sex, stroke subtype, age, weekday of admission, NIHSS, [c]no information about year of certification in one regional stroke register; unknown year of certification of hospitals occurred in every register

year. We found no association between year of certification and number of QI within given target values. There is not much comparable evidence on this subject as previous studies compared certified- and non-certified stroke centers [28, 29] or different certification procedures [30]. One strength of the present analyses is the large number of patients analyzed. Data are routinely checked for plausibility, but coding errors at hospital level cannot be ruled out. Because in Germany participation in the ADSR is mandatory only for SUs and in specific regions, we decided not to compare quality of SU care between hospitals with and without SUs, in order to avoid bias due to most an overrepresentation of hospitals with SU care in the dataset and, thus, makes comparisons with centers not providing SU care difficult

Overall from 180,887 stroke patients, 82.4% were directly admitted to a SU. There seems to be still room for quality improvement regarding the proportion of stroke patients admitted to a SU. Our data contains only information on the admission of a SU. It is possible that patients were transferred from a normal ward to a SU during hospital stay. Unfortunately, this information was not included in our dataset.

The process of admission to a SU might be affected by selection bias as severely affected patients e.g. with intracerebral or subarachnoid hemorrhage are more likely to be admitted to intensive care units or neurosurgical departments. In addition, but unlikely to affect our results relevantly, we might underestimate the entire proportion of patients being treated on a SU, while secondary admissions during the hospital stay were not recorded.

Conclusions

Our data indicate a high quality of acute SU care in Germany according to predefined quality indicators. The influence of documented structural characteristics on adherence to evidence-based quality indicators was low. However, there might be still room for quality improvement left regarding the proportion of stroke patients admitted to a SU.

Abbreviations

ADSR: German Stroke Register Study Group (Arbeitsgemeinschaft Deutscher Schlaganfall Register); DSG: German Stroke Society (Deutsche Schlaganfall Gesellschaft); GLMM: Generalized linear mixed models; ICH: Intracerebral hemorrhage; IQR: Interquartile range; IS: Ischemic stroke; NIHSS: National Institutes of Health Stroke Scale; QI: Quality indicator; RCTs: Randomized clinical trials; SD: Standard deviation; SDSH: German Stroke Foundation (Stiftung Deutsche Schlaganfall-Hilfe); SU: Stroke unit; TIA: Transient ischemic attack

Acknowledgements

The authors thank all participating hospitals participating in the regional registers of the ADSR. The following stroke registers participate in the German Stroke Registers Study Group (ADSR). The following stroke registers participate in the German Stroke Registers Study Group (ADSR): Bavaria stroke register: Dr. med. M. Eßer; Baden-Württemberg stroke register: S. Rode; Berlin Stroke Register: Dr. med. B. Hoffmann, Berlin Medical Association, Dr. Georg Walter Vivantes Klinikum am Friedrichshain; Stroke Register Hamburg: R. Hohnhold, EQS-Hamburg Landesgeschäftsstelle Qualitätssicherung [regional office for quality assurance]; Stroke Register Hesse: A. Reihs; Stroke Register of Northwest Germany: M. Kalic; Stroke Register Rhineland-Palatinate: Dr. med. S.

Dienlin; Stroke Register Schleswig-Holstein: Prof. Dr. med H. Raspe; Erlangen Stroke Register: Prof. Dr. med. P. Kolominsky-Rabas MBA; Technical committee of the ADSR: Dr. med. I. Bruder, Dr. med. S. Dienlin, Dr. med. M. Eßer, Prof. Dr. med. P. Heuschmann, Dr. med. B. Misselwitz, A. Reihs.

Funding
Parts of the data pooling exercise were financially supported within the framework of the FP7 program by the European Union European Implementation Score collaboration [EIS]; No. 223153. There was no financial or other support by other third parties for the working process or manuscript preparation.

Author's contributions
SH analysis and interpretation of the data, drafting the manuscript; SW drafting the manuscript; VR analysis of the data; KB, DN, IB, HCK, GS, BM, AJ, CB, CM, OB, and PH data collection and revising the manuscript; PUH analysis and interpretation of the data, drafting the manuscript. All authors read and approved the final manuscript.

Competing interests
SH, VR, DN, IB, BM, AJ, CB, CM, OB, and PH declare that they have no competing interests; SW receives research support from the German Ministry of Research and Education; KB has received within the last 10 years completely investigator-initiated research funding as principal or coordinating investigator in the areas of stroke, depression and subclinical atherosclerosis, multimorbidity and health services research, diabetes, multiple sclerosis and for the German National Cohort from the German Ministry of Research and Technology (BMBF). For the conduction of an investigator initiated clinical register for multiple sclerosis he has received a grant from the German Competence Net Multiple Sclerosis with funds from Biogen Idec. For the conduction (2007-2014) of a study on the course of Restless Legs Syndrome he has received unrestricted grants to the University of Muenster from the German Restless Legs Society and Boehringer Ingelheim Pharma, Mundipharma Research, Neurobiotec, Roche Pharma, UCB Germany, UCB Switzerland and Vifor Pharma; HCK serves as an auditor in the certification process of stroke units and is a member of the certification committee of the DSG; GS reports unrestricted education grants from Bayer Health Care, Biotronic, Boehringer Ingelheim, Biogen Idec, Bracco, Bristol-Myers Squibb, Grifols, Pfizer, Philips, Genzyme, Merck Serono, Noras, Novartis, Takeda, Teva, UCB, HOCOMA, Braun, Shire, Talecris, Sanofi Aventis, MSD, Meda, Desitin, Krauth + Timmermann; PUH reports grants from the European Union (within EIS) during study conduct; from the German Ministry of Research and Education, Charité, Berlin Chamber of Physicians, German Parkinson Society, University Hospital Würzburg, Robert-Koch-Institute, Charité–Universitätsmedizin Berlin (within MonDAFIS; MonDAFIS is supported by an unrestricted research grant to the Charité from Bayer), University Göttingen (within FIND-AFrandomized; FIND-AFrandomized is supported by an unrestricted research grant to the University Göttingen from Boehringer-Ingelheim), and University Hospital Heidelberg (within RASUNOA-prime; RASUNOA-prime is supported by an unrestricted research grant to the University Hospital Heidelberg from Bayer, BMS, Boehringer-Ingelheim, Daiichi Sankyo), outside submitted work.

Author details
[1]Institute of Clinical Epidemiology and Biometry (ICE-B) Würzburg, Josef-Schneider-Str. 2 / D7, 97080 Würzburg, Germany. [2]Comprehensive Heart Failure Center, University of Würzburg, Straubmühlweg 2a, 97078 Würzburg, Germany. [3]Quality Assurance Project"Stroke Register Northwest Germany", Institute of Epidemiology and Social Medicine, University of Münster, Albert-Schweitzer-Campus 1, Gebäude D3, 48149 Münster, Germany. [4]Department of Neurology, Vivantes Klinikum Neukölln, Berlin, Rudower Straße 48, 12351 Berlin, Germany. [5]Office for Quality Assurance in Hospitals (GeQiK) Stuttgart at Baden-Wuerttembergische Hospital Federation, Stuttgart, Birkenwaldstr. 151, 70191 Stuttgart, Germany. [6]Vivantes Klinikum im Friedrichshain, Berlin, Landsberger Allee 49, 10249 Berlin, Germany. [7]Department of Neurology, Asklepios Klinik Nord, Hamburg,, Tangstedter Landstraße 400, 22417 Hamburg, Germany. [8]Institute of Quality Assurance Hesse (GQH), Frankfurter Str. 10, 65760 Eschborn, Germany. [9]Quality Assurance in Stroke Management in North Rhine–Westphalia, Medical Association North Rhine, Tersteegenstr. 9, 40474 Düsseldorf, Germany. [10]Institute of Quality Assurance Rhineland-Palatinate / SQMed, Wilhelm-Theodor-Römheld-Straße 34, 55130 Mainz, Germany. [11]Quality Association for Acute Stroke Treatment Schleswig-Holstein (QugSS), Institute of Social Medicine and Epidemiology, University of Lübeck, Ratzeburger Allee 160, 23538 Lübeck, Germany. [12]German Stroke Society, Berlin, Reinhardtstr. 27C, 10117 Berlin, Germany. [13]Bavarian Permanent Working Party for Quality Assurance, Munich, Westenriederstr. 19, 80331 Munich, Germany. [14]Clinical Trial Center Würzburg, University Hospital Würzburg, Josef-Schneider-Str. 2 / D7, 97080 Würzburg, Germany.

References
1. Stroke Unit Trialists' Collaboration. Organised inpatient (stroke unit) care for stroke. Cochrane Database Syst Rev 2013; 9:CD000197. Epub 2013/09/13.
2. Bray BD, Ayis S, Campbell J, Hoffman A, Roughton M, Tyrrell PJ, et al. Associations between the organisation of stroke services, process of care, and mortality in England: prospective cohort study. BMJ. 2013;346:f2827.
3. Langhorne P, Lewsey JD, Jhund PS, Gillies M, Chalmers JW, Redpath A, et al. Estimating the impact of stroke unit care in a whole population: an epidemiological study using routine data. J Neurol Neurosurg Psychiatry. 2010;81(12):1301–5.
4. Turner M, Barber M, Dodds H, Dennis M, Langhorne P, Macleod MJ. The impact of stroke unit care on outcome in a Scottish stroke population, taking into account case mix and selection bias. J Neurol Neurosurg Psychiatry. 2015;86(3):314–8.
5. Walter A, Seidel G, Thie A, Raspe H. Semi-intensive stroke unit versus conventional care in acute ischemic stroke or TIA - a prospective study in Germany. J Neurol Sci. 2009;287(1-2):131–7.
6. Wiedmann S, Heuschmann PUH, Hill MD. Organized stroke care: Germany and Canada. In: Norrving B, editor. Oxford Textbook of Stroke and Cerebrovascular Disease. 1st ed. New York, NY: Oxford University Press; 2014. p. 270–8.
7. Nabavi DG, Ossenbrink M, Schinkel M, Koennecke HC, Hamann G, Busse O. Revised certification criteria for regional and national stroke units in Germany. Nervenarzt. 2015;86:978–88.
8. LGA InterCert GmbH. Stroke Units Zertifizierung. Landesgewerbeanstalt (LGA) TÜV Rheinland web page. http://www.lga-intercert.com/branchen/medizin-und-gesundheitswesen/stroke-units-zertifizierung/. Accessed 26 Sept 2016.
9. Krogias C, Bartig D, Kitzrow M, Weber R, Eyding J. Trends of hospitalized acute stroke care in Germany from clinical trials to bedside. Comparison of nation-wide administrative data 2008-2012. J Neurol Sci. 2014;345(1-2):202–8.
10. Scholten N, Pfaff H, Lehmann HC, Fink GR, Karbach U. Thrombolysis for acute stroke–a nationwide analysis of regional medical care. Fortschr Neurol Psychiatr. 2013;81(10):579–85.
11. Heuschmann PU, Berger K. International experience in stroke registries: German Stroke Registers Study Group. Am J Prev Med. 2006;31(6 Suppl 2):S238.
12. Wiedmann S, Heuschmann PU, Hillmann S, Busse O, Wietholter H, Walter GM, et al. The quality of acute stroke care- an analysis of evidence-based indicators in 260 000 patients. Dtsch Arztebl Int. 2014;111(45):759–65.
13. Nabavi DG, Ringelstein EB, Faiss J, Kessler C, Rother J, Busse O. Regional and national stroke units in Germany: amended certification criteria. Nervenarzt. 2012;83(8):1039–52.
14. Ringelstein EB, Busse O, Ritter MA. Current concepts of Stroke Units in Germany and Europe. Schweiz Arch Neurol Psychiatr. 2011;162(4):155–60.
15. Heuschmann PU, Busse O, Wagner M, Endres M, Villringer A, Rother J, et al. Frequency and Care of Stroke in Germany. Aktuelle Neurol. 2010;37(7):333–40.
16. Baird AE, Dambrosia J, Janket S, Eichbaum Q, Chaves C, Silver B, et al. A three-item scale for the early prediction of stroke recovery. Lancet. 2001; 357(9274):2095–9.
17. Candelise L, Gattinoni M, Bersano A, Micieli G, Sterzi R, Morabito A. Stroke-unit care for acute stroke patients: an observational follow-up study. Lancet. 2007;369(9558):299–305.

18. Rudd AG, Hoffman A, Down C, Pearson M, Lowe D. Access to stroke care in England, Wales and Northern Ireland: the effect of age, gender and weekend admission. Age Ageing. 2007;36(3):247–55.
19. McKinney JS, Deng Y, Kasner SE, Kostis JB. Comprehensive stroke centers overcome the weekend versus weekday gap in stroke treatment and mortality. Stroke. 2011;42(9):2403–9.
20. Palmer WL, Bottle A, Davie C, Vincent CA, Aylin P. Dying for the weekend: a retrospective cohort study on the association between day of hospital presentation and the quality and safety of stroke care. Arch Neurol. 2012; 69(10):1296–302.
21. Campbell JT, Bray BD, Hoffman AM, Kavanagh SJ, Rudd AG, Tyrrell PJ. The effect of out of hours presentation with acute stroke on processes of care and outcomes: analysis of data from the Stroke Improvement National Audit Programme (SINAP). PLoS One. 2014;9(2):e87946.
22. Albright KC, Savitz SI, Raman R, Martin-Schild S, Broderick J, Ernstrom K, et al. Comprehensive stroke centers and the 'weekend effect': the SPOTRIAS experience. Cerebrovasc Dis. 2012;34(5-6):424–9.
23. Albright K, Hallevi H, Raman R, Ernstrom K, Martin-Schild S, Meyer B, et al. Can comprehensive stroke centers erase the "Weekend effect"? Neurology. 2008;70(11):A18-A18.
24. Kim SC, Hong KS, Hwang SI, Kim JE, Kim AR, Cho JY, et al. Weekend admission in patients with acute ischemic stroke is not associated with poor functional outcome than weekday admission. J Clin Neurol. 2012;8(4):265–70.
25. Schwamm LH, Fonarow GC, Reeves MJ, Pan W, Frankel MR, Smith EE, et al. Get With the Guidelines-Stroke is associated with sustained improvement in care for patients hospitalized with acute stroke or transient ischemic attack. Circulation. 2009;119(1):107–15.
26. Svendsen ML, Ehlers LH, Ingeman A, Johnsen SP. Higher stroke unit volume associated with improved quality of early stroke care and reduced length of stay. Stroke. 2012;43(11):3041–5.
27. Reeves MJ, Gargano J, Maier KS, Broderick JP, Frankel M, Labresh KA, et al. Patient-Level and Hospital-Level Determinants of the Quality of Acute Stroke Care. A Multilevel Modeling Approach. Stroke. 2010; Epub 2010/10/23.
28. Johnson AM, Goldstein LB, Bennett P, O'Brien EC, Rosamond WD. Compliance with acute stroke care quality measures in hospitals with and without primary stroke center certification: the North Carolina Stroke Care Collaborative. J Am Heart Assoc. 2014;3(2):e000423.
29. Stradling D, Yu W, Langdorf ML, Tsai F, Kostanian V, Hasso AN, et al. Stroke care delivery before vs after JCAHO stroke center certification. Neurology. 2007;68(6):469–70.
30. Fonarow GC, Liang L, Smith EE, Reeves MJ, Saver JL, Xian Y, et al. Comparison of performance achievement award recognition with primary stroke center certification for acute ischemic stroke care. J Am Heart Assoc. 2013;2(5):e000451.

Isolated non-traumatic, non-aneurysmal convexal subarachnoid hemorrhage in a patient with Evans syndrome

Anna Misyail Abdul Rashid[1] and Mohamad Syafeeq Faeez Md Noh[2*]

Abstract

Background: Non-traumatic, spontaneous subarachnoid hemorrhage occurs in approximately 85% of cases where there is a ruptured saccular aneurysm. An additional 10% of cases arise from non-aneurysmal peri-mesencephalic hemorrhages.

Case presentation: We report a rare case of a young female, with underlying Evans syndrome, who was initially thought to have non-hemorrhagic stroke, eventually diagnosed having isolated non-traumatic, non-aneurysmal convexal subarachnoid haemorrhage.

Conclusions: Spontaneous non-traumatic, non-aneurysmal convexal subarachnoid hemorrhage is a rare entity - of which there are multiple possible etiologies.

Keywords: Evans syndrome, Subarachnoid haemorrhage (SAH)

Background

Classically, non-traumatic subarachnoid hemorrhage (SAH) is known to occur mostly in association with underlying aneurysm [1]. The hemorrhage is seen, whether via computed tomography (CT) or magnetic resonance imaging (MRI), in the basal cisterns. Spontaneous SAH occurring in the convexal region of the brain is a rare entity. Multiple etiologies have been attributed – these include vascular and non-vascular causes [2]. We describe a young female presenting to our center, with underlying Evans syndrome, initially misdiagnosed as suffering from acute non-hemorrhagic stroke; only to be eventually diagnosed with an acute isolated non-traumatic, non-aneurysmal convexal SAH via MRI and diagnostic cerebral angiography.

Case presentation

A 39-years-old lady, with underlying Evans syndrome under Hematology follow up presented to our center with acute onset right sided hemiparesis, associated with facial asymmetry. On examination, she was afebrile. Neurological assessment revealed a power of 3/5, with brisk reflexes. Sensation was reduced on the affected side. There were no ocular manifestations. Cerebellar signs were absent. Blood investigations, including coagulation profile, were unremarkable except for slight thrombocytopenia of 120×10^9/L (normal range 150–400 $\times 10^9$/L). Urgent plain brain CT, done a few hours after symptoms onset, revealed left high parietal region cerebral edema (HU of 50–70), with no evidence of hemorrhage (Fig. 1A). A contrasted study done the following day revealed no additional findings (Fig. 1B). A decision was made to pursue MRI, 2 days post symptom onset, due to the non-specific findings on CT. Left high parietal region low signal intensities on gradient echo (GRE) sequence, with corresponding high signal intensities seen on pre-contrast fluid-attenuated inversion recovery (FLAIR) sequence confirmed an acute SAH (Fig. 1C, D). Contrasted T2 FLAIR sequence showed accompanying lepto- and pachymeningeal enhancement (Fig. 1E). Additionally, a few small intra-parenchymal acute hemorrhages were also noted. MR angiography (MRA) and MR venography (MRV) were negative. A diagnostic cerebral angiography was pursued the following 2 weeks, despite the MRA being negative. This revealed a left sided A3 aneurysm, measuring approximately

* Correspondence: msf.mdnoh@gmail.com
[2]Department of Imaging, Faculty of Medicine and Health Sciences, Universiti Putra Malaysia, Level 3, 43400 Serdang, Selangor, Malaysia
Full list of author information is available at the end of the article

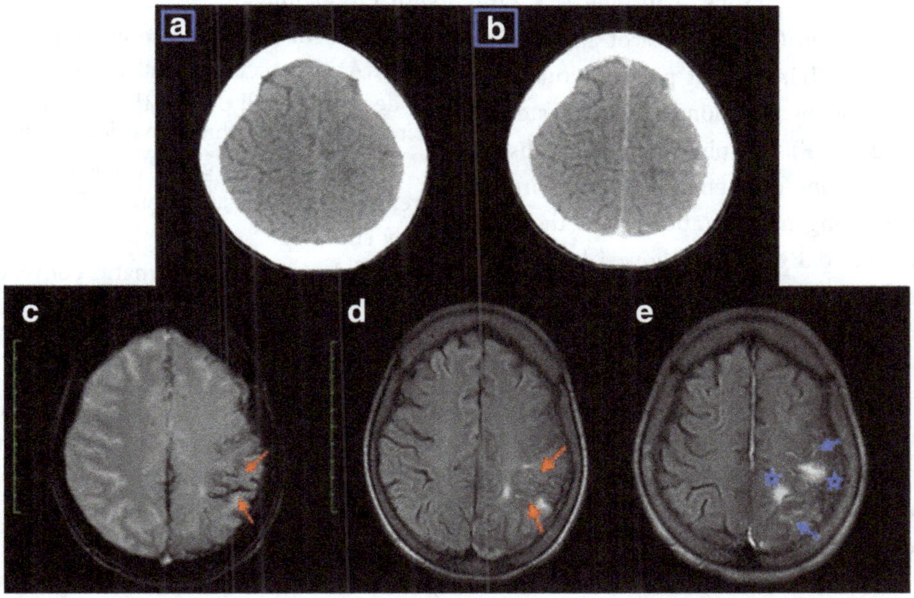

Fig. 1 Axial CT images at the high parietal region, plain (1**a**) and contrasted (1**b**) showing; 1**a** – left high parietal region cerebral edema is present, with no evidence of haemorrhage. 1**b** – Contrast is seen opacifying the sulci, but otherwise no additional findings were evident. Axial MRI images; GRE (1**c**), pre-contrast FLAIR (1**d**), and T2 FLAIR post gadolinium (1**e**), sequences at the high parietal region showing; 1**c** – Hypointense signal of the affected region (arrows) with corresponding hyperintensity on FLAIR (1**d**) confirming acute convexal SAH. 1**e** – Areas of pachy- and leptomeningeal enhancement, with small foci of haemorrhage; indirect signs of vasculitis

3.3 mm in its widest dimension (Fig. 2A, B), with no features to suggest hemorrhage. The location of this aneurysm did not correspond to the region of the focal convexal subarachnoid hemorrhage – and concluded to be an incidental finding. Patient was treated conservatively, and gradually improved with steroid therapy.

Discussion and conclusions

We report a rare case of a spontaneous isolated, non-traumatic, non-aneurysmal SAH in a young lady with underlying Evans syndrome – which is a rare haematological disorder of unknown frequency characterized by simultaneous or sequential development of autoimmune hemolytic anemia (AIHA) and immune thrombocytopenia (ITP), with or without immune neutropenia [3]. She was initially diagnosed 5-year prior the current presentation, when she came with complaints of intermittent, episodic bruising and bleeding, with anemic symptoms. Coombs test, and immunoglobulin G (IgG) done in a different center, was positive. Bone marrow aspiration was not pursued.

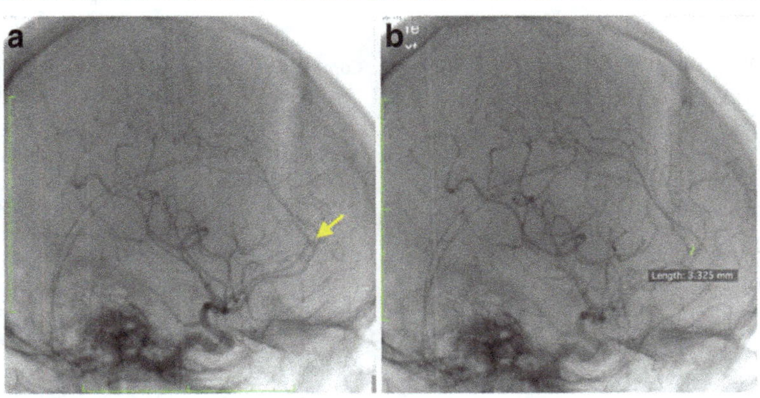

Fig. 2 Diagnostic cerebral angiography images (2**a**, 2**b**) showing; 2**a** – the left sided non-hemorrhaging A3 aneurysm. 2**b** – The aneurysm measured 3.3 mm in its widest diameter, with no other features to suggest haemorrhage

Initially described in 1951, Evans syndrome is a rare clinical entity; occurring in 0.8% to 3.7% of all patients diagnosed with ITP or AIHA at first presentation. This disorder is associated with conditions such as systemic lupus erythematosus (SLE), lymphoproliferative disorders, and primary immune-deficiencies. Patients are at increased risk of bleeding manifestations, and the first line management is steroid therapy, followed by second line pharmacotherapy, rituximab, or splenectomy; when patients do not respond to steroid therapy [3].

Isolated acute non-traumatic convexal SAH are known to be caused by multiple etiological factors; whether vascular (i.e. venous thrombosis, vasculitides) or non-vascular (i.e. abscess, tumors) [1]. Kumar et al. retrospectively reviewed 29 consecutive patients with non-traumatic convexal SAH, and concluded that amyloid angiopathy was frequent in patients aged over 60-years-old, whereas in those younger, a reversible vasoconstriction syndrome is a common cause [4].

Convexal SAH, if present, may appear as an area of slight sulcal hyperattenuation. However, in circumstances where the CT findings are barely visible or nonspecific, MRI is a better option. Useful sequences would include FLAIR, GRE T2, diffusion weighted imaging (DWI), 3D time of flight (TOF) MRA, contrast enhanced venography, and pre- as well as post-gadolinium T1-weighted imaging [2]. We were only able to visualize left high parietal cerebral edema on plain and contrasted CT; thus we proceeded with the above mentioned sequences on our MRI examination.

Interestingly, this revealed an acute SAH at the involved region with small foci of intraparenchymal haemorrhage; manifesting as hyperintensity on FLAIR sequence with corresponding hypointensity on GRE sequence, and accompanying lepto- and pachymeningeal enhancement – which are indirect features of vasculitis. Michel et al. [3] in their study inferred that immune thrombocytopenia occurring in the setting of Evans syndrome may lead to bleeding manifestations. A single predictive factor, eg, thrombocytopenia poorly correlates with bleeding risk in ITP; as this is likely multifactorial [5]. Taking into account the patient's underlying Evans syndrome, as well as indirect features of vasculitis on MRI, we concurred that in our case, MRI finding of isolated convexal SAH was likely the complication [6]. Confirmatory biopsy was not pursued as patient was not keen.

Our experience with this case portrays the additional value of MRI compared to CT; especially when dealing with rare, equivocal cases. However, due to the relative superiority of diagnostic cerebral angiography compared to MRA in detecting small intracerebral aneurysms [7], we decided to still pursue the examination, despite MRA being negative – which revealed an incidental finding of a non-hemorrhaging left sided A3 aneurysm. This strengthened our suspicion – Evans syndrome, as the likely etiology.

Isolated acute non-traumatic convexal SAH is a rare entity, with multiple possible etiological factors. Ruptured aneurysms, being the most common cause of SAH, needs to be excluded as part of the diagnostic workup. The presence of a rare disorder, such as seen in our case, complicates patient management. MRI with select sequences, complemented by diagnostic cerebral angiography prove to be powerful tools in assessment and diagnosis of equivocal cases – thus enabling proper patient management and treatment.

Abbreviations

AIHA: Autoimmune haemolytic anemia; CT: Computed tomography; DWI: Diffusion weighted imaging; FLAIR: Fluid-attenuated inversion recovery; GRE: Gradient echo; ITP: Immune thrombocytopenia; MRA: Magnetic resonance angiography; MRI: Magnetic resonance imaging; MRV: Magnetic resonance venography; SAH: Subarachnoid haemorrhage; SLE: Systemic lupus erythematosus; TOF: Time of flight

Acknowledgements

Not applicable

Funding

None

Authors' contributions

MSF drafted the manuscript and was responsible for overall content, images, and literature review. AM examined the patient and obtained the clinical history. Both authors read and approved the manuscript for publication.

Competing interests

The authors declare that they have no competing interests.

Author details

[1]Department of Medicine, Faculty of Medicine and Health Sciences, Universiti Putra, Serdang, Malaysia. [2]Department of Imaging, Faculty of Medicine and Health Sciences, Universiti Putra Malaysia, Level 3, 43400 Serdang, Selangor, Malaysia.

References

1. Marder CP, Narla V, Fink JR, et al. Subarachnoid haemorrhage: beyond aneurysms. AJR. 2014;202:25–37.
2. Cuvinciuc V, Viguier A, Calviere L, et al. Isolated acute nontraumatic cortical subarachnoid haemorrhage. Am J Neuroradiol. 2010;31:1355–62.

3. Michel M, Chanet V, Dechartres A, et al. The spectrum of Evans syndrome in adults: new insight into the disease based on the analysis of 68 cases. Blood. 2009;
4. Kumar S, Goddeau RP, Selim MH, et al. Atraumatic convexal subarachnoid haemorrhage. Neurology 2010.
5. Neunert CE. Individualized treatment for immune thrombocytopenia: predicting bleeding risk. Semin Hematol. 2013;50:S55–7.
6. Rossi CM, Di Comite G. The clinical spectrum of the neurological involvement in vasculitides. J Neurol Sci. 2009;285:13–21.
7. Okahara M, Kiyosue H, Yamashita M, et al. Diagnostic accuracy of magnetic resonance angiography for cerebral aneurysms in correlation with 3D-digital subtraction angiographic images, a study of 133 aneurysms. Stroke. 2002;33: 1803–8.

16

Cigarette smoking is an independent risk factor for post-stroke delirium

Tae Sung Lim, Jin Soo Lee, Jung Han Yoon, So Young Moon, In Soo Joo, Kyoon Huh and Ji Man Hong*

Abstract

Background: Post-stroke delirium is a common problem in the care of stroke patients, and is associated with longer hospitalization, high short-term mortality, and an increased need for long-term care. Although post-stroke delirium occurs in approximately 10 ~ 30% of patients, little is known about the risk factors for post-stroke delirium in patients who experience acute stroke.

Methods: A total of 576 consecutive patients who experienced ischemic stroke (mean age, 65.2 years; range, 23–93 years) were screened for delirium over a 2-year period in an acute stroke care unit of a tertiary referral hospital. We screened for delirium using the Confusion Assessment Method. Once delirium was suspected, we evaluated the symptoms using the Korean Version of the Delirium Rating Scale-Revised-98. Neurological deficits were assessed using the National Institutes of Health Stroke Scale at admission and discharge, and functional ability was assessed using the Barthel Index and modified Rankin Scale at discharge and 3 months after discharge.

Results: Thirty-eight (6.7%) patients with stroke developed delirium during admission to the acute stroke care unit. Patients with delirium were significantly older (70.6 vs. 64.9 years of age, $P = .001$) and smoked cigarettes more frequently (40% vs. 24%, $P = .033$) than patients without delirium. In terms of clinical features, the delirium group experienced a significantly higher rate of major hemispheric stroke (55% vs. 26%, $P < .001$), exhibited poorer functional performance at discharge and 3 months after discharge, and stayed in hospital significantly longer. Independent risk factors for delirium were older age, history of cigarette smoking, and major hemispheric stroke.

Conclusion: Abrupt cessation of cigarette smoking may be a risk factor for post-stroke delirium in ischemic stroke patients. The development of delirium after stroke is associated with worse outcome and longer hospitalization.

Keywords: Post-stroke delirium, Ischemic stroke, Acute stroke, Smoking

Background

Delirium is an acute confusional state characterized by decreased attention, an altered level of consciousness, and decreased cognitive function including impairment of memory and thought processes [1]. Substantial numbers of delirium cases are caused by systemic inflammation due to an infection or surgery in patients with predisposing risk factors, such as an old age, head trauma, stroke, or underlying dementia [2]. Delirium occurs in 10 ~ 48% of patients during admission and results in poorer functional outcome(s), lower quality of life, and longer hospitalization [3, 4]. Although the exact pathophysiology of delirium is not well understood, decreased acetylcholine and increased dopamine levels are believed to be important factors in this process [5].

Ischemic stroke is caused by an occlusion of the cerebral arteries, which may lead to neurological deficit. Presently, admission to a dedicated stroke care unit is the standard treatment for acute stroke care, and is associated with a long-term benefit in neurological and functional outcomes [6]. However, admission to such an unfamiliar environment for stroke patients and an abrupt cessation of cigarette and alcohol use could induce delirium [7]. Few studies, however, have investigated these variables as risk factors for post-stroke delirium.

The present study evaluated retrospective data from ischemic stroke patients in an acute stroke care unit over a 2-year period to identify the risk factors for post-stroke delirium.

* Correspondence: dacda@hanmail.net
Department of Neurology, School of Medicine, Ajou University, 5 San, Woncheon-dong, Yongtong-gu, Suwon-si, Kyunggi-do 442-749, Republic of Korea

Methods

Subjects and delirium screening

We screened a total of 589 consecutive ischemic stroke patients who were admitted to an acute stroke unit over a 2-year period. Of these patients, 13 were transferred out of the unit within 48 h and, thus, were excluded from further study, yielding a total of 576 patients who were enrolled in the present retrospective study. All patients were evaluated using brain computed tomography (CT) and magnetic resonance imaging (MRI); 28 patients showed negative results after brain magnetic resonance diffusion-weighted imaging.

Delirium was screened daily during admission using the Confusion Assessment Method (CAM) [8]. The diagnosis of delirium was based on the following four features: (i) acute onset and a fluctuating course; (ii) inattention; (iii) disorganized thinking; (iv) an altered level of consciousness. Once delirium was suspected, we evaluated the symptoms using the Korean Version of the Delirium Rating Scale-Revised-98 (K-DRS-R-98), which quantifies multiple parameters, such as the sleep-wake cycle, perception, hallucinations, delusions, mood, language, thought process, psychomotor behavior, orientation, attention, imprinting, short-term memory, and visuospatial orientation [9]. All items were scored on a 4-point scale, resulting in a total score range of 0 to 39.

Definition of variables

We divided all stroke patients into 5 groups based on the modified Oxfordshire Community Stroke Project criteria, which included major hemispheric, minor hemispheric (subcortical), lacunar, brainstem/cerebellar, and non-classified syndromes [10]. We recorded right, left, and bilateral hemispheric involvement. Cigarette smoking was defined as current smoking of any number of cigarettes. Daily alcohol use was defined as consuming more than 3 standard drinks per day. Infection during admission to the stroke unit was defined as a body temperature >38.5 °C [11]. Metabolic derangement was defined as follows: sodium <130 or >150 mmol/L; glucose <2.8 or >14 mmol/L; an estimated glomerular filtration rate <30 mL/min; calcium <2 or >2.75 mmol/L; and oxygen saturation <90% [11]. Neurological deficits were assessed using the National Institutes of Health Stroke Scale (NIHSS) at admission and discharge, and functional ability was assessed using the Barthel Index (BI) and modified Rankin Scale (mRS) at discharge and 3 months after discharge. Follow-up data at 3 months after discharge were available for 414 patients.

Statistics

The Student's t-test and chi-square test were used to compare differences between patients with and without delirium. Logistic regression analysis was performed with delirium occurrence as the dependent variable to analyze independent risk factors and calculate odds ratios (OR). All statistical analyses were performed using SPSS version 18.0 (SPSS Inc., Chicago, IL, USA).

Results

A total of 576 ischemic stroke patients were investigated. The characteristics of these patients are summarized in Table 1. Among them, 368 patients (63.9%) were male and 25% ($n = 144$) were cigarette smokers. The average NIHSS at admission was 5.5 (range 0–29). The comparison between patients with and without post-stroke delirium is shown in Table 2. Thirty-eight of 576 patients (6.7%) developed delirium during admission to the acute stroke care unit. Compared with patients without delirium, patients with delirium were significantly older (70.6 vs. 64.9 years of age, $P = .001$) and smoked cigarettes more frequently (40% vs. 24%, $P = .033$). In terms of clinical features, the delirium group had a significantly higher rate of major hemispheric stroke (55% vs. 26%, $P < .001$), and showed a worse modified Rankin score at discharge (2.5 vs. 1.7, $P = 0.01$) and at 3 months after discharge (2.3 vs. 1.4, $P = .018$) (Fig. 1). The length of hospitalization was longer in patients with delirium (13.3 days vs. 10.7 days, $P = .049$). The univariate and multivariate logistic regression analyses are shown in Table 3. In the multivariate analysis of risk factors for delirium, independent risk factors for delirium were older age (OR = 1.05), cigarette smoking (OR = 2.8), and major hemispheric stroke (OR = 4.8) after adjustment for age, sex and alcohol use.

Discussion

To our knowledge, the present study was the first to identify cigarette smoking as a risk factor for post-stroke delirium. Our 2-year retrospective study suggests that older age, history of cigarette smoking, and major hemispheric stroke are independent risk factors for post-stroke delirium, which is associated with a poorer functional outcome and longer hospitalization.

Table 1 Characteristics of the 576 patients with ischemic stroke

Characteristics	Values
Age, y, mean (range)	65.2 (23–93)
Male sex (%)	368 (63.9)
Hypertension (%)	382 (66.3)
Diabetes (%)	210 (36.5)
Cigarette smoking (%)	144 (25)
Daily alcohol use (%)	35 (6.1)
Underlying dementia (%)	11 (1.9)
NIHSS at admission, mean (range)	5.5 (0–29)
Delirium (%)	38 (6.7)

NIHSS National Institutes of Health Stroke Scale

Table 2 Comparison between patients with and without post-stroke delirium

	Delirium ($n = 38$)	No delirium ($n = 538$)	p-value
Demographics			
Age (SD), y	70.6 (9.3)	64.9 (13.4)	0.001*
Male sex (%)	28 (73)	339 (63)	0.409
Hypertension (%)	29 (76)	353 (65)	0.215
Diabetes (%)	18 (47)	192 (36)	0.164
Smoking (%)	15 (40)	129 (24)	0.049*
Daily alcohol use (%)	5 (13)	30 (5)	0.072
Underlying dementia (%)	0 (0)	11 (2)	1.000
Clinical features			
Involved hemisphere			0.751
Right (%)	16 (42)	194 (36)	
Left (%)	16 (42)	268 (49)	
Bilateral (%)	5 (13)	49 (9)	
Stroke syndrome			<0.001*
Major hemispheric (%)	21 (55)	140 (26)	
Minor hemispheric (%)	3 (8)	76 (14)	
Lacunar syndrome (%)	5 (13)	169 (31)	
Brainstem-cerebellum (%)	2 (5)	84 (16)	
Infection during admission (%)	2 (5)	18 (3)	0.637
Metabolic derangement (%)	8 (21)	87 (16)	0.433
NIHSS at discharge (SD)	5.0 (5.0)	3.5 (5.9)	0.142
BI at discharge (SD)	73.8 (29.0)	83.2 (29.0)	0.065
mRS at discharge (SD)	2.5 (1.6)	1.7 (1.6)	0.010*
Inpatient mortality (%)	0 (0)	4 (1)	1.000
Hospitalization period (SD), d	13.3 (7.0)	10.7 (8.0)	0.049*
BI 3 months after discharge (SD)	79.0 (34.5)	89.5 (25.0)	0.247
mRS 3 months after discharge (SD)	2.3 (1.6)	1.4 (1.5)	0.018*

NIHSS National Institutes of Health Stroke Scale, *BI* Barthel index, *mRS* modified Rankin scale, * p-value < 0.05

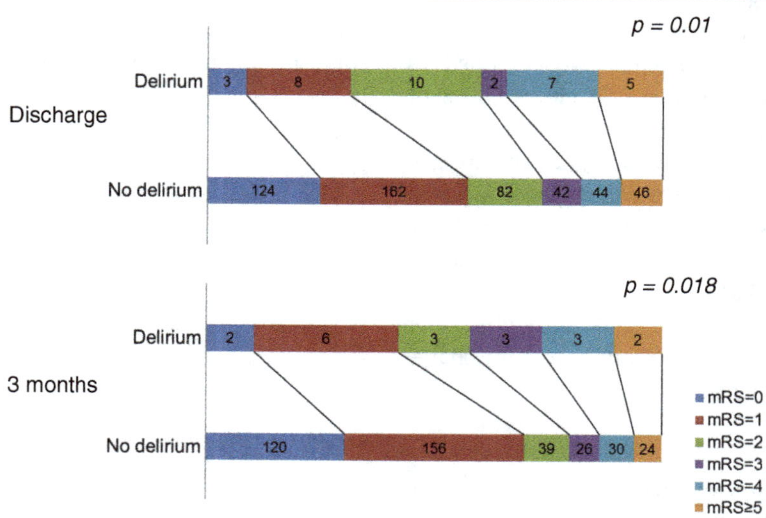

Fig. 1 Modified Rankin Scale (mRS) at discharge and 3 months after discharge

Table 3 Multivariate logistic regression analysis of risk factors for delirium

	Univariate analysis		Multivariate analysis	
	p-value	OR (95% CI)	*p*-value	OR (95% CI)
Age	0.011*	1.038 (1.008 ~ 1.068)	0.004*	1.048 (1.015 ~ 1.081)
Male sex	0.197	1.631 (0.776 ~ 3.428)	0.194	1.748 (0.753 ~ 4.060)
Hypertension	0.182	1.689 (0.783 ~ 3.643)		
Diabetes	0.151	1.622 (0.838 ~ 3.140)		
Cigarette smoking	0.036*	2.068 (1.048 ~ 4.081)	0.015*	2.764 (1.215 ~ 6.289)
Daily alcohol use	0.068	2.566 (0.934 ~ 7.045)	0.345	1.722 (0.558 ~ 5.317)
Right hemispheric involvement	0.377	1.381 (0.674 ~ 2.830)		
Stroke syndrome (ref. lacunar syndrome)				
Major hemispheric	0.001*	5.070 (1.864 ~ 13.791)	0.003*	4.781 (1.711 ~ 13.356)
Minor hemispheric	0.698	1.334 (0.311 ~ 5.726)	0.809	1.199 (0.275 ~ 5.221)
Brainstem-cerebellum	0.227	1.988 (0.652 ~ 6.063)	0.294	1.831 (0.592 ~ 5.664)

* p-valu e < 0. 05

Cigarette smoking was an independent risk factor for post-stroke delirium after adjustment for age, sex, and alcohol use. Although the exact mechanism of the contribution of cigarette smoking to delirium has yet to be elucidated, abrupt cessation of smoking and withdrawal of nicotinic stimulation has been postulated [7]. A recent systematic review suggested that current research evidence is insufficient to determine whether cigarette smoking is a risk factor for delirium [12]. However, there have been no systematic reviews to investigate post-stroke delirium cases with a relatively higher incidence of smoking. In contrast to cigarette smoking, alcohol consumption was not associated with delirium. This finding was consistent with previous studies that also reported no relationship [13, 14]. In clinical practice, alcohol withdrawal syndromes are usually considered in the management of patients with stroke, but cigarette withdrawal is not. Further studies are needed to ascertain the relationship between cigarette smoking, its proper management, such as the nicotine patch, and post-stroke delirium.

The incidence of post-stroke delirium in the present study was 6.7%, which was lower than that reported in previous studies [4]. This lower incidence is possibly due to the younger age of the stroke cohort in the present study. The mean age of the patients in the present study was 65.2 years, which is more than 7 years younger than that reported in recently published studies [11, 13]. The lower incidence of delirium in this young study cohort corresponds well with a study that had a mean age of 57.3, and reported a delirium incidence of 13%, which was significantly lower than other studies that were conducted at that time [14]. Younger age also affected the lower incidence of dementia in this population, as we could not find a significant association between preexisting dementia and post-stroke delirium. Another explanation for the lower incidence of delirium is our inclusion of patients who experienced only ischemic stroke. Previous studies report that post-stroke delirium is more frequent in hemorrhagic stroke than ischemic stroke [14, 15].

Our results suggest that major hemispheric stroke was another independent risk factor for post-stroke delirium. This finding is also consistent with previous studies [13, 16, 17]. However, other clinical factors, such as a high initial NIHSS and right hemispheric stroke, were not identified in the present study. These variables were associated with delirium in some studies [13, 14], but not in other studies [15, 18]. In previous studies, cortical involvement and subsequent decreased cortical function, such as neglect syndrome or aphasia, were important in the pathogenesis of post-stroke delirium [14, 16, 19, 20]. Our study cohort had a higher proportion of patients who experienced lacunar stroke and, in this particular population, the high NIHSS was not the result of cortical dysfunction, but motor-sensory dysfunction, which was not associated with delirium.

Patients with delirium exhibited poorer functional outcome at discharge and experienced longer hospitalization. In addition, the long-term outcome at 3 months after discharge was worse in the delirium group. These findings are consistent with the results of many previous studies [4]. Compared with our study, a recent review and meta-analysis evaluating the outcomes of acute stroke patients with delirium reported higher inpatient mortality (OR = 4.7) and a hospital stay that was 9 days longer [4]. We did not report high inpatient mortality because the overall mortality rate was very low (0.7%) due to the number of patients with a low stroke severity. Longitudinal follow-up of these patients regarding their long-term mortality and morbidity that includes their post-stroke dementia status is needed to elucidate the long-term effect of delirium in young patients who experience low severity stroke.

The present study had limitations stemming from its retrospective design. First, pre-stroke cognition was not measured using a structured questionnaire. Instead, we included the patient history of dementia diagnosis for analysis. Second, anticholinergic medication(s) was not recorded, and the use of this medication could be associated with delirium [17]. Furthermore, a prospective studies involving a structured questionnaire to assess pre-stroke cognition and medication use, and treatment trials involving cholinesterase inhibitors [21, 22] are warranted.

Conclusions

A history of cigarette smoking before stroke may be a risk factor for post-stroke delirium, most likely due to abrupt cessation of smoking, especially in young patients who experience a low severity stroke. The development of delirium after stroke was associated with a worse outcome and longer hospitalization.

Abbreviations

BI: Barthel index; CAM: Confusion assessment method; CT: Computed tomography; K-DRS-R-98: Korean version of the delirium rating scale-revised-98; MRI: Magnetic resonance imaging; mRS: Modified rankin scale; NIHSS: National institutes of health stroke scale

Acknowledgments

Not applicable.

Funding

This work was supported by grants from the Korea Health Technology R&D Project through the Korea Health Industry Development Institute (KHIDI), funded by the Ministry of Health & Welfare (HI14C1967) to Tae Sung Lim.

Authors' contributions

TSL performed the study, acquired data, conducted statistical analyses and drafted the manuscript. JSL, JHY, SYM, ISJ, and KH helped provide data, interpreted the data, and checked the final version of the manuscript. JMH conceptualized the study design, analyzed and interpreted the data, wrote and revised the manuscript. All authors read and approved the final manuscript.

Competing interests

Not applicable.

References

1. Inouye SK, Westendorp RG, Saczynski JS. Delirium in elderly people. Lancet. 2014;383(9920):911–22.
2. van Gool WA, van de Beek D, Eikelenboom P. Systemic infection and delirium: when cytokines and acetylcholine collide. Lancet. 2010;375(9716):773–5.
3. Francis J, Martin D, Kapoor WN. A prospective study of delirium in hospitalized elderly. JAMA. 1990;263(8):1097–101.
4. Shi Q, Presutti R, Selchen D, Saposnik G. Delirium in acute stroke: a systematic review and meta-analysis. Stroke. 2012;43(3):645–9.
5. Maldonado JR. Neuropathogenesis of delirium: review of current etiologic theories and common pathways. Am J Geriatr Psychiatry. 2013;21(12):1190–222.
6. Trialists'Collaboration SU. Organised inpatient (stroke unit) care for stroke. Cochrane Database Syst Rev. 2013;9:CD000197.
7. Lucidarme O, Seguin A, Daubin C, Ramakers M, Terzi N, Beck P, Charbonneau P, du Cheyron D. Nicotine withdrawal and agitation in ventilated critically ill patients. Crit Care. 2010;14(2):R58.
8. Inouye SK, Van Dyck CH, Alessi CA, Balkin S, Siegal AP, Horwitz RI. Clarifying confusion: the confusion assessment method: a new method for detection of delirium. Ann Intern Med. 1990;113(12):941–8.
9. Lee Y, Ryu J, Lee J, Kim H-J, Shin IH, Kim J-L, Trzepacz PT. Korean version of the delirium rating scale-revised-98: reliability and validity. Psychiatry Invest. 2011;8(1):30–8.
10. Bamford J, Sandercock P, Dennis M, Burn J, Warlow C. A prospective study of acute cerebrovascular disease in the community: the Oxfordshire community stroke project–1981-86. 2. Incidence, case fatality rates and overall outcome at one year of cerebral infarction, primary intracerebral and subarachnoid haemorrhage. J Neurol Neurosurg Psychiatry. 1990;53(1):16–22.
11. Miu DK, Yeung JC. Incidence of post-stroke delirium and 1-year outcome. Geriatr Gerontol Int. 2013;13(1):123–9.
12. Hsieh SJ, Shum M, Lee AN, Hasselmark F, Gong MN. Cigarette smoking as a risk factor for delirium in hospitalized and intensive care unit patients. A systematic review. Ann Am Thorac Soc. 2013;10(5):496–503.
13. Oldenbeuving AW, de Kort PL, Jansen BP, Algra A, Kappelle LJ, Roks G. Delirium in the acute phase after stroke: incidence, risk factors, and outcome. Neurology. 2011;76(11):993–9.
14. Caeiro L, Ferro JM, Albuquerque R, Figueira ML. Delirium in the first days of acute stroke. J Neurol. 2004;251(2):171–8.
15. Gustafson Y, Olsson T, Eriksson S, Asplund K, Bucht G. Acute confusional states (delirium) in stroke patients. Cerebrovasc Dis. 1991;1(5):257–64.
16. Sheng AZ, Shen Q, Cordato D, Zhang YY, Chan Y, Kam D. Delirium within three days of stroke in a cohort of elderly patients. J Am Geriatr Soc. 2006; 54(8):1192–8.
17. Carin-Levy G, Mead GE, Nicol K, Rush R, van Wijck F. Delirium in acute stroke: screening tools, incidence rates and predictors: a systematic review. J Neurol. 2012;259(8):1590–9.
18. Shih H, Huang W, Liu C, Tsai T, Lu C, Lu M, Chen P, Tseng C, Jou S, Tsai C. Confusion or delirium in patients with posterior cerebral arterial infarction. Acta Neurol Taiwanica. 2007;16(3):136.
19. Dahl M, Rønning O, Thommessen B. Delirium in acute stroke–prevalence and risk factors. Acta Neurol Scand. 2010;122(s190):39–43.
20. McManus J, Pathansali R, Hassan H, Ouldred E, Cooper D, Stewart R, Macdonald A, Jackson S. The course of delirium in acute stroke. Age Ageing. 2009;38(4):385–9.
21. Klimiec E, Dziedzic T, Kowalska K, Szyper A, Pera J, Potoczek P, Slowik A, Klimkowicz-Mrowiec A. PRospective Observational POLIsh Study on post-stroke delirium (PROPOLIS): methodology of hospital-based cohort study on delirium prevalence, predictors and diagnostic tools. BMC Neurol. 2015;15:94.
22. Oldenbeuving AW, de Kort PL, Jansen BP, Kappelle LJ, Roks G. A pilot study of rivastigmine in the treatment of delirium after stroke: a safe alternative. BMC Neurol. 2008;8:34.

Daily repetitive sensory stimulation of the paretic hand for the treatment of sensorimotor deficits in patients with subacute stroke

Jan C. Kattenstroth[1†], Tobias Kalisch[1,2†], Matthias Sczesny-Kaiser[2], Wolfgang Greulich[3], Martin Tegenthoff[2] and Hubert R. Dinse[1,2,4*]

Abstract

Background: Repetitive sensory stimulation (RSS) adapts the timing of stimulation protocols used in cellular studies to induce synaptic plasticity. In healthy subjects, RSS leads to widespread sensorimotor cortical reorganization paralleled by improved sensorimotor behavior. Here, we investigated whether RSS reduces sensorimotor upper limb impairment in patients with subacute stroke more effectively than conventional therapy.

Methods: A single-blinded sham-controlled clinical trial assessed the effectiveness of RSS in treating sensorimotor deficits of the upper limbs. Patients with subacute unilateral ischemic stroke were randomly assigned to receive standard therapy in combination with RSS or with sham RSS. Patients were masked to treatment allocation. RSS consisted of intermittent 20 Hz electrical stimulation applied on the affected hand for 45 min/day, 5 days per week, for 2 weeks, and was transmitted using custom-made stimulation-gloves with built-in electrodes contacting each fingertip separately. Before and after the intervention, we assessed light-touch and tactile discrimination, proprioception, dexterity, grip force, and subtasks of the Jebsen Taylor hand-function test for the non-affected and the affected hand. Data from these quantitative tests were combined into a total performance index serving as primary outcome measure. In addition, tolerability and side effects of RSS intervention were recorded.

Results: Seventy one eligible patients were enrolled and randomly assigned to receive RSS treatment ($n = 35$) or sham RSS ($n = 36$). Data of 25 patients were not completed because they were transferred to another hospital, resulting in $n = 23$ for each group. Before treatment, sensorimotor performance between groups was balanced ($p = 0.237$). After 2 weeks of the intervention, patients in the group receiving standard therapy with RSS showed significantly better restored sensorimotor function than the control group (standardized mean difference 0.57; 95% CI -0.013–1.16; $p = 0.027$) RSS treatment was superior in all domains tested. Repetitive sensory stimulation was well tolerated and accepted, and no adverse events were observed.

(Continued on next page)

* Correspondence: Hubert.dinse@rub.de
†Equal contributors
[1]Institute for Neuroinformatik, Neural Plasticity Lab, Ruhr-University of Bochum, Bochum, Germany
[2]Department of Neurology, University Hospital Bergmannsheil, Ruhr-University Bochum, Bochum, Germany
Full list of author information is available at the end of the article

(Continued from previous page)

Conclusions: Rehabilitation including RSS enhanced sensorimotor recovery more effectively than standard therapy alone. Rehabilitation outcome between the effects of RSS and standard therapy was largest for sensory and motor improvement; however, the results for proprioception and everyday tasks were encouraging warranting further studies in more severe patients.

Keywords: Neurorehabilitation, Neuroplasticity, Sensorimotor, Stroke, Repetitive sensory stimulation

Background

Sensorimotor impairment resulting from cerebral dysfunction has substantial physical, psychological, and social implications. However, according to a 2014 Cochrane review, no high-quality evidence is available to support interventions currently used as part of routine practice [1]. Triggered by substantial progress in understanding the neuroplasticity mechanisms underlying learning and rehabilitation [2, 3], numerous alternative strategies have been suggested and tested, many of which showed a moderate quality of evidence such as constraint-induced movement therapy, robot-assisted therapy, mirror therapy, central and peripheral nerve stimulation, and virtual reality approaches [1, 3–6]. There is growing evidence that high doses of intervention are more beneficial than low doses. However, rehabilitation outcome is often limited [1, 7].

Recent work in healthy human subjects demonstrated that intensive training may not be necessary to induce behavioral improvement; however, it can be effectively acquired using a complementary approach in which plasticity processes are driven in response to exposure to repetitive sensory stimulation (RSS) [8, 9]. RSS is an approach that targets the cortical areas that represent the site of sensory stimulation to facilitate the development of neuroplastic processes. For example, a few hours of RSS in healthy participants has been demonstrated to alter cortical maps and cortical excitability representing the sites of the RSS stimulation [10, 11]. This becomes possible through the use of long-term potentiation-like sensory stimulation protocols [12, 13].

Despite different backgrounds and rationales for use, the concept of sensory stimulation protocols to induce neuroplasticity processes has attracted substantial interest and is currently being investigated and applied in many laboratories; however, different laboratories use different terms and different stimulation protocols [9, 13–19]. From our perspective, the rationale behind RSS is using the broad knowledge of brain plasticity to design specific sensory stimulation protocols in humans to induce synaptic plasticity to alter perception and behavior. The concept is to translate protocols that induce plasticity at the cellular level, such as long-term potentiation (LTP) and long-term depression (LTD), into sensory stimulation protocols [8, 20]. Central to using RSS is its ability to drive and facilitate neuroplasticity processes [2, 3], a property shared by central stimulation methods such as intracortical microstimulation, transcranial direct current stimulation, and transcranial magnetic stimulation [21–24].

In cellular research, high-frequency stimulation is used to induce LTP, whereas low-frequency stimulation evokes LTD [25, 26]. In the present study, we used a LTP-like protocol consisting of intermittent high-frequency tactile stimulation, which has been used before in healthy subjects to drive improvements in tactile perceptual abilities [12] parallel to cortical reorganization. To explain the changes evoked by RSS, this specific form of stimulation was suggested to evoke LTP-like plasticity processes in the cortical regions representing the stimulated skin sites [8, 27]. As a result, synaptic transmission is altered and cortical processing is remodeled, facilitating the reactivation of the cortical tissue that has preserved some functionality. The behavioral outcome of these processes is reflected in behavioral recovery. Evidence from studies in healthy subjects demonstrated far-reaching cortical remodeling including changes in cortical excitability, expansion of cortical representational areas, and enhanced functional connectivity between the somatosensory and motor cortex [10, 11, 28–30]. Accordingly, the background behind RSS as used in this study differs from electrical mesh-glove stimulation or electrical therapeutic stimulation, although these procedures have been reported to have a beneficial outcome on cortical excitability or muscular strength. In contrast to whole hand stimulation [31, 32], stimulating the tips of the fingers, which are the most densely innervated, allows a very specific targeting of somatosensory cortical representational areas. In fact, available imaging and EEG (electroencephalography) data from healthy participants provide supporting evidence that RSS selectively activates areas in somatosensory and motor areas representing the fingers and the hand [10, 11, 28, 33].

Various forms of electrical stimulation exist that are currently used in rehabilitation with mixed results [1, 34–38]. For each of these approaches, a wide range of stimulation parameters are in use, and the underlying mechanisms mediating beneficial effects remain largely to be clarified. FES (functional electrical stimulation) is applied to induce contraction of muscles to support motor action. On the other hand, so-called therapeutic electrical stimulation methods are applied to improve performance after the termination of stimulation, such as NMES (neuromuscular electrical stimulation), EMG (electromyography) -triggered electrical stimulation (EMG-ES), and TENS (transcutaneous electrical nerve stimulation). While TENS was introduced for pain treatment, effects observed after NMES and EMG-ES are assumed to be related to repetitive muscle contractions. Accordingly, as described above, the underlying principle and the aimed target of RSS differs from that of FES, NMES, or TENS.

The effects of RSS protocols have been extensively explored in both healthy young and elderly adults. When applied to the fingers, substantial improvements in the tactile, haptic, proprioceptive, and sensorimotor performance parallel to cortical reorganization were demonstrated [10, 12, 14, 15, 28, 39]. The effectiveness of this form of learning is assumed to arise from using stimulation protocols optimized to alter synaptic transmission and efficacy [8, 9]. While a number of studies used RSS or variants of this approach in patients with subacute or chronic stroke, RSS has yet to be implemented in routine clinical practice. So far, available studies indicate mixed effects in the treatment of upper limb impairment [16–18, 27, 39–43]. These mixed results of sensory stimulation come from the fact that sensory stimulation as method is poorly defined. Sensory stimulation approaches employ various forms of stimulation and testing parameters, as well as quite varying treatment times ranging from single applications to long-term treatment. This almost certainly causes large variability in outcome parameters. From our view, a significant advantage of repetitive stimulation is its passive nature, which does not require active subject participation, making the intervention substantially easier to implement and more acceptable to the individual.

Therefore, here we aimed to address whether in routine clinical practice, repetitive stimulation reduces sensorimotor deficits following stroke more effectively than conventional therapy. Based on our previous data about the effectiveness of RSS [10, 14, 15, 28, 39–41], we hypothesized that the standard therapy with RSS is superior to standard therapy with sham RSS. Because stroke can affect diverse aspects of sensorimotor abilities, we undertook a broad objective behavioral assessment evaluating the sensory, proprioceptive, sensorimotor, and motor functions. In addition, we aimed to find out tolerability, acceptance, and possible side-effects of the glove-applied RSS intervention.

Methods

Study design

This randomized single-blinded sham-controlled clinical trial was designed as a proof-of-concept study evaluating the effectiveness, safety, and compliance. We recruited 71 patients with subacute ischemic stroke with contralateral sensorimotor impairment from the HELIOS rehabilitation clinic in Hagen Ambrock, Germany. The study was done in accordance with the ethical principles from the Declaration of Helsinki. It was approved by the Ethics Committee of Ruhr-University of Bochum. All patients provided verbal and written informed consent before participating. The trial was retrospectively registered January 31, 2012 under DRKS00003515 (https://www.drks.de/drks_web/navigate.do;jsessionid=AEE2585CCB82A22A2B285470B37C47C8?navigationId=results). Recruitment had started June 15, 2010, lasting until December 31, 2012).

Patients

The main inclusion criteria were age of 40–70 years, a diagnosis of unilateral subacute ischemic stroke, i.e., a left or right medial cerebral artery infarction with contralateral sensorimotor deficits of the upper limbs 3 to 4 weeks post-ictus. Also, patients should have low levels of spasticity, and stimulation perception thresholds of at least 20 mA. All patients were right-handed. Patients with mild transient ischemic stroke lasting fewer than 24 h, hemorrhagic stroke, and carotid artery dissection, history of cerebrovascular disease, wearing a pacemaker, aphasia, or cognitive impairment that prevented completion of the assessment were excluded. Patients were recruited with the help of physio- and occupational therapists at the rehabilitation clinic. The most relevant criteria patients did not meet were spasticity and paresis. Because of difficulties with patient enrollment, we widened the age criterion to patients aged 30 to 90 years.

Randomization and masking

Patients were randomly assigned to either the target or control group using block randomization. The selection was performed using a computer-generated random list of numbers. Randomization sequence was accessible to assessors of the main outcome parameters only. No attempts were made to balance for gender or the side of the stroke. The patients and assessors of clinical tests (modified Rankin Scale, National Institutes of Health Stroke Scale, modified Barthel Index, Medical Research Council Scale, Frenchay Arm Test, and Wolf Motor Function Test) were masked to the treatment allocation. There was no masking for assessors of the main outcome parameters. Individual RSS intervention was conducted and monitored by therapists, who had received a detailed instruction in handling RSS procedures. Table 1 shows the baseline characteristics of the study patients.

Procedures

Interventions were commenced 3.5 weeks (median) after stroke. Patients allocated to the control group received the same standard stroke rehabilitation as patients allocated to the intervention (RSS) group. Patients received RSS with standard rehabilitation therapy (physio- and ergotherapy) or sham RSS with standard therapy (control). In case of sham RSS, patients assumed a subthreshold treatment, although zero mA was applied. RSS treatment was applied independent of the schedule of the standard therapy. Total RSS-treatment time for both groups was 2 weeks (10 days).

Interventions

RSS and sham RSS were applied for 45 min daily on the affected hand of the patients from both treatment groups. The stimulation sequence was the same as described previously [12] and consisted of 20-Hz bursts for 1.4 s with 5-s inter-train intervals, and a ramp/fall time of 0.3 s and 0.2 ms pulse width. The pulse trains were delivered with 2-channel stimulation devices. To account for innervation of the fingers, the stimulation for the predominantly median nerve-innervated fingers d1-d3 (the thumb, index, and middle finger) and the predominantly ulnar nerve-innervated fingers d4 and d5 (ring and little finger) was separately controlled and delivered. The pulses were transmitted by custom-made stimulation gloves that had built-in electrodes (1 × 4 cm) located on the first and third segment of each finger (cathode proximal). In the RSS group, the intensity of the stimulation was set individually at the highest values that the patient could easily tolerate for an extended period, but without reaching pain levels. For sham RSS, the same stimulation parameters and the same stimulation gloves were used, except for the stimulation intensity, which was set at zero mA.

Table 1 Demographic and baseline characteristics

	RSS group (n = 23)	Sham RSS group (*n* = 23)
Sex		
• Male	18 (78%)	16 (70%)
• Female	5 (22%)	7 (30%)
Age (years)	64 (34–86)	59 (43–89)
White ethnic origin	23	23
Lesion side (Rt./Lt.)	9/14	13/10
Handedness (R/L/A)	23//	23//
mRS	3.35 ± 0.71	3.26 ± 0.75
NIHSS	5.48 ± 3.22	5.17 ± 2.23
mBI	64.8 ± 34.59	66.5 ± 34.23
MRCA	3.73 ± 2.68	3.98 ± 1.49
FAT	3.48 ± 6.19	3.50 ± 5.99
WMTF	11.76 ± 16.43	11.56 ± 14.91

depicts demographic and baseline characteristics. Data are mean (±SD) or number (%). Abbreviations: Lesion side (Rt./Lt.) = right hemisphere/left hemisphere; Handedness (R/L/A) = right handed, left handed, ambidextrous; mRS = modified Rankin Scale; NIHSS = National Institutes of Health Stroke Scale; mBI = modified Barthel Index; MRCA = Medical Research Council Scale; FAT = Frenchay Arm Test; WMTF = Wolf Motor Function Test

The standard rehabilitation therapy consisted of individualized programs depending on the degree and nature of patients' sensorimotor impairment. Occupational therapy was applied according to the concepts of Bobath, Affolter, and Perfetti. ADL training (activities of daily living) consisted of self-care tasks such as bathing and showering, dressing, self-feeding, food preparation, and personal hygiene. Cognitive therapy and activation training were offered to facilitate the recovery for independent living. Special and curative education included pottery-making to foster the skills and abilities of patients, and to prepare them for coping with confinement.

To characterize the upper extremity performance of the patients prior to the study, we used several clinical scales closely related to the performance of tasks in everyday life: the modified Rankin Scale (ranging 0 to 6, 0 no symptoms), National Institutes of Health Stroke Scale (ranging 0 to 42, 0 no symptoms), modified Barthel Index (ranging 0 to 100, 100 no symptoms), Medical Research Council Scale (ranging 0 to 5, 5 no symptoms), Frenchay Arm Test (ranging 0 to 5, 5 no symptoms), and 15 tasks of the Wolf Motor Function Test (ranging 0 to 15, 15 no symptoms). According to these scales, patients were characterized by slight to moderate to severe moderate disability. All patients had some sensory loss of various degrees.

Objective assessment of sensorimotor behavior

To quantify the behavior objectively, the following tests were performed before and after the end of treatment for the affected and the non-affected limbs. The term non-affected is meant to indicate the limb contralateral to the site of stroke, which does not exclude potential changes in performance. Testing was performed in one session with breaks in between, total time varied between 60 and 90 min.

Tactile performance

Touch thresholds were evaluated by probing the fingertips of the left and right index finger with von Frey filaments (Marstocknervtest, Marburg, Germany) [27, 44]. The test kit contained 16 different filaments calibrated to forces ranging from 0.25–294 mN in the logarithmic scale. We used a staircase procedure during which patients were required to close their eyes and report when they perceived an indentation of the skin on their fingertips. The applied forces, starting with a noticeable stimulus, were decreased in a stepwise manner until the subjects no longer perceived the stimulus (lower boundary) and then increased until the stimulus was perceived again (upper boundary). This procedure was repeated 5 times resulting in 10 values that were averaged to provide the touch threshold.

The grating orientation task (GOT) was tested in 2 alternative forced-choice paradigms [27, 45]. A set of nine custom-made hemispherical plastic domes with gratings cut into their surfaces, i.e., parallel ridges and grooves of equal widths for each dome, were applied to the tip of the index finger using a holder with a calibrated spring (150 mN) to enable constant application force. The width of the ridges and grooves (spatial frequency) varied from 0.5 to 9.5 mm. Each dome was presented 20 times. Immediately after touching the plastic domes, patients were asked to report the perceived orientation. The grating discrimination threshold was defined as the level at which 75% of the responses were correct and was determined by interpolating between the groove widths with 75% correct responses. The performance at this level was midway between chance and perfect performance.

Nine-hole peg test (9-HPT)

To measure upper extremity fine motor performance (dexterity), we used the 9-HPT, a brief standardized quantitative test of the upper extremity function [46]. We measured the time needed separately for placing the pegs in and out of holes.

Grip strength

Grip strength was measured 3 consecutive times for each hand with a Jamar hand dynamometer (Sammons Preston Inc., Bolingbrook, IL). Subjects were asked to stand up and hold the dynamometer with the arms parallel to the body [47]. The final results were the average across 3 trials.

Jebsen-Taylor hand function test (JTHFT)

For the assessment of the functional hand motor skills, we used JTHFT [48]. Three of the 7 JTHFT subtests were performed: (1) picking up small objects and placing them in a can (SOP); (2) picking up small objects with a teaspoon and placing them in a can (FEED); and (3) stacking checkers (STACK). The performance was evaluated based on the time needed to complete each subtest.

Joint position sense (JPS) assessment

The JPS assessment was conducted using the "Bochum Joint Position Sense Assessment" (BJPSA) as reported previously [39]. Patients were asked to compare lightweight polystyrene balls of different diameters held in the affected hand to a reference ball held in their non-affected hand, and to report, without visual information, if the tested ball located in the affected hand was larger, smaller, or equal in volume. In 3 consecutive subtests, the complete set of polystyrene balls (diameters: 3 cm, 5 cm, 6 cm, 7 cm, 8 cm, 10 cm, and 12 cm) were compared to a small reference (diameter 5 cm), mid-sized reference (diameter 7 cm), and large-sized reference (diameter 12 cm). The performance was assessed by calculating the number of errors (ERRnumb, a total of 21 decisions) and the weight of errors (ERRweight, calculated as the volume difference between the reference and test object). Previous studies showed that ERRweight and ERRnumb are independent parameters characterizing the joint position sense [39].

Outcomes

The primary outcome was the sensorimotor performance (total performance index – TPI) as obtained by a combination of 10 different quantitative objective tests shown in Tables 3 and 4, which were performed before and after the end of treatment for both the affected and the non-affected limb: touch thresholds, acuity threshold (grating orientation task thresholds), dexterity using 9-HPT, grip strength, and proprioceptive functions according to JPS assessment and subtests of JTHFT: picking up small objects and placing them in a can (SOP), picking up small objects with a teaspoon and placing them in a can (FEED), and stacking checkers (STACK).

To compare and average performances across all tests and all subjects in both groups, we calculated the normalized performance indices (IP) [49]. This approach has been used by Engeneer et al. some years ago to combine performance data across different tasks that have different dimensions which cannot be averaged [50]. In addition, pooling the performance obtained for each single task into a single total performance index increases statistical power. IPs were calculated for each subject and each test. IP was calculated using the formula $(wp\text{-}ip)/(wp\text{-}bp)$, where for a given test independent of a specific time point of measurement wp is the worst performance of all subjects, ip is the individual performance, and bp is the best performance of all subjects. IPs ranged between 1 and 0, where the best IP was 1, and the worst was 0. The total performance index (TPI) was calculated by averaging IP data across all 10 tests performed.

The secondary outcome measures were the performances in the 4 domains covering similar functional domains. For the "Sensory" domain, IP data from the touch threshold and 2-point discrimination tests were averaged. For the "Motor" domain, the IP data from the grip strength and the 9-HPT were averaged. For the "Proprioception" domain, IP data from the number and weight of errors of the JPS tests were averaged. For the

"Everyday" domain, IP data from the 3 JTHFT subtests were averaged.

The tertiary outcomes were self-reported assessments of patients from both groups on adverse effects were administered after the completion of treatment including the questions: "was RSS pleasant or unpleasant?" and "what was the type of sensation evoked by RSS?" The user feedback obtained by a custom-made questionnaire included the ease of use, perceived sensations during RSS, positive and negative aspects of RSS, willing to continue using after release from the hospital, and willing to recommend to others.

Post-assessments were conducted within the week directly after completing the 10 days of treatments (mean 2.9 ± 1.4 days).

Statistical analysis

Data were checked for normal distribution using Shapiro-Wilk test. Descriptive statistics were compiled. Normally distributed data were reported as the mean and standard deviation (SD). We used Student's t-test to detect the differences between the 2 groups after the intervention. For statistical evaluation of the demographic and baseline characteristics, we used Student's t- and Chi-square tests. Moreover, we computed effect sizes according to Cohen's d, and confidence intervals. As early intervention with RSS following a stroke has not yet been tested, sample size and power calculation was therefore based on effect sizes in the range of 0.4 to 0.8 obtained in previous studies on sensory and dexterity performance [27], unpublished data, as well as data from elderly age-matched healthy participants [51], which using an alpha of < .05 and a power of 80% resulted in a sample size of 32 per group. To accommodate the possible drop outs, we selected a sample size of 70. All calculations were performed using Microsoft Excel 2010 and SPSS version 18.0 and higher.

Results

Participants

We screened 143 patients with ischemic stroke for eligibility. Seventy-one of these patients were enrolled and randomly assigned to either the standard therapy with RSS (35 patients) or the control group receiving standard therapy with sham RSS (36 patients; see Fig. 1). Seventy-two were excluded (54 not meeting inclusion criteria, 18 refused to participate). In the RSS group, 23 of 35 patients completed the treatment; a similar proportion (23 of 36 patients) completed the treatment in the sham RSS group. Twelve (RSS group) and 13 patients (sham RSS group) did not complete their assigned treatment because they were transferred to another hospital or daycare. This transfer was solely caused by organizational reasons or personal reasons of the patients. The patients transferred showed no particularities and were within the range documented for the successfully treated patients according to the age, type of infarct, and severity of behavioral impairment. The data of 46 patients ($n = 23$ each group) were assessed for further statistical analysis. All patients received all interventions per protocol.

The baseline demographic and clinical characteristics were not statistically significantly different in both groups (Table 1). Both groups were balanced for age and gender. Most importantly, prior to the intervention, there were no differences in the clinical tests: the modified Rankin Scale, National Institutes of Health Stroke Scale, modified Barthel Index, Medical Research Council

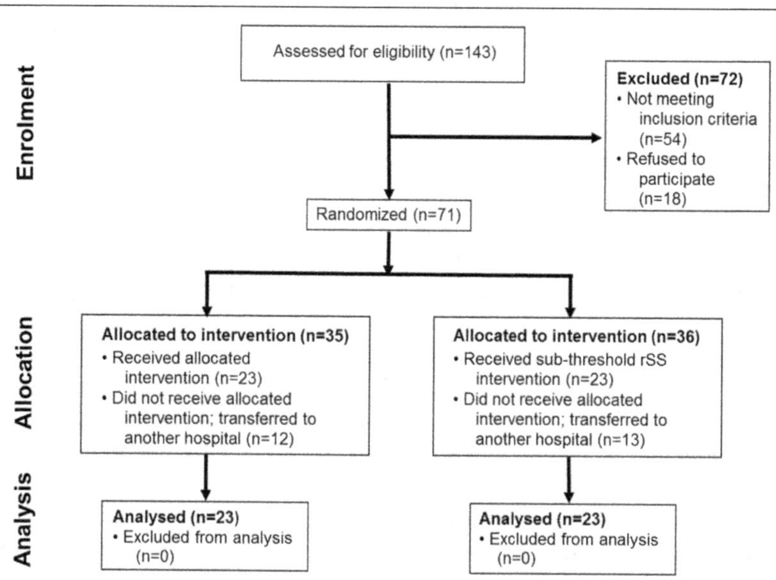

Fig. 1 Consort flow diagram

Scale, Frenchay Arm Test, and Wolf Motor Function Test. Furthermore, no significant differences were found in the averaged total performance at baseline.

Stimulation-glove: Acceptance and side effects

The glove-based RSS treatment was well tolerated, and no negative side-effects were recorded. The average stimulation intensity was 10.4 ± 3.87 mA for the median nerve-innervated fingers, and 6.7 ± 3.46 mA for the ulnar nerve-innervated fingers. The sensations perceived during RSS were rated neutral to pleasant. The ease of use was reported as uncomplicated, possibly because in all cases, therapists assisted putting on the stimulation gloves. About two-third of the patients group were interested in continuing using RSS glove-treatment later in their homes.

Average sensorimotor performance: Total performance score

As the first step in providing an overview of the effects of RSS versus sham RSS, we calculated the total performance index based on the performance of all 10 tests applied. An IP of 0 indicates the worst performance, characterized by the patient not being able to perform the task. An IP of 1 indicates the best performance observed for the non-affected limb. Accordingly, an IP of 0.5 indicates that the performance of the patient was at about 50%. The patients in both groups showed improvement; however, the beneficial effects were 2-fold higher in the RSS group compared to the sham RSS group (RSS: 22.9% gain from 0.56 to 0.68, $p < 0.00005$; sham RSS: 10.0% gain from 0.64 to 0.70, $p < 0.05$; the pre-post differences were significant between both groups using Student's t-test; one-sided $p = 0.027$). While 17 out of 23 patients (74%) in the RSS group improved their performance by more than 0.05 points on the TPI scale, only 10 out of 23 patients (43%) in the sham RSS group showed such an improvement. Calculating the Standardized Mean Difference (SMD) revealed an effect size of 0.54 for RSS versus sham RSS therapy. The differential effectiveness was also apparent in the effect size calculated separately for each group, which was 0.55 for the RSS and 0.28 for the sham RSS groups.

To analyze how the positive effects were distributed across the more severe or, less severe patients, we subdivided the data according the median of the total performance index of both groups into more (TPI < 0.6; RSS $n = 12$; sham RSS $n = 9$) and less (TPI > 0.6; RSS $n = 11$; sham RSS $n = 14$) affected patients. For the RSS therapy, we found a pre-post improvement of 0.17 ± 0.04 ($p = 0.001$; 47.5% improvement) for the more severe patient subgroup and 0.07 ± 0.02 ($p = 0.0005$; 10.3% improvement) for the less severe patient subgroup. In contrast, for those receiving sham RSS, we found a pre-post improvement for the more severe patient subgroup of 0.08 ± 0.05 ($p = 0.132$; 23.6% improvement) and 0.04 ± 0.02 ($p = 0.042$; 5.6% improvement) for the less severe subgroup. These data indicate that the RSS therapy was particularly efficient in the more severe group of patients.

Performance gain in the sensory and motor domains

Next, we analyzed how the effects of treatment were distributed across the four domains characterizing sensorimotor performance. Table 2 shows the pre- and post-IPs together with percent change and effect size for the 4 domains "sensory," "motor," "proprioception," and "everyday tasks." This breakdown of performance and performance gain into separate areas of sensorimotor performance showed that only the RSS therapy evoked significant improvement in all 4 domains indicative of a wide-range effectiveness targeting sensorimotor functions. In contrast, although the standard therapy resulted in measurable gains, only the changes in the performance of sensory and motor domains were significantly enhanced.

The raw performance values for each of the 10 subtests performed are listed in Tables 3 ab and 4. Both treatment groups showed distinct improvement in the performance. However, while 9 out of 10 subtests in the RSS group showed significant improvement post-treatment, only 1 out of 10 subtests improved significantly in the standard treatment group.

Discussion

We demonstrated that the combined treatment of sensorimotor deficits in patients with subacute stroke using RSS in combination with standard therapy was superior to standard therapy with sham RSS. We used a broad range of quantitative assessments of sensorimotor performance to investigate the therapeutic potential of RSS, consisting of intermittent high-frequency tactile stimulation in combination with standard rehabilitation therapy. An advantage of RSS was observed in all domains tested evaluating sensory, motor, and proprioceptive as well as everyday task performance. Although sham RSS had positive effects in all 10 assessments used, only 1 in 10 showed significant improvement, while in the RSS group 9 of 10 tests showed significant improvement. The superior efficiency of the RSS therapy was mirrored in the effect sizes for the RSS and sham RSS (Cohen's d). Although overall less patients could be analyzed than originally planned, we still could obtain significant differences between treatment groups. This was possible because of pooling the performance obtained for each single task into a single total performance index, which increased statistical power.

Table 2 Mean normalized performance index pre and post standard therapy with RSS and sham RSS

	Standard therapy with RSS					Standard therapy with sham RSS					Group difference
	pre	post	% gain	Cohens d	t-test	pre	post	% gain	Cohens d	t-test	t-test
Sensory	0.51 ± 0.24	0.68 ± 0.24	33.39	0.72	$p = 0.0004$	0.65 ± 0.23	0.70 ± 0.25	6.95	0.18	$p = 0.034$	$p = 0.0044$
Motor	0.50 ± 0.28	0.63 ± 0.24	27.26	0.52	$p = 0.0001$	0.54 ± 0.31	0.64 ± 0.28	17.42	0.31	$p = 0.030$	$p = 0.087$
Proprio	0.84 ± 0.12	0.88 ± 0.10	4.87	0.37	$p = 0.022$	0.87 ± 0.10	0.89 ± 0.07	2.40	0.25	$p = 0.318$	$p = 0.220$
everyday	0.50 ± 0.41	0.65 ± 0.36	30.63	0.40	$p = 0.012$	0.55 ± 0.39	0.68 ± 0.30	23.79	0.38	$p = 0.194$	$p = 0.419$

depicts mean (±SD) normalized performance index pre and post therapy effects of standard therapy with RSS ($N = 23$) and with sham RSS (N = 23) for the 4 domains tested. Mean (SD) normalized performance index pre and post therapy for the affected side are shown

Table 3 Raw data standard therapy with RSS vs. sham RSS – affected side

	standard therapy with RSS				standard therapy with sham RSS				
	PRE	POST	Cohens d	t-test pre-post	PRE	POST	Cohens d	t-test pre-post	t-test group difference
a									
Frey (mN)	87.73 ± 130.36	34.77 ± 85.75	0.48	0.035	48.91 ± 93.94	34.20 ± 83.72	0.17	0.318	0.083
GOT (mm)	7.50 ± 1.84	6.23 ± 2.26	0.61	<0.001	6.42 ± 2.31	5.95 ± 2.45	0.20	0.135	0.023
9-hole in (sec)	146.09 ± 90.24	108.83 ± 87.45	0.42	0.001	136.09 ± 95.38	95.87 ± 86.76	0.44	0.002	0.441
9-hole out (sec)	61.57 ± 85.69	27.65 ± 49.05	0.49	0.034	58.48 ± 85.92	44.00 ± 77.92	0.18	0.387	0.195
Grip strength (kg)	15.55 ± 10.77	20.18 ± 12.26	0.40	0.001	20.44 ± 13.56	21.28 ± 10.90	0.07	0.601	0.026
JTHFT Picking objects (sec)	65.24 ± 48.38	47.72 ± 44.93	0.38	0.034	54.20 ± 40.64	33.60 ± 28.78	0.58	0.106	0.386
JTHFT Feeding (sec)	73.91 ± 48.26	52.40 ± 47.50	0.45	0.031	68.55 ± 46.91	56.25 ± 49.71	0.25	0.327	0.286
JTHFT Stacking (sec)	51.03 ± 52.78	38.10 ± 49.72	0.25	0.295	40.069 ± 52.23	31.23 ± 48.19	0.19	0.500	0.442
b									
Frey (mN)	1.67 ± 1.95	1.66 ± 3.12	0.01	0.979	1.66 ± 4.38	1.46 ± 2.60	0.06	0.604	0.645
GOT (mm)	5.15 ± 2.53	4.61 ± 2.57	0.21	0.135	4.14 ± 2.07	3.98 ± 2.06	0.08	0.273	0.543
9-hole in (sec)	23.14 ± 6.95	20.23 ± 4.84	0.49	0.01	21.43 ± 8.72	20.43 ± 7.78	0.12	0.159	0.232
9-hole out (sec)	9.0 ± 2.45	8.14 ± 1.83	0.40	0.062	8.30 ± 2.87	8.22 ± 2.45	0.03	0.833	0.547
Grip strength (kg)	32.90 ± 8.63	34.75 ± 9.47	0.20	0.105	35.21 ± 11.43	34.60 ± 10.58	0.06	0.494	0.481
JTHFT Picking objects (sec)	12.60 ± 4.03	12.74 ± 3.52	0.04	0.973	12.12 ± 5.37	11.99 ± 4.56	0.03	0.759	0.373
JTHFT Feeding (sec)	16.08 ± 6.25	14.66 ± 4.51	0.26	0.269	16.09 ± 10.07	14.38 ± 6.84	0.20	0.172	0.649
JTHFT Stacking (sec)	4.07 ± 1.23	3.67 ± 1.22	0.32	0.298	3.64 ± 1.47	3.35 ± 1.01	0.23	0.136	0.354

JHTFT Jepsen Taylor hand function test

a and b depict the effects of standard therapy with RSS and standard therapy with sham RSS for all 8 unilateral tests used (N = 23 each). Mean (±SD) raw performance values (dimensions indicated in the left columns) pre- and post-therapy for the affected (a) and not affected (b) arm are shown

Table 4 Raw data standard therapy with RSS vs. sham RSS – bilateral task JPS = Joint Position Sense

	standard therapy with RSS				standard therapy with sham RSS				
	PRE	POST	Cohens d	t-test pre-post	PRE	POST	Cohens d	t-test pre-post	t-test group difference
JPS Number of Errors	4.53 ± 4.52	3.90 ± 2.46	0.34	0.072	4.00 ± 2.67	3.53 ± 2.03	0.22	0.509	0.304
JPS Weight of Errors	205.95 ± 223.91	119.60 ± 210.35	0.37	0.0075	148.52 ± 152.34	108.90 ± 123.46	0.27	0.204	0.136

depicts the effects of standard therapy with RSS and standard therapy with sham RSS for the bilateral task testing the Joint Position Sense (N = 23 each). Mean (±SD) raw performance values (dimensions indicated in the left columns) pre- and post-therapy are shown

RSS treatment using finger-tip stimulation gloves

For treatment, patients were equipped with custom-made stimulation gloves that had built-in electrodes contacting the first and third segment of each finger, enabling clearly defined stimulation of the fingertips. Accordingly, the gloves used employ a profoundly different strategy than the so-called mesh gloves or whole hand stimulation approaches, where the entire hand is diffusely stimulated. As stimulation thresholds vary between the median and ulnaris nerves innervating the fingers, a 2-channel stimulation device allowed for the separate adjustment of the stimulation intensities. We did not observe adverse events. All patients tolerated the gloves without problems. The evoked sensations on the fingers and hand were described as tickling or massaging. To exclude the possibility that offering a new therapy might bias patients [52], we used a sham protocol to control for the effects of RSS. This procedure allowed the use of the stimulation gloves in the control group without actual stimulation. Compared to a waiting group without employing the stimulation glove, our procedure can be regarded as more conservative in that it most likely preserves possible placebo effects mediated by using a new stimulation device.

RSS effects on sensory and motor function

The largest gains were observed for sensory functions, which was not unexpected when using a sensory stimulation protocol. On the other hand, the improvement in the sensory functions was rather limited in the control group receiving standard therapy (33.3% vs. 6.9%). This latter finding fits with previous studies that reported that following motor rehabilitation, beneficial effects on pure sensory functions are small. Given that learning and re-learning skilled motor behavior requires largely intact somatosensory input processing, it is conceivable that when the sensation is corrupted, motor recovery is corrupted as well. It has, therefore, been assumed that patients with somatosensory deficits following stroke experience more persistent motor impairment than those without such deficits [5].

The RSS group improved not only sensory functions to a greater extent than the sham RSS group alone but also motor recovery, which was similarly better in the RSS group (27.2% vs. 17.4%). The effectiveness of RSS in improving motor function was also demonstrated for healthy adults and elderly individuals [51, 53, 54]. However, how RSS affects the motor system requires further research. It is assumed, for example, that the transfer of beneficial effects to sensorimotor behavior is based on the interconnections between the somatosensory and motor cortex [55, 56], which in turn elicits reorganization in the motor cortex. Moreover, dexterity tasks, such as the pegboard task, require intact tactile inputs for fine manipulation. In such cases, the net motor behavior is dependent on working tactile functions. We, therefore, assume that a combination of task-inherent tactile-motor requirements together with motor cortex reorganization results in the motor recovery observed following RSS.

In the present study, no follow-up assessment was planned; however, outcome measures were obtained within the week following the 10 days of treatment. However, other studies employing RSS treatment have shown that in patients with chronic stroke, restoration effects were fully preserved in a 4-week follow-up [41].

It should be noted that comparable beneficial effects have been reported following RSS applied alone, without any parallel standard therapy. In patients with chronic stroke, improvement in the sensory and motor abilities was reported following 4 weeks of RSS treatment [41]. In patients with chronic brain injury where the cerebrovascular dysfunctions dated as far back as 13 years, the application of RSS for up to 76 weeks showed substantial improvements in the sensory and motor abilities [27].

Comparison with other therapeutic measures

Most rehabilitation strategies for upper extremity stroke patients target motor recovery. However, among the many sources that contribute to incomplete recovery, poor recovery of somatosensation might play a crucial role. There is agreement that intact afferent sensory information is not only crucial for tactile and haptic but also for motor performance [7, 57]. As a consequence, maintained compromised sensory abilities further complicate motor function recovery. According to a recent systematic review on upper extremity motor recovery, more than 10 different forms of interventions had been reviewed including fitness training or physical fitness training, repetitive task training, electrostimulation, biofeedback, force and position feedback, bilateral training, constraint-induced movement therapy, or mental practice with motor imagery [5]. SMDs for a 95% CI differed widely ranging from 0.09 for upper limb high intensity training to 0.84 for mental practicing with motor imagery, or 0.47 for electrostimulation (arm function) and 0.12 hand function (cf. 0.57 as found in our present study). A similar difference for hand and arm function was found following constraint-induced movement therapy (0.17 vs. 0.73). As the authors concluded, these data indicate that large amount of research is still required to define much more clearly the interventions that carry most benefits.

Implication for everyday life

An issue of substantial relevance is the question in how far improvements that can be measured in a laboratory or clinical surrounding are transferable into everyday life, which constitutes the major challenge of all intervention strategies. In a recent case study with patients with chronic brain injuries, comparable effect sizes for gains of sensorimotor performance as reported here were obtained using RSS treatment [27]. One patient reported subjectively improved sensations when touching object surfaces with the fingers, which had not been possible before the intervention. In contrast, another patient showed improvements in all investigated aspects of sensorimotor performance, but reported little impact on changes of everyday life activity of the affected extremity. It is conceivable that this patient got used to not involving the affected hand and arm, a phenomenon captured in the concept of "compensatory learned non-use of the affected limb" [58, 59]. As a consequence, such individuals might not be able to recognize gains of sensorimotor performance induced by an intervention although they can be demonstrated under laboratory conditions. Given that, further investigations are necessary to improve therapeutic programs to facilitate re-using affected limbs.

Comparing affected and non-affected side

A detailed analysis of the baseline performance and treatment effects of the non-affected side were beyond the scope of this study. However, after the 2 weeks of treatment, patients of both groups improved their performance to a variable degree. Further studies are needed to investigate in how far this improvement is due to mere task learning and practicing. Alternatively, it is conceivable that neural reorganization of the stroke-affected cortical sites also mediated behavioral changes of the contralateral limb.

Strengths and limitations

Overall this study is limited by the substantial number of patients that were transferred to other hospitals, which thus could not participate in the study. After 2 weeks of the intervention, patients in the group receiving standard therapy with RSS showed better restored sensorimotor function than the control group as indicated by significant differences in the total performance index. However, when comparing group differences for the data obtained for each of the ten different tasks, only 2 tasks (2-point discrimination and grip strength) were significantly different, although the within group pre-post comparisons indicated much stronger benefits for the RSS therapy. This discrepancy is most likely due to the huge interindividual variability. It is conceivable that having included the additional patients that had been transferred to other locations, the resulting higher statistical power would have revealed significant differences for the other tasks as well. Despite the fact that both groups were statistically balanced, the patients in the standard therapy group with sham RSS were slightly less affected. It is therefore possible that the degree of affectedness might impose some influence on the overall outcome of this study. However, the recorded beneficial effects of the RSS group will inform future trials. The main strength of this study is that we assessed a broad range of parameters characterizing sensorimotor behavior objectively, and reported the effects of RSS and sham RSS not only separately for these markers, but that we combined them into domains characterizing diverse aspects of sensorimotor behavior. Another limitation is that we did not include patients with more severe impairments. This, together with larger samples sizes to accommodate the high interindividual variability present in this group of subacute stroke patients, is recommended in future trials.

Conclusion

This randomized sham-controlled clinical study demonstrated that application of RSS using an LTP-like protocol in combination with standard therapy enhances a broad range of sensorimotor performances of the upper limb in patients with subacute stroke over a treatment period of only 2 weeks. Furthermore, this outcome was superior to the effects observed with the standard therapy alone. Patients tolerated the RSS treatment well, as well as the RSS application using a custom-made stimulation glove. Further studies are needed to obtain more detailed insight into the mechanisms underlying this approach. In addition, future trials will have to explore effectiveness in more severe patients, and additional beneficial effects might be obtained when using RSS as a priming procedure before behavioral training. Independent of this, the present data, when confirmed by future studies, suggest that the application of RSS combined with standard therapy might be another promising approach in the treatment of sensorimotor impairments after stroke compared to the current standard treatment practice.

Abbreviations

9-HPT: Nine-Hole Peg Test; ADL: Activities of daily living; BJPSA: Bochum Joint Position Sense Assessment; CI: Confidence intervals; d1: Thumb; d2: Index finger; d3: Middle finger; d4: Ring finger; d5: Little finger; EEG: Electroencephalography; EMG: Electromyography; ERRnumb: Number of errors (Bochum Joint Position Sense Assessment); ERRweight: Weight of errors (Bochum Joint Position Sense Assessment); FAT: Frenchay Arm Test; FEED: Picking up small objects with a teaspoon (Jebsen-Taylor Hand Function Test); FES: Functional electrical stimulation; GOT: Grating orientation task; IP: Normalized performance indices; JPS: Joint position sense; JTHFT: Jebsen-Taylor Hand Function Test; LTD: Long-term depression; LTP: Long-term potentiation; mBI: Modified Barthel Index; MRCA: Medical Research Council Scale; mRS: Modified Rankin Scale; NIHSS: National Institutes of Health Stroke Scale; NMES: Neuromuscular electrical stimulation; R/L/A: Right handed/left handed/ambidextrous; RSS: Repetitive sensory stimulation; SD: Standard deviation; SMD: Standardized mean difference; SOP: Picking up small objects (Jebsen-Taylor Hand Function Test); STACK: Stacking checkers (Jebsen-Taylor Hand Function Test); TENS: Transcutaneous electrical nerve stimulation; TPI: Total performance index; WMFT: Wolf Motor Function Test

Acknowledgements

We thank Dr. Jan Wrede for help with data management, the therapists for their commitment, and all the patients who kindly participated.

Funding

H.R.D. and M.T. acknowledge support of a SFB grant 874 (TP A1, TP A5) by the German Research Foundation (Deutsche Forschungsgemeinschaft, DFG). T.K. was supported by a Grant from FoRUM (F637–08). J.C.K. was a recipient of a stipend from the Allgemeiner Deutscher Tanzlehrerverband (ADTV). All authors had full access to all the data in the study and the corresponding author had final responsibility for the decision to submit for publication.

Authors' contributions

JCK, TK, MT, and HRD conceived the study. JCK, TK, WG, MT, and HRD designed and coordinated the study. JCK and TK collected data. JCK, TK, MSK, and HRD analysed data. JCK, TK, MSK, WG, MT, and HRD interpreted data. JCK, TK, MSK, and HRD wrote a first draft. All authors read and approved the final manuscript.

Competing interests

MT and HRD hold patents for sensory stimulation procedures (DE102012110062.4; DE102006042156B4; US 8,046,083 B2). The other authors declare that they have no competing interests.

Author details

[1]Institute for Neuroinformatik, Neural Plasticity Lab, Ruhr-University of Bochum, Bochum, Germany. [2]Department of Neurology, University Hospital Bergmannsheil, Ruhr-University Bochum, Bochum, Germany. [3]HELIOS Hospital Hagen Ambrock, Hagen, Germany. [4]Department of Neuroinformatik, Neural Plasticity Lab, Ruhr-University of Bochum, Building NB3, 44780 Bochum, Germany.

References

1. Pollock A, Farmer SE, Brady MC, et al. Interventions for improving upper limb function after stroke. Cochrane Database Syst Rev. 2014;12(11): CD010820.
2. Adams HP Jr, Nudo RJ. Management of patients with stroke: is it time to expand treatment options? Ann Neurol. 2013;74:4–10. doi: https://doi.org/10.1002/ana.23948.
3. Alonso-Alonso M, Fregni F, Pascual-Leone A. Brain stimulation in poststroke rehabilitation. Cerebrovasc Dis. 2007;24(Suppl 1):157–66.
4. Oujamaa L, Relave I, Froger J, Mottet D, Pelissier JY. Rehabilitation of arm function after stroke literature review. Ann Phys Rehabil Med. 2009;52:269–93.
5. Langhorne P, Coupar F, Pollock A. Motor recovery after stroke: a systematic review. Lancet Neurol. 2009;8:741–54.
6. Dobkin BH. Strategies for stroke rehabilitation. Lancet Neurol. 2004;3:528–36.
7. Celnik P, Hummel F, Harris-Love M, Wolk R, Cohen LG. Somatosensory stimulation enhances the effects of training functional hand tasks in patients with chronic stroke. Arch Phys Med Rehabil. 2007;88:1369–76.
8. Dinse HR, Kattenstroth JC, Gattica Tossi MA, Tegenthoff M, Kalisch T. Sensory Stimulation for Augmenting Perception, Sensorimotor Behavior and Cognition In: Segev I, Markram H, editors. Augmenting Cognition. Lausanne: EPFL Press; 2011. p. 11–39.
9. Beste C, Dinse HR. Learning without training. Curr Biol. 2013;23:R489–99.
10. Pleger B, Foerster AF, Ragert P, et al. Functional imaging of perceptual learning in human primary and secondary somatosensory cortex. Neuron. 2003;40:643–53.
11. Hoeffken O, Veit M, Knossalla F, et al. Sustained increase of somatosensory cortex excitability by tactile coactivation studied by paired median nerve stimulation in humans correlates with perceptual gain. J Physiol. 2007;584:463–71.
12. Ragert P, Kalisch T, Bliem B, Franzkowiak S, Dinse HR. Differential effects in human tactile discrimination behavior evoked by tactile high- and low-frequency stimulation. BMC Neurosci. 2008;9:9.
13. Teyler TJ, Hamm JP, Clapp WC, et al. Long-term potentiation of human visual evoked responses. Eur J Neurosci. 2005;21:2045–50.
14. Dinse HR, Kalisch T, Ragert P, Pleger B, Schwenkreis P, Tegenthoff M. Improving human haptic performance in normal and impaired human populations through unattended activation-based learning. ACM Trans Appl Perc. 2005;2:71–88.
15. Dinse HR, Kleibel N, Kalisch T, Ragert P, Wilimzig C, Tegenthoff M. Tactile coactivation resets age-related decline of human tactile discrimination. Ann Neurol. 2006;60:88–94.
16. Wu CW, Seo HJ, Cohen LG. Influence of electric somatosensory stimulation on paretic-hand function in chronic stroke. Arch Phys Med Rehabil. 2006;87: 351–7.
17. Conforto AB, Kaelin-Lang A, Cohen LG. Increase in hand muscle strength of stroke patients after somatosensory stimulation. Ann Neurol. 2002;51:122–5.
18. McDonnell MN, Hillier SL, Miles TS, Thompson PD, Ridding MC. Influence of combined afferent stimulation and task-specific training following stroke: a pilot randomized controlled trial. Neurorehabil Neural Repair. 2007;21:435–43.
19. Clapp WC, Hamm JP, Kirk IJ, Teyler TJ. Translating long-term potentiation from animals to humans: a novel method for noninvasive assessment of cortical plasticity. Biol Psychiatry. 2012;71:496–02.
20. Bliss TV, Collingridge GL. A synaptic model of memory: long-term potentiation in the hippocampus. Nature. 1993;361:31–9.
21. Elsner B, Kugler J, Pohl M, Mehrholz J. Transcranial direct current stimulation (tDCS) for improving activities of daily living, and physical and cognitive functioning, in people after stroke. Cochrane Database Syst Rev. 2016; 21;3: CD009645.
22. Hao Z, Wang D, Zeng Y, Liu M. Repetitive transcranial magnetic stimulation for improving function after stroke. Cochrane Database Syst Rev. 2013; 31(5):CD008862.

23. Plautz EJ, Barbay S, Frost SB, et al. Post-infarct cortical plasticity and behavioral recovery using concurrent cortical stimulation and rehabilitative training: a feasibility study in primates. Neurol Res. 2003;25:801–10.
24. Plow EB, Carey JR, Nudo RJ, Pascual-Leone A. Invasive cortical stimulation to promote recovery of function after stroke: a critical appraisal. Stroke. 2009; 40:1926–31.
25. Malenka RC, Bear MF. LTP and LTD: an embarrassment of riches. Neuron. 2004;44:5–21.
26. Nicoll RA, Malenka RC. Contrasting properties of two forms of long-term potentiation in the hippocampus. Nature. 1995;377:115–8.
27. Kattenstroth JC, Kalisch T, Tegenthoff M, Dinse HR. Long-term sensory stimulation therapy improves hand function and restores cortical responsiveness in patients with chronic cerebral lesions. Three single case studies. Front Hum Neurosci. 2012;6:244.
28. Dinse HR, Ragert P, Pleger B, Schwenkreis P, Tegenthoff M. Pharmacological modulation of perceptual learning and associated cortical reorganization. Science. 2003;301:91–4.
29. Ridding MC, McKay DR, Thompson PD, Miles TS. Changes in corticomotor representations induced by prolonged peripheral nerve stimulation in humans. Clin Neurophysiol. 2001;112:1461–9.
30. Freyer F, Reinacher M, Nolte G, Dinse HR, Ritter P. Repetitive tactile stimulation changes resting-state functional connectivity – implications for treatment of sensorimotor decline. Front Hum Neurosci. 2012;6:144.
31. Dimitrijević MM, Stokić DS, Wawro AW, Wun CC. Modification of motor control of wrist extension by mesh-glove electrical afferent stimulation in stroke patients. Arch Phys Med Rehabil. 1996;77:252–8.
32. Lin KC, Huang PC, Chen YT, Wu CY, Huang WL. Combining afferent stimulation and mirror therapy for rehabilitating motor function, motor control, ambulation, and daily functions after stroke. Neurorehabil Neural Repair. 2014;28:153–62. doi: https://doi.org/10.1177/1545968313508468.
33. Pleger B, Dinse HR, Ragert P, et al. Shifts in cortical representations predict human discrimination improvement. Proc Natl Acad Sci U S A. 2001;98:12255–60.
34. Wilson RD, Page SJ, Delahanty M, et al. Recovery after stroke: a randomized controlled trial comparing EMG-triggered, cyclic, and sensory electrical stimulation. Neurorehabil Neural Repair. 2016;30:978–87.
35. de Kroon JR, van der Lee JH, MJ IJ, Lankhorst GJ. Therapeutic electrical stimulation to improve motor control and functional abilities of the upper extremity after stroke: a systematic review. Clin Rehabil. 2002;16:–350, 360.
36. Farmer SE, Durairaj V, Swain I, Pandyan AD. Assistive technologies: can they contribute to rehabilitation of the upper limb after stroke? Arch Phys Med Rehabil. 2014;95:968–85.
37. Nascimento LR, Michaelsen SM, Ada L, Polese JC, Teixeira-Salmela LF. Cyclical electrical stimulation increases strength and improves activity after stroke: a systematic review. J Physiother. 2014;60:22–30. https://doi.org/10.1016/j.jphys.2013.12.002.
38. Meilink A, Hemmen B, Seelen HA, Kwakkel G. Impact of EMG-triggered neuromuscular stimulation of the wrist and finger extensors of the paretic hand after stroke: a systematic review of the literature. Clin Rehabil. 2008;22: 291–305. doi: https://doi.org/10.1177/0269215507083368.
39. Kattenstroth JC, Kalisch T, Kowalewski R, Tegenthoff M, Dinse HR. Quantitative assessment of joint position sense recovery in subacute stroke patients: a pilot study. J Rehabil Med. 2013;45:1004–9.
40. Dinse HR, Boland J, Kalisch T, et al. Repetitive sensory stimulation training in stroke. Eur J Neurol. 2008;15(Suppl. 3):400.
41. Smith P, Dinse H, Kalisch T, Johnson M, Walker-Batson D. Effects of repetitive electrical stimulation to treat sensory loss in persons poststroke. Arch Phys Med Rehabil. 2009;90:2108–11.
42. Sawaki L, Wu CW, Kaelin-Lang A, Cohen LG. Effects of somatosensory stimulation on use-dependent plasticity in chronic stroke. Stroke. 2006;37:246–7.
43. Conforto AB, Ferreiro KN, Tomasi C, et al. Effects of somatosensory stimulation on motor function after subacute stroke. Neurorehabil Neural Repair. 2010;24:263–72.
44. Semmes J, Weinstein S, Ghent L, Teuber HL. Performance on complex tactual tasks after brain injury in man: analyses by locus of lesion. Am J Psychol. 1954;67:220–40.
45. Van Boven RW, Johnson KO. The limit of tactile spatial resolution in humans: grating orientation discrimination at the lip, tongue, and finger. Neurology. 1994;44:2361–6.
46. Oxford Grice K, Vogel KA, Le V, Mitchell A, Muniz S, Vollmer MA. Adult norms for a commercially available nine hole peg test for finger dexterity. Am J Occup Ther. 2003;57:570–3.
47. Schmidt RT, Toews JV. Grip strength as measured by the Jamar dynamometer. Arch Phys Med Rehabil. 1970;51:321–7.
48. Jebsen RH, Taylor N, Trieschmann RB, Trotter MJ, Howard LA. An objective and standardized test of hand function. Arch Phys Med Rehabil. 1969;50:311–9.
49. Kattenstroth JC, Kalisch T, Holt S, Tegenthoff M, Dinse HR. Six months of dance intervention enhances postural, sensorimotor, and cognitive performance in elderly without affecting cardio-respiratory functions. Front Ag Neurosci. 2013;5:5. doi: https://doi.org/10.3389/fnagi.2013.00005.
50. Engineer ND, Engineer CT, Reed AC, et al. Inverted-U function relating cortical plasticity and task difficulty. Neuroscience. 2012;205:81–90.
51. Kalisch T, Tegenthoff M, Dinse HR. Improvement of sensorimotor functions in old age by passive sensory stimulation. Clin Interv Aging. 2008;3:673–90.
52. Krishna R, Maithreyi R, Surapaneni KM. Research bias: a review for medical students. J Clin Diagn Res. 2010;4:2320–4.
53. Kowalewski R, Kattenstroth JC, Kalisch T, Dinse HR (2012) Improved acuity and dexterity, but unchanged touch and pain thresholds following repetitive sensory stimulation of the fingers. Neural Plasticity 2012, ID 974504, doi: https://doi.org/10.1155/2012/974504
54. Ladda AM, Pfannmoeller JP, Kalisch T, et al. Effects of combining 2 weeks of passive sensory stimulation with active hand motor training in healthy adults. PLoS One. 2014;9:e84402.
55. Jones EG, Coulter JD, Hendry SH. Intracortical connectivity of architectonic fields in the somatic sensory, motor and parietal cortex of monkeys. J Comp Neurol. 1978;181:291–47.
56. Pavlides C, Miyashita E, Asanuma H. Projection from the sensory to the motor cortex is important in learning motor skills in the monkey. J Neurophysiol. 1993;70:733–41.
57. Ebied AM. The role of cutaneous sensation in the motor function of the hand. J Orthopaedic Res. 2003;22:862–6.
58. Krakauer JW. Motor learning: its relevance to stroke recovery and neurorehabilitation. Curr Opin Neurol. 2006;19:84–90.
59. Grotta JC, Noser EA, Ro T, et al. Constraint-induced movement therapy. Stroke. 2004;35:2699–701.

18

Rheumatoid meningitis presenting with a stroke-like attack treated with recombinant tissue plasminogen activator

Masashi Akamatsu, Futaba Maki*, Hisanao Akiyama, Daisuke Hara, Masashi Hoshino and Yasuhiro Hasegawa

Abstract

Background: Rheumatoid meningitis presenting with a stroke-like attack (RMSA) is a rare manifestation of rheumatoid arthritis (RA). When the patients arrive within the time-window for recombinant tissue plasminogen activator (rt-PA) infusion therapy, no diagnostic protocol has been established.

Case presentation: A 55-year-old woman was brought by ambulance to our hospital with complaints of sudden-onset dysarthria and left arm numbness. The National Institutes of Health Stroke Scale (NIHSS) score was 5, and the Alberta Stroke Program Early CT Score was 8. She was diagnosed with acute embolic stroke. At 4 h, 6 min after onset, intravenous administration of rt-PA (alteplase, 0.6 mg/kg) was started. Her neurological deficits improved rapidly, and her NIHSS score was 1. Brain MRI was then performed. There was no hemorrhagic transformation, but the MRI findings were not compatible with ischemic stroke. She had a past history of RA diagnosed 6 months earlier, and she had been treated with methotrexate (10 mg daily). She was diagnosed with RMSA, and continuous infusion of methylprednisolone 1000 mg daily was started for 3 days. The high signal intensity on the FLAIR image disappeared.

Conclusion: CT-based decision-making for rt-PA injection is reasonable, but MRI is needed for the early diagnosis of RMSA. In this case, it is particularly important that neither adverse events nor bleeding complications were observed, suggesting the safety of CT-based thrombolytic therapy in RMSA.

Keywords: Rheumatoid meningitis, Recombinant tissue plasminogen activator (rt-PA), Stroke mimics

Background

Rheumatoid vasculitis is one of the extra-articular complications of rheumatoid arthritis (RA). Although there are no reports of the exact incidence of central nervous system (CNS) complications of RA [1], they are considered relatively rare [2]. Among such complications, there have been extremely rare cases of sudden-onset focal brain dysfunction that resemble a stroke, which is known as rheumatoid meningitis presenting with a stroke-like attack (RMSA) [3, 4]. The safety of thrombolysis in patients with this stroke mimic remains uncertain. The case of a patient who, 6 months after being diagnosed with RA, was brought to our hospital as an emergency due to the abrupt onset of focal neurologic deficits and was treated with recombinant tissue plasminogen activator (rt-PA) is described.

Case presentation

A 55-year-old woman suddenly became aware of speech difficulty and left arm numbness at 11:00 pm while talking on the telephone with her daughter. She was taken to our hospital by ambulance. She was diagnosed with RA 6 months earlier, and she had been treated with methotrexate at a dose of 10 mg daily. She had a history of herpes simplex encephalitis from 30 years earlier. Her blood pressure was 155/80 mmHg, pulse rate was 80/min and regular,

* Correspondence: f2maki@marianna-u.ac.jp
Department of Neurology, St. Marianna University School of Medicine, 2-16-1 Sugao, Miyamae, Kawasaki, Kanagawa 216-8511, Japan

and temperature was 36.8 °C. ECG was normal. Her Glasgow coma scale was E4 V4 M6, and neurological examination demonstrated dysarthria, left hemiparesis, left-sided sensory impairment, and left unilateral spatial neglect. The National Institutes of Health Stroke Scale (NIHSS) score was 5. Head computed tomography (CT) showed no obvious lesions except effacement of the cortical sulci in the right parietal lobe, and the Alberta Stroke Program Early CT Score (ASPECTS), a 10-point quantitative topographic CT scan score, was 8. No arterial occlusion or stenosis was seen on CT angiography (Fig. 1). Blood tests showed a platelet count of $274 \times 10^3/\mu l$, prothrombin time International Normalized Ratio (PT-INR) of 1.07, and activated partial thromboplastin time (APTT) of 25.6 s (APTT-control 31.0 s). She was diagnosed with acute embolic stroke in the right parietal lobe, and there was no contraindication to intravenous thrombolytic therapy. At 4 h 6 min after onset, intravenous administration of rt-PA was started in accordance with the Japanese guideline (alteplase, 0.6 mg/kg) [5, 6], with an intravenous drip infusion of 30 mg of edaravone, a free radical scavenger, over a period of 30 min. Head magnetic resonance imaging (MRI) was performed at 1 h, 30 min after starting the thrombolytic therapy (Fig. 2). Diffusion-weighted imaging (DWI) demonstrated a linear high-intensity lesion in the right temporoparietal cortex. The lesion was demonstrated to be a hypodense linear lesion on the apparent diffusion coefficient (ADC) map image. This cortical lesion was seen as a high-intensity lesion on fluid-attenuated inversion recovery (FLAIR) imaging. These MRI findings were not compatible with acute ischemic stroke. Her neurological deficits improved rapidly (NIHSS score: 5 on admission, 1 at 24 h after thrombolytic therapy).

Contrast-enhanced head MRI performed on hospital day 3 found that the high signals on DWI had disappeared. However, the FLAIR image showed ribbon-like high signals in the cerebral cortex, and no contrast effect was observed (Fig. 3). In subsequent additional tests, rheumatoid factor (RF) was 85 IU/L and anti-cyclic citrullinated peptide (CCP) antibody was elevated at 223.7 U/mL, while myeloperoxidase-anti-neutrophil cytoplasmic antibodies (MPO-ANCA) and proteinase-3-anti-neutrophil cytoplasmic antibodies (PR3-ANCA) were negative. Lumbar puncture showed a cell count of 68/μL (monocytes 14, polynuclear cells 54), protein 40 mg/dL, and glucose 52 mg/dL. Single photon emission computed tomography (SPECT) performed on day 6 showed decreased accumulation in the right temporoparietal region. Spinal fluid testing performed on day 10 showed an elevated interleukin-6 (IL-6) of 271 pg/mL, but anti-CCP antibody was normal at 3.7 U/mL. Because of the elevated cerebrospinal fluid cell count and the patient's history of herpes encephalitis, she was temporarily treated with a continuous intravenous infusion of acyclovir 1500 mg/day until the polymerase chain reaction test was confirmed to be negative. The patient was finally diagnosed with RMSA. On day 16, continuous infusion of methylprednisolone 1000 mg daily was started for 3 days, and it was repeated on day 28. Her symptoms then gradually resolved, and the high signal on the FLAIR image also disappeared. The patient was discharged on day 44 with only a slight attention deficit on neurological examination.

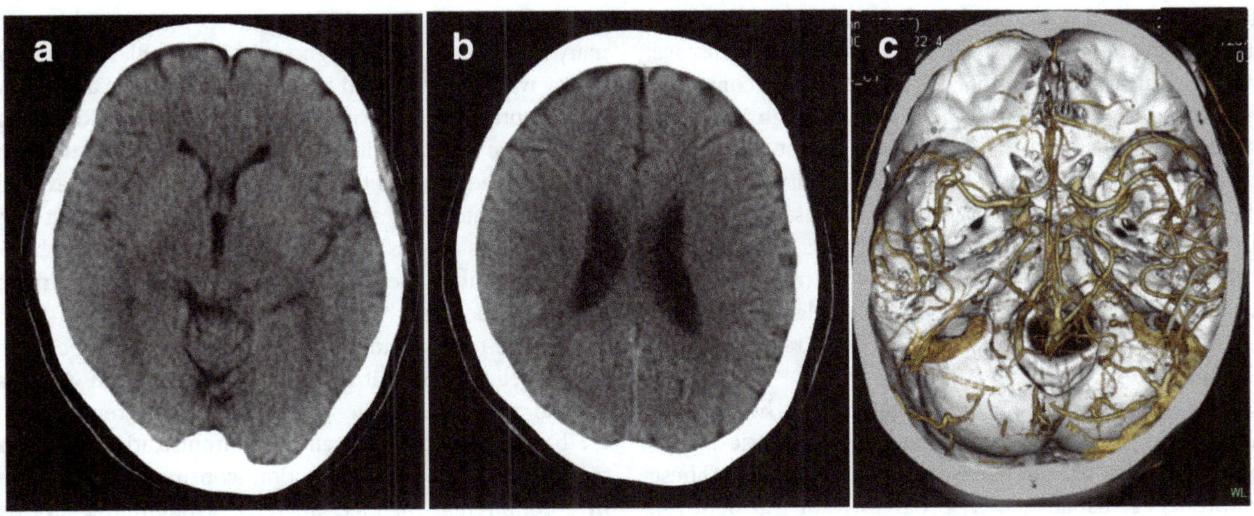

Fig. 1 Brain CT images (**a**, **b**) do not show a hypodense area at admission, but equivocal findings of effacement in the right temporoparietal region (ASPECT score, 8). CT angiography (**c**) shows no vascular occlusion or stenosis. CT = computerized tomography, ASPECTS = Alberta Stroke Program Early CT Score

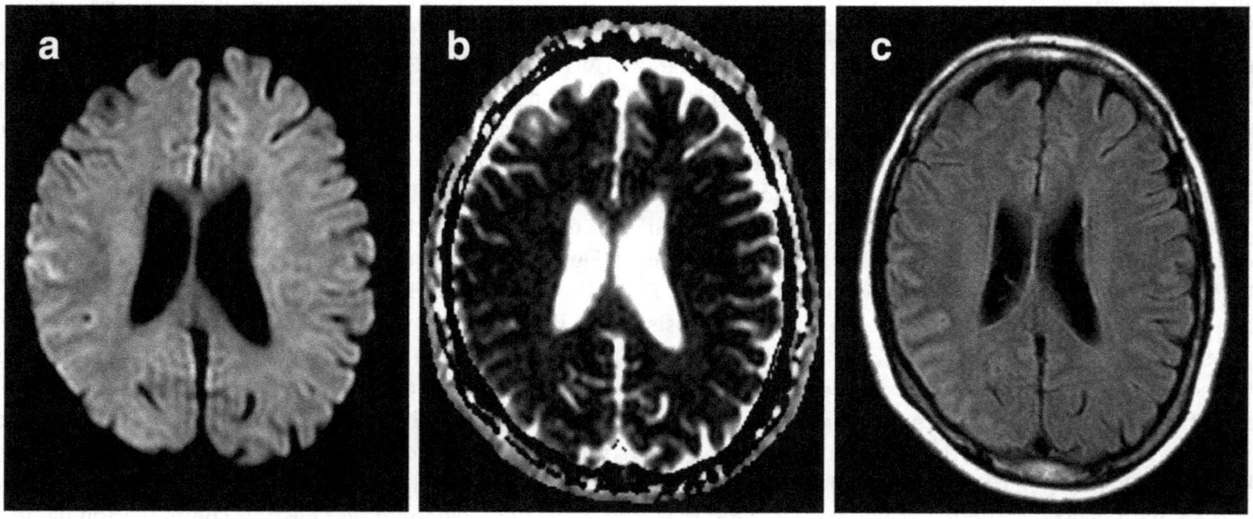

Fig. 2 MRI findings at day 1. DWI (**a**) demonstrates a linear high-intensity lesion in the right frontotemporal cortex. Reduced ADC of this lesion is seen on the ADC map (**b**), and this cortical lesion appears as a high-intensity lesion on the FLAIR image (**c**). MRI = magnetic resonance imaging, DWI = diffusion-weighted imaging, ADC = apparent diffusion coefficient, FLAIR = fluid attenuated inversion recovery

Discussion

The present patient was given a diagnosis of "definite RA" based on a score of 7 on the new 2010 American College of Rheumatology/European League Against Rheumatism (ACR/EULAR) classification criteria. Rheumatoid meningitis (RM) is defined as a condition of inflammation of the meninges or dura mater with cell infiltration. In the past, most RM cases were reported as autopsy cases, but the number of reported cases of RM has increased along with the increase in patients with long-standing disease and advances in diagnostic imaging. In many patients, RA is in the very early stage or long-term, and the disease duration is said to be ≥10 years for 50% or more [3]. The present patient presented 6 months after her diagnosis of RA, and thus was in the comparatively early stages of the disease; although the reason for that is not clear, it is consistent with earlier reports [4, 7]. In addition, although it did not correlate with her arthritic activity, the onset of RM was sudden and at a time when her RA activity was stable. There have been scattered reports of the use of intravenous steroid pulse therapy and oral steroids (1 mg/kg) [7, 8]. Even when there is improvement with treatment, caution must be taken regarding possible relapse or recurrence, but the present patient did not relapse up to 6 months later.

The neurological symptoms of RM may be hemiplegia, monoplegia, impaired consciousness, psychiatric symptoms, convulsions, and sensory impairment [9]. These symptoms are usually slowly progressive or transient [8]. However, to the best of our knowledge, there have been only two reports of patients with stroke-like attacks [10, 11]. Thus, although rare, RMSA should be included in the differential diagnosis of acute ischemic stroke presenting within the time window for thrombolytic therapy. The present patient is the first reported case of RMSA who was treated with rt-PA. MRI is helpful to differentiate it from acute ischemic stroke when it is performed on hospitalization.

The present patient's symptoms rapidly improved in the early treatment period. It is possible that the brain-protective agent, edaravone, which was co-administered with intravenous rt-PA, contributed to that improvement. Free radicals have been reported to be involved in the vasculitis and cerebral edema associated with encephalitis as well [12], and to some extent, the administration of edaravone, a free radical scavenger, makes sense. MRI and biopsy findings have primary importance in the diagnosis of RM [3, 8]. A meningeal biopsy was not performed in the present case because of the rapid improvement of symptoms. However, the MRI findings were typical for RM, with a restricted ADC at the subarachnoid space adjacent to the right frontotemporal cortex. This linear high-intensity lesion on DWI is thought to result from proteinaceous debris accumulation at the subarachnoid space adjacent to the parenchyma with meningeal lymphocytic infiltration [13].

Evidence to date indicates that endovascular procedures provide clinical benefit in selected patients with acute ischemic stroke [14–17]. Thus, there is a trend toward CT-based prompt intravenous administration of rt-PA treatment rather than more time-consuming MRI study. In a comprehensive meta-analysis, stroke-mimicking patients were found to have a significantly lower risk for intracerebral hemorrhage and systemic complications than patients with true acute ischemic stroke (risk ratio = 0.33,

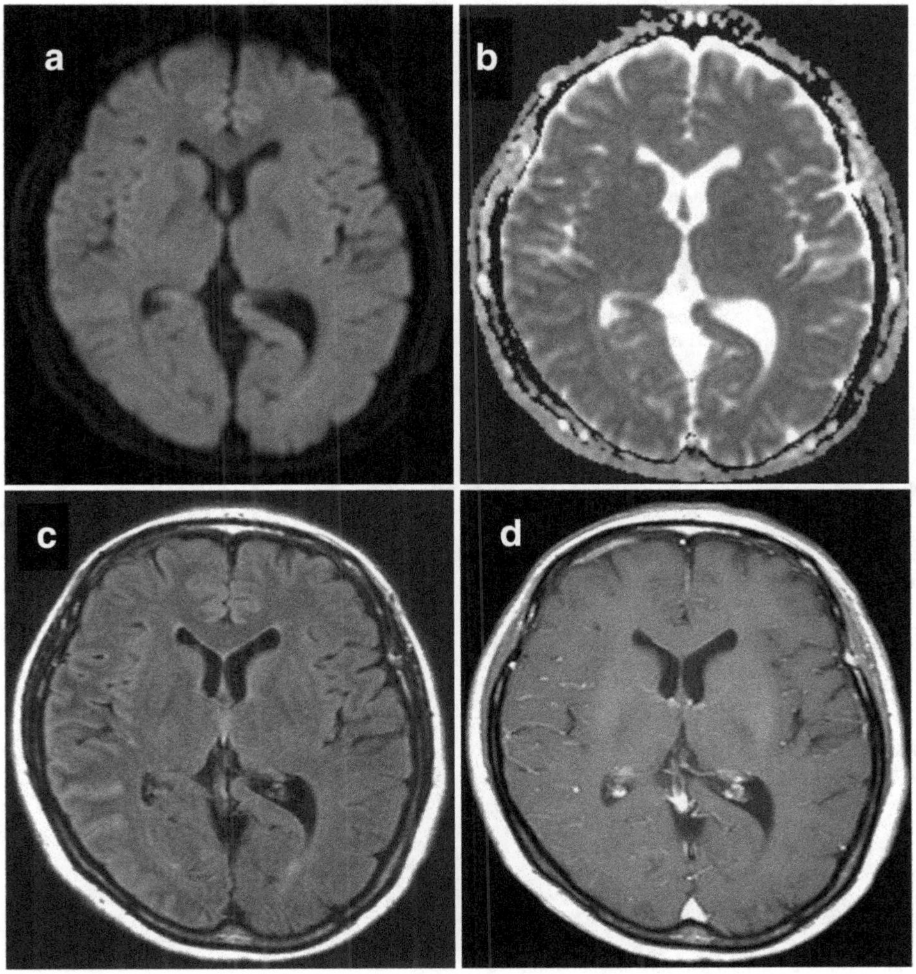

Fig. 3 MRI images at day 3. The abnormal findings at day 1 have disappeared on DWI (**a**) and the ADC image (**b**), but the high-intensity area remains on the FLAIR image (**c**) at day 3. There is no definite enhancement of the lesion on gadolinium-enhanced T1-weighted imaging (**d**). MRI = magnetic resonance imaging, DWI = diffusion-weighted imaging, ADC = apparent diffusion coefficient, FLAIR = fluid attenuated inversion recovery

95% confidence interval, 0.14–0.77; $p = 0.01$) [18]. However, if the patients with RMSA would be susceptible to hemorrhagic transformation after receiving iv-tPA, it should be better to adopt the MRI first strategy for every patients with a history of RA. In the present case, it is particularly important that neither adverse events nor bleeding complications were observed, suggesting the safety of CT-based thrombolytic therapy even in RA patients.

Abbreviations

ADC: Apparent diffusion coefficient; ASPECTS: The Alberta Stroke Program Early CT Score; CT: Computerized tomography; DWI: Diffusion weighted image; FLAIR: Fluid attenuated inversion recovery; MRI: Magnetic resonance imaging; NIHSS: National Institute of Health Stroke Scale; RA: Rheumatoid arthritis; RMSA: Rheumatoid meningitis presenting with a stroke-like attack

Authors' contributions

FM and MA contributed equally to the diagnosis and treatment of the patient and drafted the manuscript. DH and MH contributed to emergency treatment. HA contributed to checking the manuscript. YH contributed to editing and revising the manuscript and supervised this publication. All authors have read and approved the final manuscript.

Competing interests

The authors declare that they have no competing interests.

References

1. Bougea A, Anagnostou E, Konstantinos G, et al. A systematic review of peripheral and central nervous system involvement of rheumatoid arthritis, systemic lupus erythematosus, primary Sjogren's syndrome, and associated immunological profiles. Int J Chronic Dis. 2015;2015:910352.

2. Manabe Y, Narai H, Warita H, et al. Rheumatoid factor positive hypertrophic cranial pachymeningitis in association with hypopituitarism and multiple cranial nerve palsies. Intern Med. 2001;40:964–7.
3. Starosta MA, Brandwein SR. Clinical manifestations and treatment of rheumatoid pachymeningitis. Neurology. 2007;68:1079–80.
4. Magaki S, Chang E, Hammond RR, et al. Two cases of rheumatoid meningitis. Neuropathology. 2016;36:93–102.
5. Kern R, Nagayama M, Toyoda K, et al. Comparison of the European and Japanese guidelines for the management of ischemic stroke. Cerebrovasc Dis. 2013;35:402–18.
6. Mori E, Minematsu K, Nakagawara J, et al. Effects of 0.6 mg/kg intravenous alteplase on vascular and clinical outcomes in middle cerebral artery occlusion: Japan Alteplase clinical trial II (J-ACT II). Stroke. 2010;41:461–5.
7. Krysl D, Zamecnik J, Senolt L, et al. Chronic repetitive nonprogressive epilepsia partialis continua due to rheumatoid meningitis. Seizure. 2013; 22:80–2.
8. Chowdhry V, Kumar N, Lachance DH, et al. An unusual presentation of rheumatoid meningitis. J Neuroimaging. 2005;15:286–8.
9. Bathon JM, Moreland LW, DiBartolomeo AG. Inflammatory central nervous system involvement in rheumatoid arthritis. Semin Arthritis Rheum. 1989;18:258–66.
10. Bourgeois P, Rivest J, Bocti C. Rheumatoid meningitis presenting with stroke-like episodes. Neurology. 2014;82:1564–5.
11. Roy B, Uphoff DF, Silverman IE. Rheumatoid meningitis presenting with multiple Strokelike episodes. JAMA Neurol. 2015;72:1073–6.
12. Hooper DC, Kean RB, Scott GS, et al. The central nervous system inflammatory response to neurotropic virus infection is peroxynitrite dependent. J Immunol. 2001;167:3470–7.
13. Hasiloglu ZI, Asik M, Erer B, et al. Magnetic resonance imaging of rheumatoid meningitis: a case report and literature review. Rheumatol Int. 2012;32:3679–81.
14. Berkhemer OA, Fransen PS, Beumer D, et al. A randomized trial of intraarterial treatment for acute ischemic stroke. N Engl J Med. 2015; 372:11–20.
15. Goyal M, Demchuk AM, Menon BK, et al. Randomized assessment of rapid endovascular treatment of ischemic stroke. N Engl J Med. 2015; 372:1019–30.
16. Campbell BC, Mitchell PJ, Kleinig TJ, et al. Endovascular therapy for ischemic stroke with perfusion-imaging selection. N Engl J Med. 2015; 372:1009–18.
17. Saver JL, Goyal M, Bonafe A, et al. Solitaire with the intention for Thrombectomy as primary endovascular treatment for acute ischemic stroke (SWIFT PRIME) trial: protocol for a randomized, controlled, multicenter study comparing the solitaire revascularization device with IV tPA with IV tPA alone in acute ischemic stroke. Int J Stroke. 2015; 10:439–48.
18. Tsivgoulis G, Zand R, Katsanos AH, et al. Safety of intravenous thrombolysis in stroke mimics: prospective 5-year study and comprehensive meta-analysis. Stroke. 2015;46:1281–7.

19

Subarachnoid hemorrhage after transient global amnesia caused by cerebral venous congestion

Yuta Maetani[1], Masahiro Nakamori[1*], Tomoaki Watanabe[1], Hayato Matsushima[1], Eiji Imamura[1] and Shinichi Wakabayashi[2]

Abstract

Background: Transient global amnesia is reported to be caused by cerebral venous congestion. Internal jugular venous flow reversal in particular with the Valsalva maneuver leads to cerebral venous congestion. In addition, Valsalva maneuver can also induce subarachnoid hemorrhage. Transient global amnesia and subarachnoid hemorrhage might have common a pathophysiology in cerebral venous congestion.

Case presentation: We report here the case of a 57-year-old woman who twice experienced convexal subarachnoid hemorrhage just after straining at stool following an episode of transient global amnesia. Digital subtraction angiography showed left temporal congestion. Left jugular vein ultrasonography revealed reflux with the Valsalva maneuver only in acute phase, indicating transient cerebral venous congestion.

Conclusions: Subarachnoid hemorrhage followed by transient global amnesia indicates a common factor between them. Transient venous congestion is discussed in order to explain this rare phenomenon.

Keywords: Transient global amnesia, Subarachnoid hemorrhage, Cerebral venous congestion, Valsalva maneuver, Straining

Background

Transient global amnesia (TGA) is a clinical syndrome characterized by the sudden onset of reduced episodic memory. Several possibilities, such as cerebral ischemia and epileptic episode are suggested as the etiology of TGA, but the pathophysiology is still elusive. Internal jugular venous flow reversal that leads to cerebral venous congestion can contribute to TGA [1]. Particularly, the Valsalva maneuver leads to internal jugular venous flow reversal in patients with TGA [2].

Subarachnoid hemorrhage (SAH) is mainly caused by the rupture of a cerebral aneurysm or cerebral arteriovenous malformation, but sometimes the origin cannot be detected despite detailed examinations such as digital subtraction angiography (DSA). Valsalva maneuver that leads to cerebral venous congestion can also induce SAH [3].

Thus, TGA and SAH might be induced by venous congestion. However, there are few reports of the relation between TGA and SAH. Although TGA as a presentation of SAH has been reported, to the best of our knowledge, SAH after TGA has been never reported. We report the case of a patient with SAH after TGA following straining at stool.

Case presentation

A 57-year-old woman was admitted to our hospital due to sudden-onset amnesia. She had no past medical history, except for dyslipidemia, had taken no medicine, including pills and nutritional supplements. She had neither smoked nor drank. She was an elementary school teacher. Before developing amnesia, she visited another elementary school for a workshop. She did not clearly remember the situation at the onset of TGA. At the first medical examination, she

* Correspondence: mnakamori1@gmail.com
[1]Department of Neurology, Suiseikai Kajikawa Hospital, 1-1-23, Higashisendamachi, Naka-ku, Hiroshima 730-0053, Hiroshima, Japan
Full list of author information is available at the end of the article

presented with no neurologic deficit, except for amnesia. Magnetic resonance imaging (MRI), electroencephalogram, and laboratory findings were normal. We diagnosed the patient with TGA. The patient's symptom disappeared after about 6 hours. Diffusion-weighted imaging (DWI) carried out the next day revealed a high-density spot in the left hippocampus (Fig. 1), which indicated TGA. She was discharged two days after onset.

Several hours after discharge, the patient had a sudden terrible headache. The patient had strained at stool just before onset. She came back to our hospital immediately. At the time of the second admission, the patient was alert and had a blood pressure of 140/88mmHg. Her heart rate and oxygen saturation were normal. She had a throbbing headache, but exhibited no signs of neurologic deficit, including amnesia. Computed tomography (CT) and MRI revealed convexal subarachnoid hemorrhage (cSAH) in the right frontal lobe (Fig. 2a). The signal in this lesion was hyperintense on fluid-attenuated inversion recovery and T2-weighted images, and hypointense on T2* susceptibility-weighted images (Fig. 2b-d). This indicates hemorrhage and not thrombosis. There were no signs of leukoaraiosis or microbleeds on MRI and no vessel abnormalities, such as aneurysms or arteriovenous fistula/malformation on magnetic resonance angiography (MRA) (Fig. 3) and magnetic resonance venography (MRV). Laboratory findings, including those regarding the coagulating system, were normal. On day 2 of the second admission, a strong headache re-occurred when the patient strained at stool. CT and MRI revealed another cSAH in the right frontal lobe (Figs. 2e-h). There were no findings such as aneurysms, anomalies, or sinus thrombosis on DSA. However, DSA revealed hypoplastic left transvers sinus and congestion in the left temporal lobe. Left carotid artery angiography in the last part of the venous phase revealed reflux from the inferior petrosal vein into the cavernous (Fig. 4a, b). Left vertebral artery angiography revealed that hypoplastic left sinus caused venous blood flow into supplementary path, that is, the basilar venous plexus in addition to normal flow into bilateral transverse sinus (Fig. 4c, d), which indicated the left temporal venous congestion. However, perfusion-weighted imaging did not show distinct congestion in the lesion of cSAH.

Jugular vein ultrasonography revealed reflux only with the Valsalva maneuver in left internal jugular vein (Fig. 5). Reflux was confirmed according to a previous report [4]. The internal jugular venous valve was not found. The other examinations, such as electrocardiography, Holter electrocardiography, transthoracic echocardiography, carotid artery ultrasonography, leg venous ultrasonography, whole-body CT scan, and electroencephalogram were normal.

The headache steadily improved and the patient was discharged. Repeated brain imaging tests, including CT, MRI, MRA, and MRV indicated no relapse of cSAH, new lesion, reversible lesion, contraction, or thrombosis. The left internal jugular venous reflux following the Valsalva maneuver on ultrasonography disappeared four months later. Medical history and the test results are summarized in the Additional file 1.

Discussion and Conclusion

Secondary TGA is likely to be caused by stroke, epilepsy, migraine, or abnormal cerebral venous reflux. CA-1 subfield of the hippocampus is related to TGA, and is affected by hypoxemia-induced metabolic stress, β-amyloid-induced neurotoxicity, and ischemia [1]. However, the predominant hypothesis is that TGA most commonly occurs due to abnormal

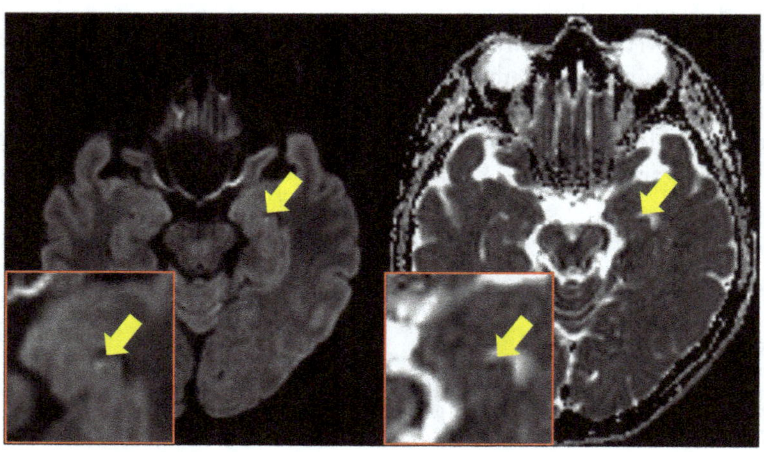

Fig. 1 Brain magnetic resonance imaging (MRI) showed a high-density spot in the left hippocampus on diffusion-weighted imaging at the first admission

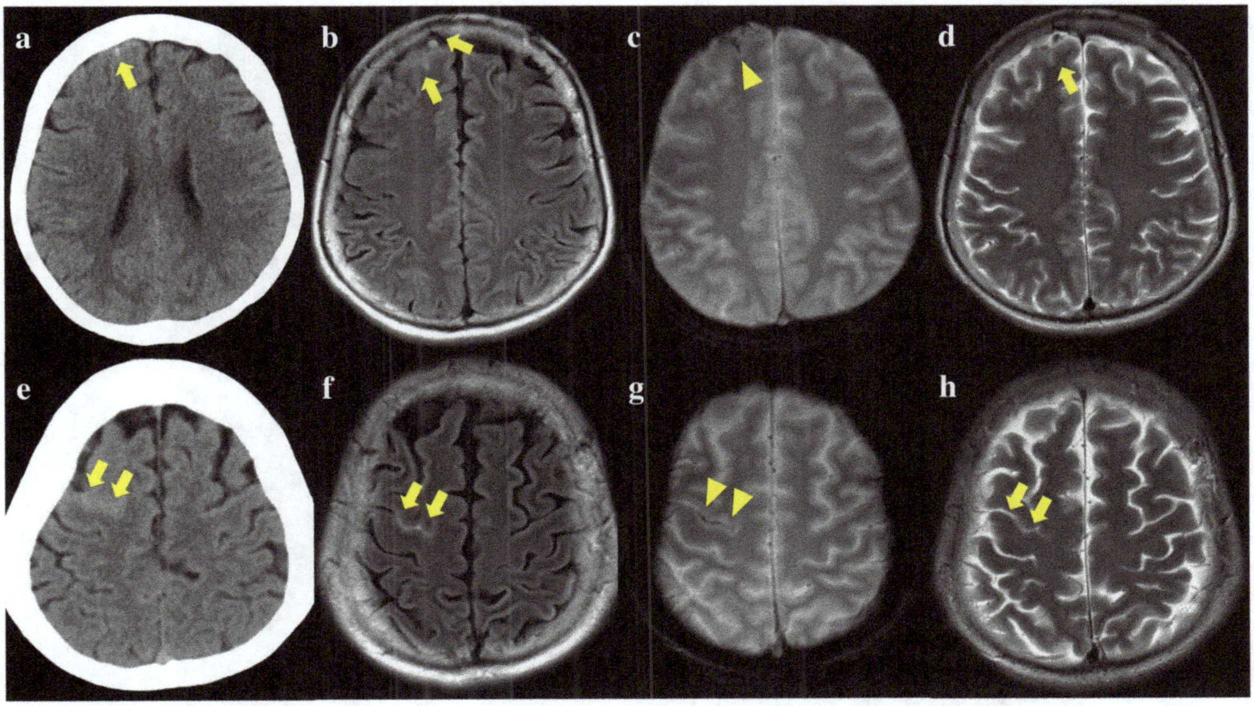

Fig. 2 Head computed tomography and magnetic resonance imaging showed twice convexal subarachnoid hemorrhage on day1 of second admission (**a-d**), on day2 of second admission (**e-h**). Lesions have high density on computed tomography (**a**, **e**), a hyperintense signal on fluid-attenuated inversion recovery (**b**, **e**) and T2-weighted image (**d**, **h**) (arrow), and a hypointense signal on T2* susceptibility-weighted image (arrow head), which indicate not thrombosis but hemorrhage

cerebral venous drainage from the temporal lobes [1, 5]. Increased intrathoracic pressure, such as that caused by Valsalva maneuver, could trigger retrograde venous flow in patients with valve incompetence in the internal jugular veins. The resulting venous congestion would preferentially affect the function of the medial temporal lobes, thus triggering the anterograde amnesia [1]. In this case, DSA showed congestion in the temporal lobe.

Internal jugular venous flow reversal and internal jugular vein valve incompetency can contribute to TGA. Although not all patients with TGA show internal jugular venous flow reversal or internal jugular vein valve incompetency, this phenomenon is more common in patients with TGA than in controls or patients with transient ischemic attack [2]. Since the Valsalva maneuver causes internal jugular venous flow reversal in patients with TGA [2], in this case, it was not clear whether the patient performed the Valsalva maneuver before the onset of TGA. A high-density spot was found in her left hippocampus on DWI and left internal jugular venous flow reversal was noted with ultrasonography only during the acute phase. This was in agreement with a diagnosis of TGA.

However, a high-density spot on DWI also indicated ischemic stroke. TGA may be associated with right-to-

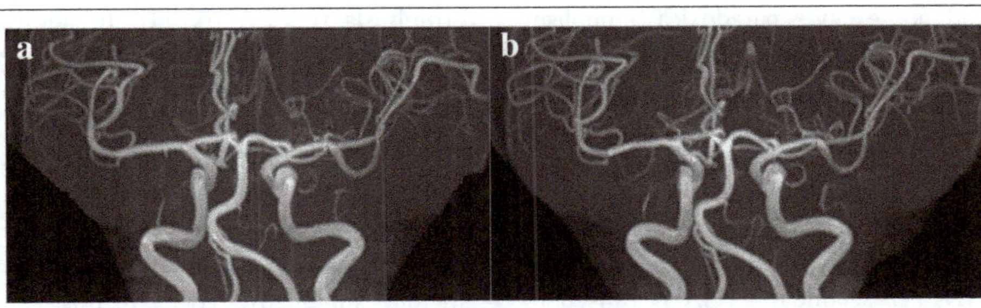

Fig. 3 Magnetic resonance angiographies (MRA) showed no signs of reversible cerebral vasoconstriction syndrome. Images are presented from (**a**) the second admission, when the patient developed convexal subarachnoid hemorrhage, (**b**) discharge from the second admission. There was no change in MRA from the first admission, when the patient developed transient global amnesia, to four months after discharge from the hospital

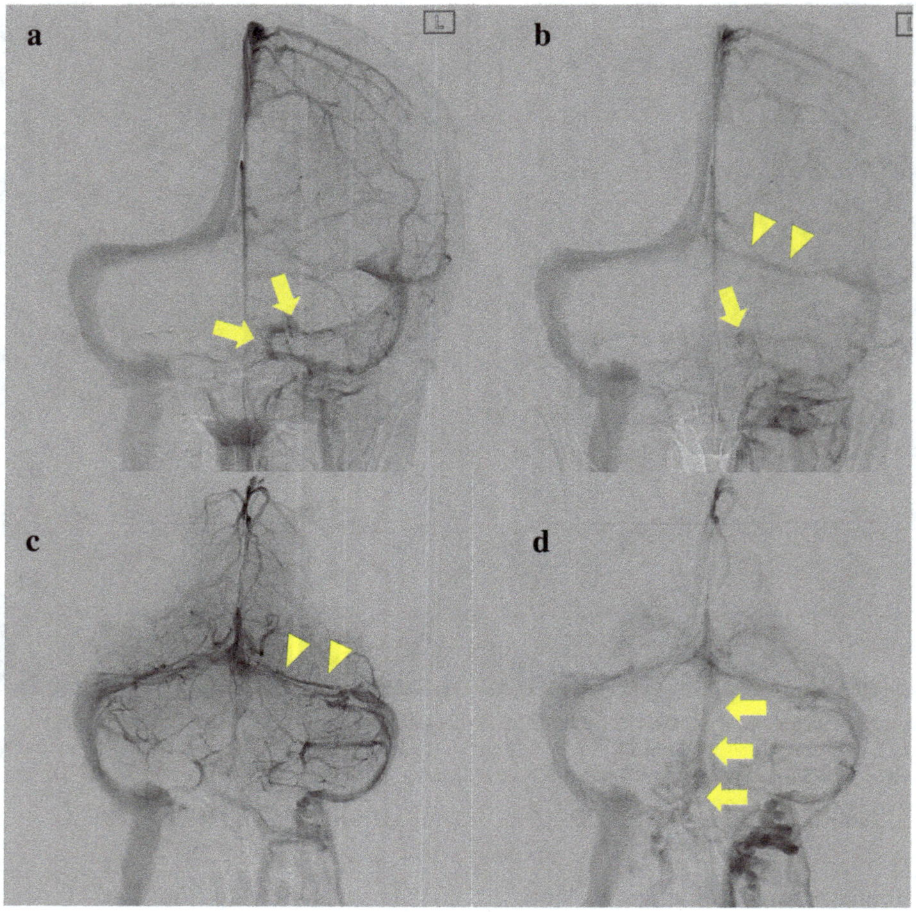

Fig. 4 Digital subtraction angiographies are shown. **a** Left carotid artery angiography in the late venous phase, (**b**) in the last part of the venous phase. **c** Left vertebral artery angiography in the early venous phase, (**d**) in the late venous phase. Cerebral venous blood flowed into inferior petrosal vein through sigmoid sinus (**a**), and subsequently flowed backward from the inferior petrosal vein into the cavernous (arrow) (**b**). Digital subtraction angiography revealed left hypoplastic transvers sinus (arrow head). Blood flow through left transvers sinus was delayed and not much due to left hypoplastic sinus (**b**, **c**). Venous blood flowed normally into bilateral transverse sinus in the early venous phase (**c**), and furthermore, into the basilar venous plexus due to left hypoplastic transverse sinus in the late venous phase (**d**)

left shunt, such as patent foramen ovale [6, 7]. We did not perform the right-to-left shunt study using transesophageal echocardiography or transcranial doppler. There were no abnormal findings such as thrombosis on leg venous ultrasonography and transthoracic echocardiography. Pulmonary arteriovenous fistula was ruled out by chest-body CT. We could not exclude paradoxical embolism, which is limitation, though results of our tests suggested that the patient was unlikely to have paradoxical embolism.

According to previous reports, TGA may not be associated with ischemic stroke. TGA patients have a much lower stroke risk than TIA patients [8]. On the other hand, the relation between TGA and SAH is not well documented [9]. Most studies reported amnesia as a presentation of SAH, i.e., secondary TGA is caused by SAH. To our knowledge, SAH after TGA has never been reported. Because TGA is a benign disease and recurrences are infrequent, the follow-up of the patients with TGA is stopped early. Thus, the relationship between TGA and SAH might be overlooked.

It is reported that cSAH may be caused by cerebral amyloid angiopathy (CAA), reversible cerebral vasoconstriction syndrome (RCVS), posterior reversible encephalopathy syndrome (PRES), or cerebral venous thrombosis (CVT) [10, 11]. In addition, patients ≤60 years frequently present a severe headache of abrupt onset with arterial narrowing on conventional angiograms, presumptively diagnosed with a primary vasoconstriction syndrome, while patients >60 years usually have temporary sensory or motor symptoms and are likely to present leukoaraiosis and/or hemispheric microbleeds and superficial siderosis on brain MRI, compatible with amyloid angiopathy [10]. In this case, CAA, RCVS, PRES, and CVT were not detected.

The Valsalva maneuver can induce SAH [3]. It is unlikely that the patient had headaches twice by chance

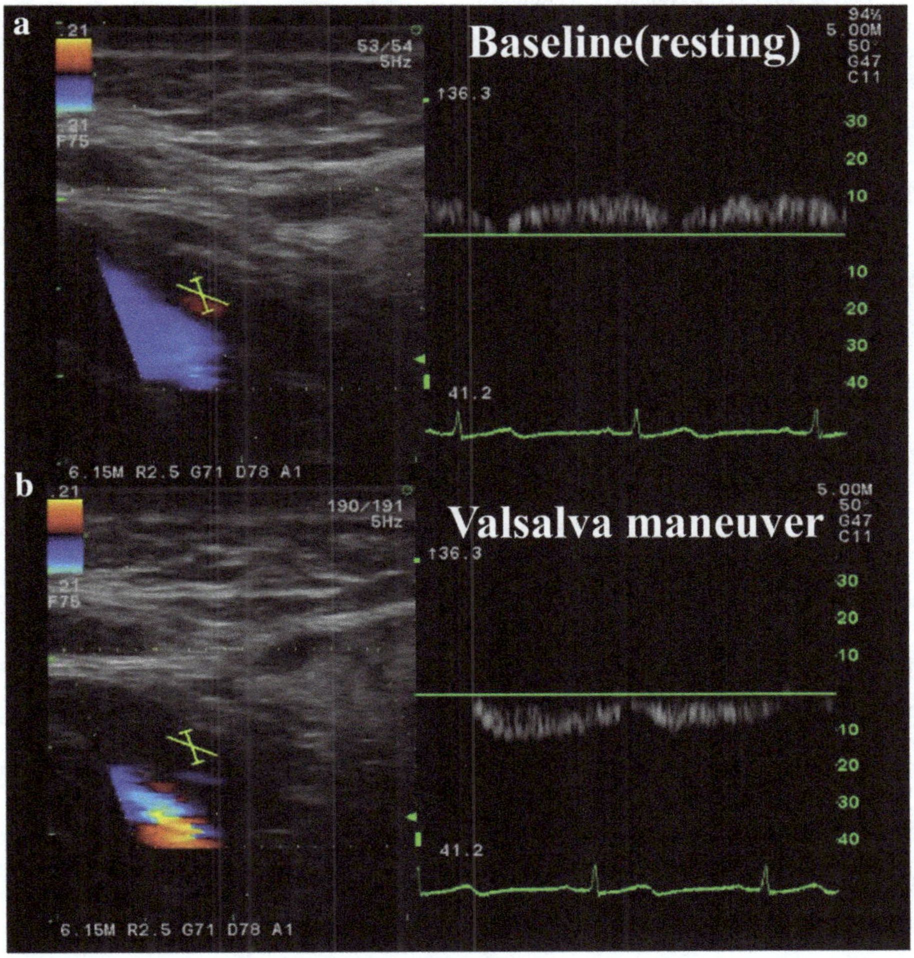

Fig. 5 Left jugular vein echo results are shown. **a** Baseline (resting), (**b**) with Valsalva maneuver. Internal jugular reflux is observed only with Valsalva maneuver in the acute phase

just after straining at stool. Four months after admission, internal jugular venous flow reversal was not observed after the Valsalva maneuver and the patient did not have a headache, which suggested that transient venous congestion occurred at the onset of cSAH. Internal jugular venous flow reversal is seen in normal individuals, although it does not always lead to the development of TGA [1]. In this case, transient internal jugular venous flow reversal induced transient aggravation of venous congestion, which might have been pathological.

For SAH caused by CVT, the leading hypothesis is that secondary venous hypertension may trigger rupture of fragile superficial veins. The superficial veins have thin walls, which contain no smooth muscle fibers or no valves. Given obstructed drainage, these veins bridging the subarachnoid and subdural spaces can store blood and regulate cerebral venous stream [12]. This phenomenon may occur in TGA patients with internal jugular venous flow reversal due to venous congestion. Patients with TGA are reported to have hypoplastic venous sinus [13]. In this case, the left transverse sinus was hypoplastic. The frontal convexal veins might have been hypoplastic and fragile, which resulted in cSAH.

It is unclear why the patient had a hemorrhage twice in the right side. Left cerebral blood could not have avoided flowing into superior sagittal sinus due to left temporal congestion, which might have resulted in secondary right cerebral hemisphere congestion. Although we attempted to prove it, perfusion-weighted imaging did not reveal distinct increased blood flow in right convexal frontal lobe. Given congestion only on the surface of brain, it is difficult to prove the congestion. Further studies are required to test this hypothesis.

Few persons develop TGA or SAH, although venous congestion is common. Disease onset might be affected by venous structural deficits, such as vein valve incompetency and vessel wall vulnerability. Transient venous congestion may also contribute to disease onset.

The mechanism of the onset in this case was unique, as straining was the trigger. TGA may be attributed to abnormal venous flow. Therefore, TGA and cSAH might share the same precipitating factor, namely transient venous congestion.

Abbreviations

CAA: Cerebral amyloid angiopathy; CSAH: Convexal subarachnoid hemorrhage; CT: Computed tomography; CVT: Cerebral venous thrombosis; DSA: Digital subtraction angiography; DWI: Diffusion-weighted imaging; MRA: Magnetic resonance angiography; MRI: Magnetic resonance imaging; MRV: Magnetic resonance venography; PRES: Posterior reversible encephalopathy syndrome; RCVS: Reversible cerebral vasoconstriction syndrome; SAH: Subarachnoid hemorrhage; TGA: Transient global amnesia

Acknowledgements

None.

Funding

The authors received no financial support for the research, authorship and/or publication of this article.

Authors' contributions

YM examined, evaluated the patient. YM and MN designed the study and wrote the draft. YM and MN contributed to the acquisition and analysis of the clinical data and the interpretation of the clinical data. TW, HM, EI and SW participated in the design of the case-report and helped to draft the manuscript. All authors read and approved the final manuscript.

Competing interests

The authors declare that they have no competing interests.

Author details

[1]Department of Neurology, Suiseikai Kajikawa Hospital, 1-1-23, Higashisendamachi, Naka-ku, Hiroshima 730-0053, Hiroshima, Japan. [2]Department of Neurosurgery, Suiseikai Kajikawa Hospital, 1-1-23, Higashisendamachi, Naka-ku, Hiroshima 730-0053, Hiroshima, Japan.

References

1. Arena JE, Rabinstein AA. Transient global amnesia. Mayo Clin Proc. 2015; 90:264–72.
2. Maalikjy Akkawi N, Agosti C, Anzola GP, Borroni B, Magoni M, Pezzini A. Transient global amnesia: a clinical and sonographic study. Eur Neurol. 2003; 49:67–71.
3. Yamakawa H, Ohe N, Yano H, Yoshimura S, Iwama T. Venous drainage patterns in perimesencephalic nonaneurysmal subarachnoid hemorrhage. Clin Neurol and Neurosurg. 2008;110:587–91.
4. Cejas C, Cisneros LF, Lagos R, Zuk C, Ameriso SF. Internal jugular vein valve incompetence is highly prevalent in transient global amnesia. Stroke. 2010; 4:67–71.
5. Lewis SL. Aetiology of transient global amnesia. Lancet. 1998;352:397–9.
6. Klötzsch C, Sliwka U, Berlit P, Noth J. An increased frequency of patent foramen ovale in patients with transient global amnesia. Analysis of 53 consecutive patients. Arch Neurol. 1996;53:504–8.
7. Anzola GP. Clinical impact of patent foramen ovale diagnosis with transcranial Doppler. Eur J Ultrasound. 2002;16:11–20.
8. Mangla A, Navi BB, Layton K, Kamel H. Transient global amnesia and the risk of ischemic stroke. Stroke. 2014;45:389–93.
9. Sandyk R. Transient global amnesia: a presentation of subarachnoid haemorrhage. J Neurol. 1984;231:283–4.
10. Kumar S, Goddeau RP Jr, Selim MH, et al. Atraumatic convexal subarachnoid hemorrhage: clinical presentation, imaging patterns, and etiologies. Neurology. 2010;74:893–9.
11. Beitzke M, Gattringer T, Enzinger C, Wagner G, Niederkorn K, Fazekas F. Clinical presentation, etiology, and long-term prognosis in patients with nontraumatic convexal subarachnoid hemorrhage. Stroke. 2011;42:3055–60.
12. Sahin N, Solak A, Genc B, Bilgic N. Cerebral venous thrombosis as a rare cause of subarachnoid hemorrhage: case report and literature review. Clin Imaging. 2014;38:373–9.
13. Bartsch T, Alfke K, Stingele R, et al. Selective affection of hippocampal CA-1 neurons in patients with transient global amnesia without long-term sequelae. Brain. 2006;129:2874–84.

20

Effect of botulinum toxin injection on length and force of the rectus femoris and triceps surae muscles during locomotion in patients with chronic hemiparesis (FOLOTOX)

Anthony Supiot[1,3,4*], Maxime Geiger[1,3,4], Djamel Bensmail[1], Phillippe Aegerter[2], Didier Pradon[1] and Nicolas Roche[1]

Abstract

Background: After stroke, spasticity of the rectus femoris (RF) and triceps surae (TS) muscles frequently alters the gait pattern. Knee flexion and ankle dorsiflexion in swing are often reduced, respectively called Stiff Knee Gait (SKG) and equinus. A preliminary uncontrolled study suggested that botulinum toxin type A (BTX-A) injections could improve muscle length and force generated during gait, improving inter-segmental coordination.
The aim of this randomised controlled study is thus to evaluate changes in the length of the RF and TS muscles during gait 1 month after either BTX-A or placebo injection in patients with chronic stroke, SKG and spastic equinus. The secondary aims are to evaluate peak length and peak force generated during gait, as well inter-segmental coordination assessed using the continuous relative phase method initially described by Barela et al. in patients with stroke.

Methods: This is a prospective, three-centre, randomised, placebo-controlled, triple blind study over 3 months with 4 visits. Forty patients will be included. During visits V1, V3 and V4, length and force generated by RF and TS during gait will be assessed using musculoskeletal models (MSM). Muscle force will also be assessed using an isokinetic dynamometer. Inter segmental coordination will be evaluated using 3D gait analysis and functional tests will be performed. During V2, patients will receive either an injection of BTX-A in the RF and TS muscles or a placebo injection of saline solution.

Discussion: We expect an increase in peak length and a decrease in peak force generated by the RF and TS muscles in the BTX-A group 1 month post injection. Moreover, we expect these parameters to be more improved in the BTX-A than the Control group. This is the first study to assess these parameters in a randomised, controlled trial using instrumented methods (isokinetic evaluation and 3D gait analysis). The results should help to improve understanding of the mechanism(s) underlying improvements in inter-segmental coordination that have been found in many previous uncontrolled studies.

Keywords: Stroke, Botulinum toxin type A, Muscle length, Motion analysis, Gait

* Correspondence: anthony.supiot@gmail.com
[1]Inserm Unit 1179, Team 3: Technologies and Innovative Therapies Applied to Neuromuscular diseases, UVSQ, CIC 805, Physiology–Functional Testing Ward, AP-HP, Raymond Poincaré Teaching Hospital, Garches, France
[3]CIAMS, University Paris-Sud, Université Paris-Saclay, 91405 Orsay Cedex, France
Full list of author information is available at the end of the article

Background

Around 85% of stroke survivors regain the capacity to walk. However the kinetic and kinematic parameters of post-stroke gait are typically altered, with a reduction in cadence, stride length and velocity [1–3]. Stiff knee gait (SKG), characterized by decreased knee flexion during swing phase [4], and equinus (reduced ankle dorsiflexion) [5] are common post-stroke gait patterns.

The loss of knee flexion during swing can be attributed to several mechanisms, including weakness of the hip flexor muscles, a reduced plantar flexion moment and inappropriate activity of part of the quadriceps muscle, particularly the Rectus Femoris (RF) [4]. The bi-articular RF is normally active during the final phase of double support (end of stance, beginning of swing) to control knee flexion. If it is inappropriately activated during swing, it restricts knee flexion during this phase [4, 6, 7].

The loss of dorsiflexion can be secondary either to weakness of the dorsiflexor muscles, particularly the Tibialis anterior (TA), or to inappropriate activity of the Triceps Surae (TS) muscles [8, 9]. Inappropriate activity of the TS reduces dorsiflexion and results in initial contact with the foot in plantar flexion.

Medical interventions to improve gait mostly target the inappropriate activity of the RF and TS. Botulinum toxin type A (BTX-A) is a common treatment to reduce muscle activity. It blocks the liberation of neurotransmitters at the presynaptic neuromuscular junction, inducing focal, transitory and reversible paralysis of the injected muscle. The effect lasts around 3 months [10].

Several uncontrolled studies have evaluated the effects of intramuscular BTX-A injection on gait, showing increases in knee flexion of 5 to 8 degrees following the treatment [6, 11, 12]. Knee flexion velocity [11] and gait velocity [6] have also been found to increase with BTX-A, along with a reduction of impairment (Stroke Impairment Assessment Set) and an improvement in gait capacity (Abiloco scale) [12]. BTX-A injection has been shown to improve coordination between the hemiparetic thigh and shank [13], associated with a reduction of compensatory behaviour in the non-hemiparetic limb [14]. In addition, a pilot study using a musculoskeletal model (SIMM ®) in 10 patients with stroke [15] showed that peak normalised RF length increased following BTX-A injection, as did peak and mean lengthening velocity. The SIMM ® musculoskeletal model can also be used to assess peak muscle force developed during gait, however this has never been done in patients with stroke.

The effectiveness of BTX-A injections in the TS has also been demonstrated. A randomised placebo-controlled study of 234 patients with stroke showed that BTX-A injection in the TS reduces passive resistance to ankle dorsiflexion (Modified Ashworth), pain, and dependence on assistive devices (orthoses and walking sticks) [5]. More recent studies have shown that BTX-A injection of the TS also increases gait speed [16, 17]. BTX-A injection combined with non-pharmacological treatments such as functional electrical stimulation, stretching and taping, increases ankle dorsiflexion in stance in adults with spastic equinus [18].

There is therefore much evidence to show that BTX-A injection in the RF or TS muscles reduces spasticity and improves gait kinematics, however the effect on length of the RF muscle has only been evaluated in one pilot study [15].

Based on the results of the pilot study by Lampire et al. [15], we hypothesise that BTX-A injection into the spastic RF and TS muscles of patients with chronic hemiparesis i) will improve peak length and mean lengthening velocity of the RF and TS and ii) will increase peak length and lengthening velocity of these muscles during gait.

Muscle force generated during gait has never been evaluated using a musculoskeletal model after BTX-A injection. Because BTX-A injection blocks transmission at the neuromuscular junction and is known to reduce muscle force evaluated by static tests, we believe it is important to evaluate the effect of BTX-A on force generated during gait. We hypothesise that force produced by the RF and TS muscles during gait will be decreased following BTX-A injection but not after the placebo injection.

The main aim of this randomised, placebo-controlled, triple blind study is to evaluate the effect of BTX-A injection in the RF and TS muscles on their peak length during gait in patients with chronic stroke.

The secondary aims are to: i) evaluate peak force generated by the RF and TS during gait following BTX-A injection, ii) evaluate changes in inter-segmental coordination during gait following BTX-A injection, iii) evaluate the impact of BTX-A injection on quality of life and iv) compare the effect of BTX-A injection with a placebo injection on the parameters specified above, in patients with chronic stroke.

The third aims are to: i) evaluate the quality of life, ii) evaluate the functional independence in motor and cognitive domains, iii) evaluate the locomotor ability.

Method/design

Ethical approval

All subjects included will provide written informed consent for participation. This study will be performed in accordance with the ethical codes of the World Medical Association and has been approved by the local ethics committee (reference number: AOM 11223-P110136 6

FOLOTOX/ 2012–003168-34 ref. CPP 12064 ClinicalTrials.gov: NCT01821573).

Study design

The study will be prospective, 3-centre, randomised, placebo-controlled and triple blinded. The total duration of the study will be 36 months. The duration of participation of each patient will be 3 months, with four visits. The patients and the injecting doctors and assistants, as well as the evaluators will be blinded to the patients' group allocations. Randomization will be carried out by computer software. During visits V1, V3 and V4 the measurements will be carried out throughout the day with breaks allowed between each (Table 1).

Participants

Patients will be recruited from routine medical consultations in the participating hospitals. For this study, stroke is defined according to the World Health Organisation as a rapid onset event of vascular origin reflecting a focal disturbance of cerebral function, excluding isolated impairments of higher function and persisting longer than 24 h [19].

Inclusion criteria

Adults over the age of 18 years with unilateral chronic stroke that occurred more than 6 months previously and who are able to walk 10 m without any assistive devices will be included. They must have a loss of peak knee flexion during the swing phase of the gait cycle due to spasticity of the RF muscle. The ankle must also remain in plantarflexion during swing due to spasticity of the TS. The severity of RF and TS spasticity of the affected limb will be determined using the Modified Ashworth Scale (MAS). Subjects will be included if they have a spasticity equal or upper of 1. Patients must give informed consent and females must be taking oral contraception.

Table 1 Tests and evaluations during each visit

Tests and evaluations	V1	V2	V3	V4
Inclusion/ exclusion criteria	X			
Informed consent	X			
Randomisation	X			
Injection BTX-A or placebo		X		
Evaluation of passive range of motion (MG)	X		X	X
Evaluation of spasticity (MAS)	X		X	X
Evaluation of strength (MRS)	X		X	X
SF 36	X		X	X
FIM	X		X	X
ABILOCO scale	X		X	X
Berg balance scale	X		X	X
Abc scale	X		X	X
Timed up and go	X		X	X
3D analysis	X		X	X
Isokinetic evaluation	X		X	X

V1 visit 1, *V2* visit 2, *V3* visit 3, *V4* visit 4, *MA* manual goniometer, *MAS* modified Ashworth, *MRC* Medical Research Council, *SF36* The Short Form (36) Health Survey, *FIM* Functional independence measure, *3D analysis* gait motion analysis. All outcome measures will be evaluated during the first visit (baseline-V1) and 1 month (V3) and 3 (V4) months after injection. All evaluations will be performed in the same order at each session in order to limit bias related to fatigue

Exclusion criteria

Participants will not be included if they have aphasia, have undergone lower limb surgery less than 6 months previously, for example muscle-tendon lengthening, ankle foot arthroplasty, RF tenotomy with or without transfer, or any surgery aimed to improve gait, if they have other diseases or pre-existing neuro-muscular disorders, if they are pregnant, if they had an injection of BTX-A less than 3 months previously, if they had a previous hypersensitive reaction to BTX-A or are taking aminoglycosides.

Randomization method

All patients included are routinely followed in the spasticity-units of the three participating centers. All will already be treated with BTX-A and will have undergone regular spasticity ratings using the MAS. Patients with spasticity of both the RF and TS will therefore be identified before the study is presented to them during visit 1. In addition, all patients will already have undergone routine 3D gait analysis as part of their management, thus the decrease in peak knee flexion and peak ankle plantarflexion in swing phase will already be documented, with the cause reported as RF and TS spasticity. Randomization will be carried out using randoWeb software (http://randoweb.aphp.fr) at the beginning of visit 2, then either BTX-A or the placebo will be injected according to group allocation. To avoid problems relating to expiration of the BTX-A, the BTX-A and placebo packs will be randomized, not the patients. A randomization list will be uploaded on a dedicated server (CleanWeb) and each patient will be attributed an injection pack number. The randomization will be block-balanced. Patients will thus be injected with either BTX-A or the placebo at visit 2.

Intervention group

Previous studies [6, 12, 15, 20] demonstrated that 200 U of BTX-A injected into the RF could improve RF length, spatio temporal gait parameters and intersegmental coordination. Pradon et al. showed that BTX-A injected in the TS (total of200 U: 75 U in each gastrocnemius and 50 U in the soleus) combined with use of an ankle foot orthosis improved gait parameters [20]. Caty et al. demonstrated that 200 U of Botulinum toxin type A (Botox) in the TS improved stiff knee gait and gait capacity [12].

The doses determined for the present study have thus been based on those studies as well as French Health Authority guidelines. Patients in the BTX-A group will receive a total of 350 units of BTX-A (Botox®, Allergan Inc). BTX-A is in powder form (BOTOX® 100 units Allergan). The BTX-A powder will dissolve with NaCl (0.9%) solution to have four syringes 1) 150 units (3 ml) for an injection in the RF in 3 points, 2) 70 units (1.4 ml) for the medial gastrocnemius in 1 point, 3) 70 units (1.4 ml) for the lateral gastrocnemius in 1 point, and 4) 60 units (1.2 ml) for the soleus in 3 points.For injection into the RF, the first point will be 5 cm below the inguinal crease, on a line between the antero-inferior iliac spine and the patella. The second point will be ten centimetres above the patella and the third on the same line, half way between the first two points [13, 15]. For injection into the triceps surea, the French Health Authority guidelines will be followed [21]. For the gastrocnemii, the injection points are on a horizontal line separating the upper 1/4 from the lower 3/4 of the lower leg. For the soleus, the proximal injection points are on a horizontal line separating the upper 2/5 and lower 3/5 of the lower leg and the distal point is on a line separating the upper 2/3 from the lower 1/3 of the lower leg.

Placebo group

For placebo group a solution of NaCl (0.9%) will use as a placebo. In addition the patients will receive identical volumes of NaCl (0.9%) that intervention group. Identically the placebo will be conditioned in four syringes: 1) 3 ml for the RF in 3 points, 2) 1.4 ml for the medial gastrocnemius in 1 point, 3) 1.4 ml for the lateral gastrocnemius in 1 point, and 4) 60 units (1.2 ml) for the soleus in 3 points. The injection points will be identical to those used for the intervention group.

All injections (both groups) will be carried out under electrostimulation guidance with a stimulation intensity of 5 mA. Visit 2, during which BTX-A or placebo injection will be performed, will be either on the same day as Visit 1 after randomisation, or within 7 days.

Blinding

In order to ensure study blinding, only the pharmacist of each centre will know the nature of the box (BTX-A or placebo). Moreover, an independent nurse will prepare the syringe in a separate room.

Clinical evaluation

All patients will undergo a comprehensive clinical evaluation. To limit inter-investigator variability, one physiotherapist in each centre will carry out all assessments. In addition, this physiotherapist will be blinded to group allocation.The clinical examination will include passive range of motion (ROM) of the hip, knee and ankle using a manual goniometer. Measurement of joint ROM will be carried out according to the protocol recommended by Clarkson [22]. Spasticity will be evaluated using the Modified Ashworth Scale (MAS) [23]. This scale has been validated for the evaluation of spasticity [24, 25] and is sensitive to change following BTX-A treatment [26]. Lastly, strength of the hip extensor, flexor and abductor, knee flexor and extensor, ankle dorsiflexor and plantarflexor muscles of the affected and non-affected lower limbs will be measured using the Medical Research Council (MRC) scale [27, 28] (Table 2).

Outcome measures

Primary aim: Outcome

The primary outcome is change in maximal length of the injected muscles during gait one month after injection of BTX-A or placebo, quantified by 3D motion analysis and a musculo-skeletal model. It will be determined by comparison of the results of the evaluations carried out at V1, V3 and V4.

Table 2 Summary of outcome measures for each study aim

Aims	Parameter evaluated	Outcome measure
First	Peak length of RF and TS during gait	3D analysis
		MSM
	Peak strength of RF and TS	Isometric evaluation
Second	Inter-segmental gait coordination	3D analysis:
		EMG analysis
		Muscle synergies
		Peak joint angles
		Peak joint torques
		Inter joint coordination
		ABILOCO scale
		TUG
		6MWT
		10MWT
		Stairs test
	Balance	Berg balance scale
		ABC scale
Third	Independence	FIM
	Quality of life	SF 36

RF rectus femoris, *TS* triceps surae, *TUG* Timed up and go test, *6MWT* Six minute walk test, *10 MWT* Ten meter walk test, *ABC scale* Activities Balance Confidence scale, *FIM* Functional independence measure, *SF 36* Short form (36) health survey, *3D analysis* gait motion analysis, *MSM* Musculoskeletal models

Musculoskeletal model

Musculoskeletal models (MSM) have been used in many studies since the 1980's [29–34] to simulate the mechanical properties of muscle contraction. This procedure has been validated, particularly for the TS muscle [35]. Kinematic, kinetic and EMG data recorded during 3D gait analysis are inputted into the model for the calculation of biomechanical muscle parameters during movement. MSM thus provide information regarding muscle function during normal and pathological gait [36–40]. SIMM® (Software for Interactive Musculoskeletal Modeling) software will be used to calculate the three biomechanical muscle properties of interest in the present study. The standard generic SIMM® model [30] uses data from the gait analysis. The model is constituted of thirteen rigid segments with seventeen degrees of freedom and each limb is made up of forty-three muscle-tendon complexes. Each complex is defined by its origin, insertion, and if necessary, by via-points in order to specify the trajectory of the muscle. SIMM® uses static optimization based on inverse dynamics, with a constraint based on the EMG envelope to calculate muscle forces.

Calculation of length

Normalized peak length will be defined as: peak muscle length during gait minus muscle length in the 'virtual' anatomical reference position, in millimetres [15]. This normalization reduces bias related to morphological differences between subjects, as well as differences related to marker placement between different visits for each patient.

Peak muscle lengthening velocity will be calculated for each gait cycle and mean peak lengthening velocity will be then calculated for each subject.

Secondary aim: Outcomes

The secondary outcomes are peak muscle force generated during gait assessed by the MSM, peak force measured during the isometric evaluation, inter-segmental coordination during gait assessed by 3D analysis, and functional tests.

Peak force during gait

Peak force developed during gait will be calculated and expressed as a percentage of body weight in order to take into account differences in the magnitude of muscle forces between subjects.

The instant of the gait cycle (as a % of the gait cycle, normalised according to the toe off) at which the peak force of each muscle occurs will be determined. A negative value indicates that the peak force occurred in stance phase, while a positive value indicates that it occurred in swing phase.

Maximal strength

A CON-TREX isokinetic dynamometer will be used to evaluate force. The physiotherapist carrying out this evaluation will be blinded to group allocation. A standardized sitting position on the dynamometer will be used with the trunk fixed by a belt to the back rest to ensure that the position is maintained throughout the test. Participants will be asked to place their hands on their thighs and to keep the upper limbs relaxed throughout the test. To avoid any mal-alignment of axes, limit compensatory body movements and eliminate the degrees of freedom of the other joints, the non-paretic lower leg will be blocked and the thigh of the tested leg will be fixed. Care will be taken to align the axes of rotation of the joints of the tested limb with the axes of rotation of the dynamometer. All settings will be noted in order to ensure the position is identical across sessions for each subject.

The peak force couple produced by the knee flexors and extensors during active movements of knee flexion and extension will be calculated, as well as the angle at which the peak force couple occurs during passive movements. An isometric evaluation of maximum force developed by the quadriceps and hamstring muscles will also be carried out with the knee flexed to 90 degrees [41].

Inter-segmental coordination during locomotion

Inter segmental coordination during gait will be analyzed using a 3-dimensional (3D) motion capture system (Motion Analysis Corporation, Santa Rosa, CA, USA, six cameras, Sampling Frequency 100 Hz) and two force plates (AMTI, Watertown, MA, USA, Sampling Frequency 1000 Hz). The trajectories of 24 markers placed on anatomical landmarks using the Helen Hayes marker set will be recorded and filtered using a fourth-order zero-lag Butter worth low-pass-filter with a 6 Hz cut off frequency.

3D Gait Analysis will be carried out during V1, V3 and V4. To limit inter-investigator variability, one operator in each centre will carry out all assessments. In addition, this operator will be in blinded to group allocation. Two conditions will be analysed: preferred and maximal walking speed. For each condition, eight trials will be recorded to ensure a minimum of ten gait cycles from both lower limbs. Boudarham et al. suggested that during 3D analysis, there is a phase of adaptation during which gait is unstable [42]. They thus suggested kinematic and kinetic analysis should be based on three to nine gait trials in patients with hemiparesis.

OrthoTrack 6.5 software (Motion Analysis Corporation, Santa Rosa, CA, USA) will be used to calculate kinematic and kinetic parameters, using Euler rotations (Grood and Suntay method) for the kinematic parameters.

Spatio-temporal parameters will be calculated for both lower limbs, including gait velocity, cadence, step and stride length, step width, and the duration of the single support phase. Kinematic and kinetic parameters will be calculated for both lower limbs for each sub-phase of the gait cycle (initial double contact phase, single support phase, final double contact phase and swing phase). The main kinematic parameters are peak flexion, extension, peak abduction, adduction, valgus/varus and rotation as appropriate for the pelvis, hips, knees and ankles. Ground reaction force and peak joint moments of the hips, knees and ankles will be calculated in the three dimensions of space.

The activity of eight muscles will also be recorded using a surface EMG system (MA311, Motion Lab Systems, Baton rouge; band-pass 15-3000 Hz): rectus femoris (RF), vastus lateralis (VL), gluteus maximus (GMax), hamstring (HAM), biceps femoris (BF), soleus (SOL), medial gastrocnemius (MG), tibialis anterior (TA). Electrode placements will follow SENIAM recommendations [43]. These muscles function in synergies to produce gait, therefore an analysis of muscle synergies will be performed. Evaluation of the coordination of lower limb segments during gait typically involves reducing all the degrees of freedom to a small number of patterns [44] that reflect the underlying neural control of gait [45]. To extract muscle synergies, we will use the model presented in Delis [46]. We will use the associated sNM3F algorithm to obtain a space-by-time modular description of EMG patterns. According to that method, modularity is defined as "linear combinations of both spatial and temporal modules". This model has been shown to unify and encompass most previous approaches and to yield a concise description of muscle patterns underlying the execution of various motor tasks. Muscle synergies will be extracted from the EMG recorded during the gait analysis (RF, VL, HAM, GAS and SOL) using spatial and temporal methods in order to evaluate changes in the pattern of muscle activity following BTX-A or placebo injection and the subsequent reduction (or not) of spasticity and force produced. The relationship between muscle force and type of synergy developed by patients will be then be evaluated.

Five functional tests will be used to evaluate the impact of any changes in intersegmental coordination on functional ability. These tests will be carried out by the blinded physiotherapist.

The Timed up and go test (TUG): This test consists of measuring the timed performance of rising from a chair, walking 3 m, turning and sitting again. The subject wears his/her usual shoes and may use his/her usual gait aid. The starting position is sitting with the back against the backrest of the chair, the arms resting on the chair arms and the gait aid within easy reach. Time begins when the subject's back is no longer in contact with the chair back and stops when the subject is sitting once again with his/her back against the chair back.

The 6 min walk test (6MWT): Subjects will be asked to walk for 6 min and the distance covered will be measured. They may slow down or stop but must resume walking as soon as possible. A standardized sentence of encouragement will be used to inform the patient of the remaining time each minute. This test will be carried out in a 30 m long, unused corridor. A cone will be placed at each end around which the subject must turn [47, 48].

Ten meter walk test (10 MWT): The time taken to walk 10 m at maximal velocity will be recorded. The patients will be asked to walk as fast as possible over a distance of 14 m. The first and last 2 m will not be counted in order to eliminate the phases of acceleration and deceleration. Subjects will wear their usual shoes and may use a gait aid. Three trials will be carried out and the average used for analysis [49, 50].

Stairs test (ST): Subjects will be asked to ascend and descend a flight of 13 stairs (15 cm high) 3 times at maximal speed, and the mean will be used for analysis. The starting point will be a line 16 cm away from the first step. After each ascent or descent, the subject will be allowed to rest. Subjects can use the handrail but only for balance, and must not pull on it. The time will begin when the first foot leaves the ground and will stop when the last foot touches the ground [51].

The berg balance scale (BBS) will be used to measure balance [52].The BBS has been developed to measure static and dynamic equilibrium in adults to detect people at risk of fall. It can also be used to identify people who can walk unaided and to predict the difficulties some individuals may encounter in everyday activities. The BBS includes 14 tests that assess static balance and dynamic equilibrium as: unipodal support trunk rotation getting up and sitting.

Third aim: Functional outcomes

Quality of life will be evaluated using the short form-36 (SF 36) [53, 54].The Functional Independence Measure (FIM) [55] will be used to evaluate functional independence in eighteen motor and cognitive domains. The FIM can be used to follow change from the beginning of rehabilitation to discharge [56]. The ABILOCO scale (a measure of locomotor ability for adults) [57] will be used to be assess locomotor ability. The test rates the individual's ability to move about effectively in his/her environment by the evaluation of thirteen tasks including simple and complex movements. The scale is sensitive to changes in walking ability [12].The ABC scale (Activities Balance Confidence) will be used assess confidence in carrying out sixteen activities of daily living both indoors and outdoors [58].

Management of adverse events

Patients will be informed about possible adverse events at the time of inclusion. If any adverse events occur, the study coordinator must be immediately contacted. Two types of adverse events will be considered.

Non-serious adverse events or effects are defined as any harmful manifestation that occurs in the subject, whether or not this manifestation is linked to any experimental element of the research or products used. Non-serious events may include: pain or burning at the injection site, injected limb pain, ecchymosis, hypertonia, muscular weakness, arthralgia, asthenia, hyperesthesia, pain, depression, insomnia, discomfort, nausea etc.

Serious adverse events or effects are any adverse event or effect that results in death, endangers life, requires hospitalization or prolongation of hospitalization, causes significant or lasting disability, or results in an anomaly or a congenital malformation. Undesirable effects whose nature, severity or evolution does not correspond to the information contained in the references recognized by the authorities are considered as serious, as are any adverse effects related to the diffusion of the BTX-A away from the injection site. Serious adverse events therefore include excessive muscle weakness, dysphagia, inhalation pneumonia, anaphylactic reactions etc.

Statistical analysis

Sample size calculation

Sample size was estimated using G*power software [59]. The input data were taken from Lampire et al. [15] who assessed the effect of BTX-A injection on length and lengthening velocity of rectus femoris during gait in chronic stroke patients). Using a two-tailed test at a threshold of 5% and a power of 80%, a sample of seventeen subjects per group was found to be necessary [60]. We therefore plan to recruit forty patients to take into account potential patients lost to follow-up. The study is currently underway. On the first of April 2018, twenty-eight participants had been included.

Statistical analysis

Data will be analysed using SAS 9.3 (Cary Inc., NorthCarolina, USA) and "R" software (v2.14 R Foundation for Statistical Computing, Vienna,Austria. http://www.R-project.org/).

Description

Patients will be described by their status: eligible, included, not included (with reason for non-inclusion), left the study, and completed evaluations, within each group and for each centre (CONSORT criteria). The data will be described according to group allocation (BTX-A or placebo) and time (visit), using the usual statistics for each type of variable.

A Chi-squared test will be used to compare the distributions of qualitative variables, and analysis of variance will be used to compare the distributions of continuous quantitative variables (the variables may be adjusted to improve the symmetry or stabilise the variance). Ordinal variables (or those that do not have a normal distribution) will be compared using the non-parametric Kruskal-Wallis test.

Analysis of primary outcome

Change in peak length of the RF and TS muscles during gait at 1 month (difference in length between V3 and V1 will be compared between groups using a Student t-test. To prevent the risk of false positives induced by multiple testing, a Bonferroni Holm correction will be applied to the p-values for peak length, peak force and peak strength [61]. The level of significance will be set at 0.05/3.

Analysis of secondary outcomes

The statistical test used for the primary outcome will also be used to evaluate the effect of BTX-A at 3 months (V4). To compare changes in the secondary criteria across visits between the two groups (change in peak length of injected muscles, joint angles, modified Ashworth score, functional scores and quality of life), repeated measures models will be used. Depending on the distribution of continuous or binary variables, mixed models or generalized estimation equations (GEE) will be used respectively. The models will include the treatment variable (BTX-A or placebo), time and interaction between time and treatment as explanatory factors. If a significant interaction is found, comparisons between both groups (BTX-A and placebo) will be carried out for each time-point using a Student t-test. In order to take in to account any effects of multiple testing, these outcomes will be considered as explanatory factors rather than determinants of the effectiveness of BTX-A.

Analysis of safety criteria

The number and percentage of patients who experience adverse expected or unexpected effects, as well as serious adverse effects relating to the active treatment will be analysed. The nature of each effect will be specified. The duration and percentages of any adverse effects following BTX-A injection will be compared with any that occur following placebo injection using non-parametric tests.

Sample analysed

Because this is a study of effectiveness, the main analysis will be carried out following intention to treat principles. The safety analysis will be carried out on all participants who received at least one injection, whatever the substance injected. For the safety analysis, participants will not be analysed according to treatment allocation, but according to the treatment actually received.

Missing, unused or invalid data

The status of the patients (included, randomised, evaluated as intention to treat, lost to follow-up, left the study or deviated from the protocol) will be described and compared for each treatment arm and centre. Patients lost to follow-up, deceased (which should be exceptional) or left the study will be censored at the date of the last information. In case of censure, the last known value of the result will be used. All missing or invalid data will be replaced by the last available data for the corresponding parameters for the patient. The "last observation carried forwards procedure" will be used. In case of a large quantity of missing data, sensitivity analysis using conditional imputation will be carried out.

Management of changes to the planned analysis

Changes or supplementary analyses could be carried out. They will be considered as "post-hoc" and will be reported as such in the analysis and publication. Any retrospective changes to the planned analysis will be validated by the Study Committee and justified in an amendment to the protocol and in the trial report.

The statistical analysis will determine if BTX-A: i) increases peak muscle length during gait; ii) reduces peak force generated; iii) improves inter-segmental coordination during gait and iv) improves performance on functional tests.The second aim is to determine whether the effects of BTX-A are maintained at V4 compared with V1, suggesting a remnant action of BTX-A.

Discussion

We expect that BTX-A injection in the RF and TS muscles will increase their length and peak lengthening velocity and decrease peak muscle force during gait 1 month, and perhaps also 3 months, after the injection. We expect to find a reduction in the spasticity of these muscles, an increase in passive knee flexion and passive ankle dorsiflexion, a decrease in knee extensor and plantarflexor muscle strength (MRC scale, and isokinetic dynamometer) and a reduction in force generated by these muscles during gait (SIMM model) in the BTX-A group. The peak force couple produced by the knee flexors/extensors during active movements (measured on the isokinetic dynamometer) should decrease, and the angle at which peak force occurs during passive movements should increase, demonstrating a decrease in spasticity. We also expect spatiotemporal gait parameters to improve, with an increase in gait velocity, cadence and stride length. Peak ankle dorsiflexion in stance and perhaps also in swing, and peak knee flexion in swing should increase. Peak plantar flexion moment in pre-swing phase may decrease. Based on the results of the pilot study by Lampire [15], we hypothesise that the length and lengthening velocity of the injected muscles will improve 1 month post injection.

We anticipate that these changes (particularly 1 month after BTX-A injection) will be associated with a concomitant increase in gait velocity during the 10-MWT and distance walked during the 6MWT, and reductions in performance time of the stairs and Timed Up and Go tests.

This is the first randomised, placebo-controlled trial using instrumented measures, such as 3D gait analysis and an isokinetic dynamometer, to evaluate the effects of BTX-A on gait parameters and force in patients with chronic stroke-related hemiparesis. We expect improvements of all the parameters studied in the BTX-A group. In contrast, we do not expect any significant improvement of any outcome measures in the placebo group.

Analysis of correlations between the different results will reveal if changes in the biomechanical properties of the injected muscles are related to improvements in kinematic and kinetic parameters and functional tests.

The results of this study will therefore increase understanding of the results of many previous un-controlled studies that have found improvements in kinematic parameters following BTX-A injection in patients with chronic hemiparesis.

Abbreviations

10MWT: Ten meter walk test; 6MWT: Six minute walk test; ABC scale: Activities balance confidence scale; ABILOCO: A measure of locomotion ability for adults; BBS scale: Berg balance scale; BTX A: Botulium toxin type A; EMG: Electromyography; GEE: Generalized estimation equation; MAS: Modified ashworth scale; MRC: Medical research council; MSM: Musculoskeletal models; RF: Rectus femoris; SKG: Stiff knee gait; ST: Stairs test; TA: Tibialis anterior; TS: Triceps surae; TUG: Timed up and go test

Acknowledgements

The authors would like to thank « Assistance Publique - Hôpitaux de Paris » for supporting this study and Johanna Robertson for translation and constructive criticism.

Funding

This study is supported by the « Département de la recherche Clinique et du développement AP-HP», Assistance Publique-Hôpitaux de Paris, Hôpital Ambroise Paré, Unité de Recherche Clinique (URC), Boulogne Billancourt, France promotor code: AOM11223,P110136, budget: 18 000 euros. The translation of the article was funded by Allergan® who employed an independent translator. Allergan® will have no access to the results.

Funding was received from Allergan® for the translation of this article. In addition, Allergan® will provide the medical supplies. The funder had no influence on the design of the protocol, and will not have any impact on data generation, statistical analyses or writing of the final manuscript.

Authors' contributions

These authors contributed equally to the design of this study: RN; PD All authors helped to draft the manuscript. All the authors read and approved the final manuscript.

Competing interests

An outcomes assessor controlled the independence of the study from its source of finance.

Author details

[1]Inserm Unit 1179, Team 3: Technologies and Innovative Therapies Applied to Neuromuscular diseases, UVSQ, CIC 805, Physiology–Functional Testing Ward, AP-HP, Raymond Poincaré Teaching Hospital, Garches, France. [2]Assistance Publique-Hôpitaux de Paris, Hôpital Ambroise Paré, Unité de Recherche Clinique (URC), Boulogne, France. [3]CIAMS, University Paris-Sud, Université Paris-Saclay, 91405 Orsay Cedex, France. [4]CIAMS, Université d'Orléans, 45067 Orléans, France.

References

1. Brandstater ME, Gowland C, Clark BM. Hemiplegic gait: analysis of temporal variables. Arch Phys Med Rehabil. 1983;64:583–7.
2. Olney SJ, Griffin MP, McBride ID. Temporal, kinematic, and kinetic variables related to gait speed in subjects with hemiplegia: a regression approach. Phys Ther. 1994;74:872–85.
3. Pinzur MS, Sherman R, Dimonte-Levine P, Trimble J. Gait changes in adult onset hemiplegia. Am J Phys Med Rehabil. 1987;66:228–37.
4. Kerrigan DC, Gronley J, Perry J. Stiff-legged gait in spastic paresis. A study of quadriceps and hamstrings muscle activity. Am J Phys Med Rehabil. 1991; 70:294–300.
5. Pittock SJ, Moore AP, Hardiman O, Ehler E, Kovac M, Bojakowski J, et al. A Double-Blind Randomised Placebo-Controlled Evaluation of Three Doses of Botulinum Toxin Type A (Dysport®) in the Treatment of Spastic Equinovarus Deformity after Stroke. Cerebrovasc Dis. 2003;15:289–300.
6. Robertson JVG, Pradon D, Bensmail D, Fermanian C, Bussel B, Roche N. Relevance of botulinum toxin injection and nerve block of rectus femoris to kinematic and functional parameters of stiff knee gait in hemiplegic adults. Gait Posture. 2009;29:108–12.
7. Kerrigan DC, Roth RS, Riley PO. The modelling of adult spastic paretic stiff-legged gait swing period based on actual kinematic data. Gait Posture. 1998;7:117–24.
8. Kim CM, Eng JJ. Magnitude and pattern of 3D kinematic and kinetic gait profiles in persons with stroke: relationship to walking speed. Gait Posture. 2004;20:140–6.
9. Knutsson E, Richards C. Different types of disturbed motor control in gait of hemiparetic patients. Brain J Neurol. 1979;102:405–30.
10. Schantz EJ, Johnson EA. Properties and use of botulinum toxin and other microbial neurotoxins in medicine. Microbiol Rev. 1992;56:80–99.
11. Stoquart GG, Detrembleur C, Palumbo S, Deltombe T, Lejeune TM. Effect of Botulinum toxin injection in the rectus Femoris on stiff-knee gait in people with stroke: a prospective observational study. Arch Phys Med Rehabil. 2008; 89:56–61.
12. Caty GD, Detrembleur C, Bleyenheuft C, Deltombe T, Lejeune TM. Effect of simultaneous Botulinum toxin injections into several muscles on impairment, activity, participation, and quality of life among stroke patients presenting with a stiff knee gait. Stroke. 2008;39:2803–8.
13. Hutin E, Pradon D, Barbier F, Gracies J-M, Bussel B, Roche N. Lower limb coordination in Hemiparetic subjects: impact of Botulinum toxin injections into rectus Femoris. Neurorehabil Neural Repair. 2010;24:442–9.
14. Simon SR. Quantification of human motion: gait analysis—benefits and limitations to its application to clinical problems. J Biomech. 2004;37:1869–80.
15. Lampire N, Roche N, Carne P, Cheze L, Pradon D. Effect of botulinum toxin injection on length and lengthening velocity of rectus femoris during gait in hemiparetic patients. Clin Biomech Bristol Avon. 2013;28:164–70.
16. Hesse S, Krajnik J, Luecke D, Jahnke MT, Gregoric M, Mauritz KH. Ankle muscle activity before and after Botulinum toxin therapy for lower limb extensor spasticity in chronic Hemiparetic patients. Stroke. 1996;27:455–60.
17. Mancini F, Sandrini G, Moglia A, Nappi G, Pacchetti C. A randomised, double-blind, dose-ranging study to evaluate efficacy and safety of three doses of botulinum toxin type a (Botox) for the treatment of spastic foot. Neurol Sci. 2005;26:26–31.
18. Baricich A, Carda S, Bertoni M, Maderna L, Cisari C. A single-blinded, randomized pilot study of botulinum toxin type a combined with non-pharmacological treatment for spastic foot. J Rehabil Med. 2008;40:870–2.
19. Stroke--1989. Recommendations on stroke prevention, diagnosis, and therapy. Report of the WHO Task Force on Stroke and other Cerebrovascular Disorders. Stroke J Cereb Circ. 1989;20:1407–31.
20. Pradon D, Hutin E, Khadir S, Taiar R, Genet F, Roche N. A pilot study to investigate the combined use of Botulinum toxin type-a and ankle foot orthosis for the treatment of spastic foot in chronic hemiplegic patients. Clin Biomech. 2011;26:867–72.
21. Bensmail D, Denormandie P, Parratte B. Guide des points d'injection de toxine botulinique de type A. à dire d'experts. Paris: Expressions santé; 2006.
22. Clarkson HM. Musculoskeletal assessment: joint motion and muscle testing. 3rd ed. Philadelphia: Wolters Kluwer/Lippincott Williams & Wilkins Health; 2013.
23. Bohannon RW, Smith MB. Interrater reliability of a modified Ashworth scale of muscle spasticity. Phys Ther. 1987;67:206–7.
24. Lin FM, Sabbahi M. Correlation of spasticity with hyperactive stretch reflexes and motor dysfunction in hemiplegia. Arch Phys Med Rehabil. 1999;80:526–30.
25. Katz RT, Rovai GP, Brait C, Rymer WZ. Objective quantification of spastic hypertonia: correlation with clinical findings. Arch Phys Med Rehabil. 1992; 73:339–47.
26. Shaw L, Rodgers H, Price C, van Wijck F, Shackley P, Steen N, et al. BoTULS: a multicentre randomised controlled trial to evaluate the clinical effectiveness and cost-effectiveness of treating upper limb spasticity due to stroke with botulinum toxin type a. Health Technol Assess. 2010;14 https://doi.org/10.3310/hta14260.
27. Paternostro-Sluga T, Grim-Stieger M, Posch M, Schuhfried O, Vacariu G, Mittermaier C, et al. Reliability and validity of the Medical Research Council (MRC) scale and a modified scale for testing muscle strength in patients with radial palsy. J Rehabil Med. 2008;40:665–71.
28. Bohannon RW. Manual muscle testing: does it meet the standards of an adequate screening test? Clin Rehabil. 2005;19:662–7.
29. Chapman AE. The mechanical properties of human muscle. Exerc Sport Sci Rev. 1985;13:443–501.
30. Delp SL, Loan JP, Hoy MG, Zajac FE, Topp EL, Rosen JM. An interactive graphics-based model of the lower extremity to study orthopaedic surgical procedures. IEEE Trans Biomed Eng. 1990;37:757–67.
31. Hatze H. A complete set of control equations for the human musculo-skeletal system. J Biomech. 1977;10:799–805.
32. Hoy MG, Zajac FE, Gordon ME. A musculoskeletal model of the human lower extremity: the effect of muscle, tendon, and moment arm on the moment-angle relationship of musculotendon actuators at the hip, knee, and ankle. J Biomech. 1990;23:157–69.
33. Pandy MG, Anderson FC. Dynamic simulation of human movement using large-scale models of the body. Phonetica. 2000;57:219–28.
34. Zajac FE. Muscle and tendon: properties, models, scaling, and application to biomechanics and motor control. Crit Rev Biomed Eng. 1989;17:359–411.
35. Arndt AN, Komi PV, Brüggemann G-P, Lukkariniemi J. Individual muscle contributions to the in vivo achilles tendon force. Clin Biomech Bristol Avon. 1998;13:532–41.
36. Anderson FC, Pandy MG. Individual muscle contributions to support in normal walking. Gait Posture. 2003;17:159–69.
37. Erdemir A, McLean S, Herzog W, van den Bogert AJ. Model-based estimation of muscle forces exerted during movements. Clin Biomech. 2007; 22:131–54.
38. Liu MQ, Anderson FC, Schwartz MH, Delp SL. Muscle contributions to support and progression over a range of walking speeds. J Biomech. 2008; 41:3243–52.
39. Neptune RR, Zajac FE, Kautz SA. Muscle force redistributes segmental power for body progression during walking. Gait Posture. 2004;19:194–205.
40. Neptune RR, Sasaki K, Kautz SA. The effect of walking speed on muscle function and mechanical energetics. Gait Posture. 2008;28:135–43.
41. Pierce SR, Johnston TE, Shewokis PA, Lauer RT. Examination of spasticity of the knee flexors and knee extensors using isokinetic dynamometry with electromyography and clinical scales in children with spinal cord injury. J Spinal Cord Med. 2008;31:208–14.

42. Boudarham J, Roche N, Pradon D, Bonnyaud C, Bensmail D, Zory R. Variations in kinematics during clinical gait analysis in stroke patients. PLoS One. 2013;8:e66421.
43. Hermens HJ, Freriks B, Merletti R, Stegeman D, Blok J, Rau G, et al. European recommendations for surface electromyography. Roessingh Res Dev. 1999;8: 13–54.
44. Ivanenko YP, Poppele RE, Lacquaniti F. Five basic muscle activation patterns account for muscle activity during human locomotion. J Physiol. 2004; 556(Pt 1):267–82.
45. Bizzi E, Cheung VCK, d'Avella A, Saltiel P, Tresch M. Combining modules for movement. Brain Res Rev. 2008;57:125–33.
46. Delis I, Panzeri S, Pozzo T, Berret B. A unifying model of concurrent spatial and temporal modularity in muscle activity. J Neurophysiol. 2014;111:675–93.
47. Lexell J, Flansbjer U-B, Holmbäck AM, Downham D, Patten C. Reliability of gait performance tests in men and women with hemiparesis after stroke. J Rehabil Med. 2005;37:75–82.
48. Eng JJ, Dawson AS, Chu KS. Submaximal exercise in persons with stroke: test-retest reliability and concurrent validity with maximal oxygen consumption. Arch Phys Med Rehabil. 2004;85:113–8.
49. Schmid A, Duncan PW, Studenski S, Lai SM, Richards L, Perera S, et al. Improvements in speed-based gait classifications are meaningful. Stroke. 2007;38:2096–100.
50. Bowden MG, Balasubramanian CK, Behrman AL, Kautz SA. Validation of a speed-based classification system using quantitative measures of walking performance Poststroke. Neurorehabil Neural Repair. 2008;22:672–5.
51. Alzahrani MA, Dean CM, Ada L. Ability to negotiate stairs predicts free-living physical activity in community-dwelling people with stroke: an observational study. Aust J Physiother. 2009;55:277–81.
52. Berg KO, Wood-Dauphinee SL, Williams JI, Maki B. Measuring balance in the elderly: validation of an instrument. Can J Public Health Rev Can Sante Publique. 1992;83:S7–11.
53. Gallien P, Adrien S, Petrilli S, Durufle A, Robineau S, Kerdoncuff V, et al. Home care and quality of life three years after stroke. Ann Réadapt Médecine Phys. 2005;48:225–30.
54. Bugge C, Hagen S, Alexander H. Measuring stroke patients' health status in the early post-stroke phase using the SF36. Int J Nurs Stud. 2001;38:319–27.
55. Dodds TA, Martin DP, Stolov WC, Deyo RA. A validation of the functional independence measurement and its performance among rehabilitation inpatients. Arch Phys Med Rehabil. 1993;74:531–6.
56. Chumney D, Nollinger K, Shesko K, Skop K, Spencer M, Newton RA. Ability of functional independence measure to accurately predict functional outcome of stroke-specific population: systematic review. J Rehabil Res Dev. 2010;47:17.
57. Caty GD, Arnould C, Stoquart GG, Thonnard J-L, Lejeune TM. ABILOCO: a Rasch-built 13-item questionnaire to assess locomotion ability in stroke patients. Arch Phys Med Rehabil. 2008;89:284–90.
58. Powell LE, Myers AM. The activities-specific balance confidence (ABC) scale. J Gerontol A Biol Sci Med Sci. 1995;50A:M28–34.
59. Faul F, Erdfelder E, Lang A-G, Buchner A. G* power 3: a flexible statistical power analysis program for the social, behavioral, and biomedical sciences. Behav Res Methods. 2007;39:175–91.
60. Julious SA, McIntyre NE. Sample sizes for trials involving multiple correlated must-win comparisons. Pharm Stat. 2012;11:177–85.
61. Holm S. A simple sequentially Rejective multiple test procedure. Scand J Stat. 1979;6:65–70.

Time spent lying, sitting, and upright during hospitalization after stroke

Ole Petter Norvang[1,2*], Anne Hokstad[1,3], Kristin Taraldsen[1], Xiangchun Tan[1], Stian Lydersen[4], Bent Indredavik[1,3] and Torunn Askim[1,3]

Abstract

Background: Early mobilization has been an important part of acute stroke unit treatment. However, early and intense mobilization within the first 24 h post stroke may cause an unfavorable outcome. Recently, objective measurements using body-worn sensors have been applied, enabling continuous monitoring of physical activity in the hospital setting. This study aimed to use body-worn sensors to quantify the amount of physical activity and how activity levels changed over time during hospitalization in patients with acute stroke. We also wanted to investigate which factors were associated with upright and sitting activity.

Methods: This was a prospective study including patients admitted to hospital within seven days after onset of stroke. Physical activity was measured by two sensors (ActivPALs from PAL Technologies Ltd., Glasgow, UK), one attached on sternum and one on the thigh of the unaffected side, monitoring continuously from inclusion until discharge. Data were processed in Matlab R 2015B and provided information about daily time in lying, sitting, and upright positions, and daily average duration of sitting and upright bouts. A linear mixed model was used to analyze changes over time.

Results: 58 patients were included (31 women, mean (SD) age; 75.1 (12.0)). Patients were hospitalized for 12.1 (7.6) days and had a mean score on the National Institute of Health Stroke Scale of 6.2 (5.5) points. Time spent sitting and time spent upright increased per day during hospitalization by 22.10 min (95% Confidence interval (CI): 14.96, 29.24) and 3.75 min (95% CI: 1.70, 5.80) respectively. Increased time upright was associated with improved Modified Rankin Scale scores (− 38.09 min, 95% CI: -61.88, − 14.29) and higher Short Physical Performance Battery scores (6.97 min, 95% CI: 1.99, 11.95), while prolonged bouts of sitting were associated with more severe stroke (4.50 min, 95% CI: 0.80, 8.19), and older age (1.72 min, 95% CI: 0.20, 3.26).

Conclusions: Patients increased their daily time spent sitting and upright during the initial hospital stay after stroke. Prolonged bouts of sitting were associated with older age and more severe strokes. Hence future research should investigate the benefit of interventions aimed at breaking up sitting time after stroke.

Keywords: Stroke, Early rehabilitation, Accelerometer, Physical activity

* Correspondence: olepn@ntnu.no
[1]Department of Neuromedicine and Movement Science, Faculty of Medicine and health science, NTNU - Norwegian University of Science and Technology, Trondheim, Norway
[2]Clinical Services, Department of Physiotherapy, St Olavs Hospital, Trondheim University Hospital, NO-7006 Trondheim, Norway
Full list of author information is available at the end of the article

Background

One of the core elements of care for dedicated comprehensive stroke units is acute medical treatment combined with early rehabilitation [1–3]. Early rehabilitation with mobilization out of bed during hospitalization has shown to be associated with better functional outcomes for patients after stroke [4–8]. This may reduce the loss of muscle mass, increase muscle strength [6, 9], avoid complications [3, 4, 10], exploit the plasticity of the brain [11], improve neurological functioning [12], and improve gait function [13]. Although time spent out of bed early after stroke varies significantly between hospitals [14–16], the amount of physical activity is generally low during hospital stays [17, 18].

Optimal timing and intensity of early mobilization is, however, not clear, as previous studies have shown an association between mobilization within the first 24 h and a negative trend towards increased dependency [12, 19] and increased mortality [20]. On the other hand, short and frequent mobilizations have been associated with improved outcome [21].

Most studies of physical activity during hospitalization have been single-day observational studies during daytime hours. Recently, objective measurements using body-worn single sensor activity monitors have been applied, enabling continuous monitoring of physical activity over time [22, 23]. So far, only a few studies have used activity monitors to distinguish between different activities in the acute phase for stroke patients [24]. In one of these studies, Strømmen et al. (2014) found significantly increased activity in the lower extremities for hospitalized stroke patients from the first day until discharge [25]. The increased activity was significantly associated with lower severity of stroke, whereas decreased activity was found with increasing age [25]. However, the study did not discriminate between times spent in different positions, which is crucial when measuring physical activity in the acute phase after stroke. Applying two single sensors from the ActivPAL sensor system, one on the chest and one on the thigh, makes it possible to quantify the amount of time spent in different positions. This method has previously been proved valid for stroke patients [26].

The main aim of this study was to describe the amount of time spent in lying, sitting and upright (standing or walking) positions early after stroke and how these activity levels changed during the hospital stay, both regarding total time per day and duration for each mobilization. Another aim was to examine which factors were associated with total time and bouts of sitting and upright activity. Our primary hypothesis was that patients would gradually increase time spent in an upright position, and thereby increase the duration of each upright bout.

Method

Design

This study used a prospective observation design, measuring physical activity continuously with two activity monitors for three to seven consecutive days during hospitalization.

Study setting

All patients were treated in an evidence-based comprehensive stroke unit that emphasizes a multidisciplinary approach and early rehabilitation. The treatment focused on independence in daily life. All patients, regardless of participation, received routine medical treatment, including rehabilitation, in accordance with Norwegian guidelines for treatment and rehabilitation after stroke [27].

Study population

Patients were recruited during three time periods, October–December 2013, May–December 2014, and March–August 2016. Patients admitted to Trondheim University Hospital, Norway, with diagnosed first ever or recurrent acute ischemic or hemorrhagic stroke were eligible for inclusion if the onset of stroke had been within seven days, they spoke fluent Norwegian, and if they gave written consent. In line with the Norwegian regulations for informed consent, patients who were unable to consent were included if their next of kin not opposed participation. Patients with terminal illness, other health conditions severely affecting their ability to walk, or expected discharge within three days after inclusion were excluded.

Measurements

The ActivPAL Professional sensor system (from PAL Technologies Ltd) consists of a three-axis accelerometer that collects continuous data with a sampling frequency of 10 Hz, and with a battery capacity of up to 14 days. The primary outcome for this study was whether time spent lying, sitting or upright changed during the hospital stay. It has previously been shown that this activity monitor provides valid data for time spent lying, sitting, standing and walking [28, 29] and that placement on the thigh and sternum provides good validity for postures and transitions compared to video observations [26]. The 24-h period was measured from the time the activity monitors were attached. Duration of sitting bouts was estimated according to the following ratio: time spent in sitting/number of transitions from lying to sitting, while duration of upright bouts was estimated correspondingly. A time threshold for transitions was set at 1.5 s to eliminate unreliable event records.

The Short Physical Performance Battery (SPPB) (ranging from 0 to 12, where 12 is the best score) was used to assess physical function. The test consists of three different mobility tasks, and has been found to be both valid and reliable for assessing physical function amongst elderly people [30]. Gait speed was calculated based on the walking task of the SPPB. An experienced nurse or physiotherapist performed the test.

Global function was defined using the Modified Rankin Scale (mRS) (ranging from 0 to 6, where 0 is normal function and 6 denotes death) [31] at admission and after the first day in hospital. The mRS measures independence in activities of daily living.

The National Institutes of Health Stroke Scale (NIHSS) was used to measure severity of the stroke. The scale is widely used and has proved both valid and reliable [32].

Both mRS and NIHSS were scored by an experienced clinician within the first day after the patient's admission and recorded together with age, gender, number of days from first symptom to admission date, and number of days at the hospital, which were collected from the medical record.

Procedure

All patients accepting participation had two ActivPAL activity monitors attached, one at the sternum and one at the unaffected thigh, to distinguish between lying, sitting and upright position. If neither of the lower extremities were affected by the stroke, the activity monitor was attached to the right thigh. Patients were instructed to follow the standard rehabilitation routines without paying attention to the equipment. Both activity monitors were removed 14 days post stroke unless the patient had been discharged earlier. Data from the activity monitors were transferred via a USB docking station, and processed in Matlab R2015 B. The valid body and leg data had an individual start and stop time defined and used to measure a count for a full 24-h day, and the activity was coded in reference to the body position. To distinguish the different positions, data from the two sensors were synchronized and recoded according to body position (lying, sitting, and upright).

State durations were calculated by accumulating time intervals for lying, sitting, and upright and state transitions between these positions per 24-h measurement. Time upright was calculated by merging time standing and time walking. A validation procedure was performed to control for possible time drifting of the sensors.

Statistical analysis

Demographic data were reported as mean values and standard deviation (SD) for all patients, and for three subgroups categorized by time from onset of symptoms to inclusion. Baseline characteristics were compared for those included within the first two days after stroke, those included 3 to 4 days after stroke and those included 5 to 7 days after stroke. This was done using a one-way ANOVA or Kruskal-Wallis test, depending on normality of residuals, which was judged by visual inspection of Q-Q plots. To assess changes in activity levels, we used linear mixed models (LMM) with time sitting, time upright, duration of sitting bouts and duration of upright bouts, respectively, as dependent variables, patients as random factor, and days since stroke as covariate. Next, we included the following covariates, one at a time: NIHSS, age, gender, mRS pre-stroke, mRS one day post stroke, and SPPB. Because the time spent lying, sitting and upright totaled 24 h, only time spent sitting and upright were used in the mixed model analysis. Two-sided p-values less than 0.05 were considered statistically significant, and 95% confidence intervals (CI) are reported where relevant. Statistical analyses were done in SPSS 23.

Results

The flow of patients is shown in Fig. 1. Of the 105 patients who met the inclusion criteria, 47 were excluded, mainly because of early discharge.

Fifty-eight patients (31 female) were included in the analysis. Patient characteristics are presented in Table 1. Mean (SD) time from onset of symptoms to inclusion was 2.6 (1.7) days, and patients wore the activity monitors for 5.8 (1.5) days. The NIHSS score was 6.2 (5.0) points. Those included 4–7 days after symptom onset showed significantly lower scores on NIHSS as compared to those included within the first 24 h ($p = 0.002$).

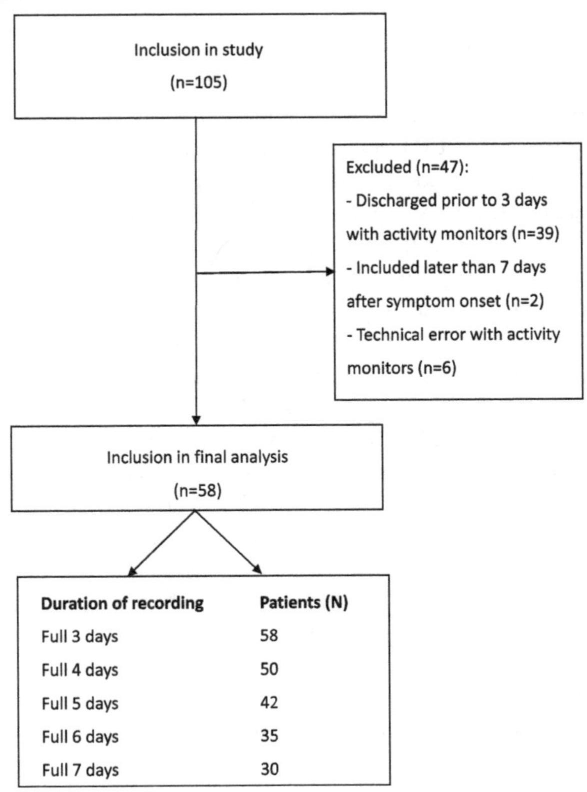

Fig. 1 Flow chart

Table 1 Demographic data for included patients ($N = 58$)

	Included 0–2 days from symptoms ($n = 19$)	Included 3–4 days from symptoms ($n = 24$)	Included 5–7 days from symptoms ($n = 15$)	Total ($n = 58$)
Female gender, *n* (%)	11 (57.9)	11 (45.8)	9 (60.0)	31 (53.5)
Age (years)	72.9 (10.0)	76.6 (13.1)	75.3 (12.1)	75.1 (12.0)
Monitoring days	5.8 (1.6)	5.8 (1.6)	6.0 (1.3)	5.8 (1.5)
Days hospitalized	10.6 (4.6)	10.0 (4.6)	12.6 (5.5)	12.1 (7.6)
Days from stroke to inclusion	0.9 (0.3)	2.4 (0.5)	5.0 (1.3)	2.6 (1.7)
NIHSS when admitted	8.4 (4.4)	8.4 (4.4)	4.6 (6.8)	6.2 (5.0)
Median (IQR)	7.0 (6.0–13.0)	4.0 (3.0–7.0)	3.0 (2.0–5.0)	5.0 (3.0–8.0)
Stroke severity groups, *n* (%)				
Mild (NIHSS < 8)	13 (68.4)	19 (79.2)	14 (93.3)	46 (79.1)
Moderate (NIHSS 8–16)	6 (31.6)	5 (20.8)	0 (0.0)	11 (19.0)
Severe (NIHSS > 16)	0 (0.0)	0 (0.0)	1 (6.7)	1 (1.7)
mRS prior to stroke	1.6 (1.1)	1.6 (1.1)	1.2 (0.9)	1.7 (1.2)
Median (IQR)	1.0 (1.0–2.0)	2.0 (2.0–3.0)	1.0 (1.0–2.0)	2.0 (1.0–2.3)
mRS when admitted	4.1 (0.5)	4.1 (0.5)	4.1 (0.7)	4.1 (0.7)
Median (IQR)	4.0 (4.0–4.0)	4.0 (4.0–5.0)	4.0 (4.0–4.0)	4.0 (4.0–4.3)
Gait speed (m/s)	1.7 (1.6)	1.5 (0.9)	1.2 (1.2)	1.5 (1.2)
SPPB	5.1 (3.8)	5.1 (3.8)	3.9 (3.5)	4.4 (3.5)
Median (IQR)	5.0 (1.0–7.0)	3.5 (2.0–7.0)	4.0 (0.0–7.0)	4.0 (1.0–7.0)

Mean (SD) unless otherwise stated
NIHSS National Institute of Health Stroke Scale, *mRS* modified Rankin Scale, *SPPB* Short Physical Performance Battery

No other significant differences were found for the baseline variables.

Figure 2 illustrates the combinations of activities for each day, showing an increase in time spent out of bed during the hospital stay. Time spent upright remained low throughout the observation period.

Results from the LMM analysis (Table 2) show a daily increase in time spent sitting of 22.10 min ($p < 0.001$) and 3.75 min upright ($p < 0.001$). Adjusted for time, we found that decreasing time spent upright was associated with increasing dependency, measured by mRS the first day after stroke ($p = 0.002$). An association was also found between time spent upright and physical function showing an increase of 6.97 min upright for every point increase on SPPB ($p = 0.007$). Neither severity of stroke nor age significantly influenced changes in overall physical activity.

Although not significant, LMM analysis indicated a daily increased duration of 4.32 min for each sitting bout ($p = 0.051$). Adjusted for time, this increase in time was associated with both a higher NIHSS score ($p = 0.018$) and increasing age ($p = 0.028$).

Discussion

In this study, we found that stroke patients increased their time spent sitting and upright during the initial hospital stay, with a corresponding decrease in time spent in a lying position. The duration of sitting bouts also increased over time, while the duration of upright bouts remained constant. Furthermore, overall increased time spent upright was associated with increasing independency (mRS) and improved physical function (SPPB), while prolonged sitting bouts were associated with higher age and more severe stroke.

Despite a statistically significant increase in time spent upright during the hospital stay, we may ask whether an estimated 3.75 min's more upright activity per day was a clinically significant change. This means that time spent

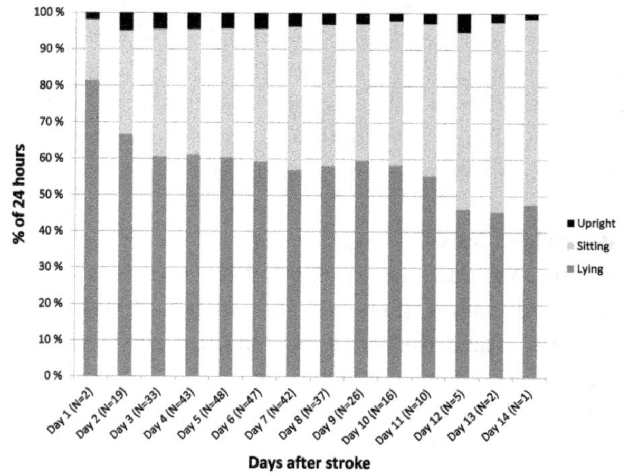

Fig. 2 Percentage of time spent in different positions within every 24 h

Table 2 Linear mixed model regression with activity level as dependent variable

Covariate	Time sitting (minutes)			Time upright (minutes)			Duration of bouts in sitting (minutes)			Duration of bouts in upright (minutes)		
	Coefficient	95% CI	*p*-value	Coefficient	95% CI	*p*-value	Coefficient	95% CI	*p*-value	Coefficient	95% CI	*p*-value
Time stroke to inclusion (days)[a]	22.10	14.96, 29.24	< 0.001	3.75	1.70, 5.80	< 0.001	4.32	−0.25, 8.66	0.051	0.14	−0.08, 0.36	0.212
NIHSS	0.19	−10.53, 10.91	0.972	−2.34	−5.97, 1.28	0.201	4.50	0.80, 8.19	0.018	−0.08	−0.35, 0.19	0.547
Age (years)[b]	3.09	−1.26, 7.44	0.160	−0.47	−1.99, 1.04	0.534	1.72	0.20, 3.26	0.028	−0.08	−0.19, 0.03	0.133
Female gender[b]	− 35.23	− 141.08, 70.60	0.508	−12.55	−48.93, 23.83	0.492	21.10	−16.95, 59.14	0.271	−0.90	−3.52, 1.71	0.493
mRS_pre strole[b]	− 2.48	−47.02, 42.06	0.912	1.72	−13.60, 17.03	0.823	9.52	−6.39, 25.43	0.236	0.09	−1.00, 1.19	0.867
mRS_post stroke[b]	− 66.98	−140.22, 6.27	0.072	−38.09	−61.88, − 14.29	0.002	6.83	− 20.29, 33.96	0.616	−0.73	−2.57, 1.11	0.432
SPPB	12.21	−2.92, 27.33	0.111	6.97	1.99, 11.95	0.007	−3.23	−8.78, 2.33	0.250	0.18	−0.20, 0.55	0.358

[a]Unadjusted
[b]Adjusted for days since stroke

upright will increase by almost 40 min during a 10-day hospital stay. A previous study has shown that every 5-min increase in time spent in bed was associated with a 4% deterioration on the mRS score three months later [6]. Hence, the daily increase in time spent upright could potentially have a great impact on functional recovery over time.

On the other hand, we found no association between stroke severity and time spent out of bed. This finding might be explained by the fact that activity measures during hospitalization also mirror the mobilization routines in the wards [33], showing that patients are mobilized out of bed as soon as they are medically approved, independent of the patients' ability to mobilize themselves.

The duration of each sitting bout also increased by more than 4 min per day during the hospital stay. More surprisingly, the increased duration of sitting bouts was associated with higher age and more severe stroke, while no associations were found for bouts in upright activity. These findings might be explained by the ability of less affected and younger patients to change position more often by themselves. This is interesting because it adds further knowledge to the ongoing debate regarding the intensity of early mobilization. Also, clinicians should be aware that patients with the most severe strokes who are not able to move independently are at increased risk of sedentary behavior, which might be harmful, thereby increasing the risk of poor outcome [6].

Our results show that stroke patients on average spend a significant proportion of each 24 h in a lying position (Fig. 2). Considering the 24-h monitoring, patients would normally spend at least 30% of the time sleeping. Still, patients spent almost 30% of the remaining time in bed. This corresponds with the high amount of time spent lying previously reported early after stroke [14, 17, 25]. One factor that could influence the low overall activity amongst our participants is the exclusion of those expected to be discharged within three days after inclusion, as these patients are likely to be more active. However, as we aimed to study change in physical activity over time, patients with short monitoring time had to be excluded.

The major strength of the present study was the prospective study design with continuous monitoring of activity, from two activity monitors, over 24 h for several days during the hospital stay. This allowed us to discriminate between lying, sitting and upright positions, which is of major importance in the acute phase after stroke. The use of such a protocol has been validated in the stroke population earlier, showing a high accuracy compared to video observation [26]. In contrast to observation of activity by, for example, behavioral mapping during daytime hours, usually for 9–10 h [7, 14, 17], continuous monitoring will account for out-of-bed time during 24 h. It is also a strength that all included patients received evidence-based treatment in a comprehensive stroke unit combining acute medical treatment and early rehabilitation. Therefore, we know that our patients were mobilized according to recommendations in the national and international guidelines [27, 34], increasing the validity of the study.

A limitation of this study was the wide window for inclusion, ranging from one to seven days post stroke. This criterion was chosen for practical reasons, as recruitment was delayed during weekends and because the diagnosis was delayed in some patients (if the MR images were inconclusive or if patients were not admitted to hospital immediately after the first stroke symptoms). Nevertheless, apart from a significant difference in NIHSS between early and late admission to hospital, indicating that patients with the most severe symptoms are admitted to hospital earlier, we found no significant differences in the demographic data at baseline. However, the variation in time from onset of stroke to inclusion is accounted for in the LMM analysis. Our prolonged recruitment period (2013–2016), with three different time periods may also have influenced our results. The same routines were, however, applied for all stroke patients in the acute stroke treatment in the time periods. Therefore, all included patients, regardless of when they were recruited, should have received treatment focused on early rehabilitation. Another limitation is the lack of possibility to draw a causal relationship between the clinical parameters and the activity categories. Our secondary analysis indicate that the clinical parameters were influencing the activity levels. However, it is also possible to reverse this relationship, and to argue that the activity levels might influence the clinical parameters. Hence, it is important to have this possible bilateral relationship in mind when interpreting the results. Finally, the accelerometers used in this project do not discriminate between active and passive mobilization, and based on our inclusion criteria, mobilization may have been conducted with or without support from another person. This could influence both length and frequency of mobilization, as an active mobilization is naturally more tiring for the patient. However, in a comprehensive stroke unit, hospital staff are trained to activate stroke patients as soon as medically accepted, to encourage active rehabilitation. This means that even though some patients receive more support than others, all patients should be challenged according to their functional level.

Clinical implications

Our study supports previous findings showing that stroke patients spend most of their time in a lying or sitting position [7, 17, 25, 28], during hospitalization. The association between increased time spent upright and improved function indicates a need to pay specific attention to patients who depend on support to be able to transfer to an upright position to ensure frequent and short periods in upright activity throughout their hospital stay as recommended [21]. As older and more severely affected stroke patients may not be able to change position as often as independent patients, hospital staff also should pay extra attention to these patients when mobilizing them to a sitting position, to reduce sedentary time and avoid complications.

Conclusion

This study showed that time spent in sitting and upright positions increased throughout the hospital stay in patients admitted to hospital following a stroke. We found that these changes were associated with improved physical function and a higher degree of independence. There was also an increased duration of bouts spent sitting during hospitalization, with longer bouts associated with increasing age and more severe strokes. Future research should focus on defining the optimal dose of activity in the acute phase in order to improve function in the long term after stroke.

Abbreviations

CI: Confidence Interval; IQR: Inter Quartile Range; LMM: Linear Mixed Model; MRS: Modified Rankin Scale; NIHSS: National Institute of Health Stroke Scale; SD: Standard Deviation; SPPB: Short Physical Performance Battery

Acknowledgements

We would like to thank the Department of Stroke for collaboration throughout the project. We would also thank the ongoing Norwegian Cognitive impairment after stroke (Nor-COAST) study for helpful collaboration in recruiting patients. Finally, we would like to thank patients and their families who agreed to participate in our study.

Funding

OPN was funded during the data collection by the Liaison Committee between the Central Norway Regional Health Authority and the University Colleges.

Authors' contributions

AH and TA planned the study. AH and OPN recruited, and AH and OPN tested patients. BI was medically responsible for the included patients. OPN, KT, and XT planned and processed data. OPN, SL, and TA performed the statistics by analyzing the data. OPN and TA interpreted the results. The manuscript was written by OPN and TA. All authors critically reviewed and approved the manuscript before it was submitted.

Authors' information

OPN (MSc) works as a physiotherapist at Clinical Services, Trondheim University Hospital and as a PhD student at the Norwegian University of Science and Technology (NTNU) in the Geriatric, Movement and Stroke (GeMS) group, Department of Neuromedicine and Movement Science, Faculty of Medicine and health science. AH (PhD) works as a medical doctor at The Norwegian Heart and Lung Patient Organization (LHL), Trondheim, Norway and as a researcher at Department of Neuromedicine and Movement Science, Faculty of Medicine and health science, NTNU. KT is a postdoctoral fellow with GeMS, Department of Neuromedicine and Movement Science, Faculty of Medicine and health science. XT works as a senior engineer with GeMS, Department of Neuromedicine and Movement Science, Faculty of Medicine and health science. SL is a professor in medical statistics at Regional Centre for Child and Youth Mental Health and Child Welfare, Department of Mental Health, Faculty of Medicine and health science, NTNU. BI is head of the Stroke Unit at St. Olavs University Hospital and Adjunct Professor at the Department of Neuromedicine and Movement Science, Faculty of Medicine and health science, NTNU. TA is a professor at the Department of Neuromedicine and Movement Science, Faculty of Medicine and health science, NTNU.

Competing interests

The authors declare that they have no competing interests.

Author details

[1]Department of Neuromedicine and Movement Science, Faculty of Medicine and health science, NTNU - Norwegian University of Science and Technology, Trondheim, Norway. [2]Clinical Services, Department of Physiotherapy, St Olavs Hospital, Trondheim University Hospital, NO-7006 Trondheim, Norway. [3]Clinic of Medicine, Department of Stroke, St. Olavs Hospital, Trondheim University Hospital, Trondheim, Norway. [4]Regional Centre for Child and Youth Mental Health and Child Care, Department of Mental Health, Faculty of Medicine, NTNU - Norwegian University of Science and Technology, Trondheim, Norway.

References

1. Langhorne P, Pollock A. What are the components of effective stroke unit care? Age Ageing. 2002;31:365–71.
2. Organised inpatient (stroke unit) care for stroke. The Cochrane database of systematic reviews. 2013:Cd000197. doi: https://doi.org/10.1002/14651858.CD000197.pub3.
3. Indredavik B, Bakke F, Slørdahl S, Rokseth R, Håheim L. Treatment in a combined acute and rehabilitation stroke unit which aspects are most important? Stroke. 1999;30:917–23.
4. Ingeman A, Andersen G, Hundborg HH, Svendsen ML, Johnsen SP. Processes of care and medical complications in patients with stroke. Stroke. 2011;42:167–72. https://doi.org/10.1161/STROKEAHA.110.599738.
5. Chippala P, Sharma R. Effect of very early mobilisation on functional status in patients with acute stroke: a single-blind, randomized controlled trail. Clin Rehabil. 2016;30:669–75. https://doi.org/10.1177/0269215515596054.
6. Askim T, Bernhardt J, Salvesen O, Indredavik B. Physical activity early after stroke and its association to functional outcome 3 months later. J Stroke Cerebrovasc Dis. 2014;23:e305–12. https://doi.org/10.1016/j.jstrokecerebrovasdis.2013.12.011.
7. Hokstad A, Indredavik B, Bernhardt J, Langhammer B, Gunnes M, Lundemo C, et al. Upright activity within the first week after stroke is associated with better functional outcome and health-related quality of life: a Norwegian multi-site study. J Rehabil Med. 2016;48:280–6. https://doi.org/10.2340/16501977-2051.
8. Yagi M, Yasunaga H, Matsui H, Morita K, Fushimi K, Fujimoto M, et al. Impact of rehabilitation on outcomes in patients with ischemic stroke: a Nationwide retrospective cohort study in Japan. Stroke. 2017;48:740–6. https://doi.org/10.1161/STROKEAHA.116.015147.
9. English C, McLennan H, Thoirs K, Coates A, Reviews BJ. Loss of skeletal muscle mass after stroke: a systematic review. Int J Stroke. 2010;5:395–402. https://doi.org/10.1111/j.1747-4949.2010.00467.x.
10. Herisson F, Godard S, Volteau C, Le Blanc E, Guillon B, Gaudron M. Early sitting in ischemic stroke patients (SEVEL): a randomized controlled trial. PLoS One. 2016;11:e0149466. https://doi.org/10.1371/journal.pone.0149466.
11. Murphy TH, Corbett D. Plasticity during stroke recovery: from synapse to behaviour. Nat Rev Neurosci. 2009;10:861–72. https://doi.org/10.1038/nrn2735.
12. Sundseth A, Thommessen B, Ronning OM. Outcome after mobilization within 24 hours of acute stroke: a randomized controlled trial. Stroke. 2012; 43:2389–94. https://doi.org/10.1161/STROKEAHA.111.646687.
13. Cumming TB, Thrift AG, Collier JM, Churilov L, Dewey HM, Donnan GA, et al. Very early mobilization after stroke fast-tracks return to walking: further results from the phase II AVERT randomized controlled trial. Stroke. 2011;42: 153–8. https://doi.org/10.1161/STROKEAHA.110.594598.

14. Bernhardt J, Chitravas N, Meslo IL, Thrift AG, Indredavik B. Not all stroke units are the same: a comparison of physical activity patterns in Melbourne, Australia, and Trondheim, Norway. Stroke. 2008;39:2059–65. https://doi.org/10.1161/STROKEAHA.107.507160.
15. Wellwood I, Langhorne P, McKevitt C, Bernhardt J, Rudd A, Wolfe C. An observational study of acute stroke care in four countries: the European registers of stroke study. Cerebrovasc Dis. 2009;28:171–6. https://doi.org/10.1159/000226116.
16. Hokstad A, Indredavik B, Bernhardt J, Ihle-Hansen H, Salvesen O, Seljeseth YM, et al. Hospital differences in motor activity early after stroke: a comparison of 11 Norwegian stroke units. J Stroke Cerebrovasc Dis. 2015;24:1333–40. https://doi.org/10.1016/j.jstrokecerebrovasdis.2015.02.009.
17. Askim T, Bernhardt J, Loge AD, Indredavik B. Stroke patients do not need to be inactive in the first two-weeks after stroke: results from a stroke unit focused on early rehabilitation. Int J Stroke. 2012;7:25–31. https://doi.org/10.1111/j.1747-4949.2011.00697.x.
18. Bernhardt J, Dewey H, Thrift A, Donnan G. Inactive and alone: physical activity within the first 14 days of acute stroke unit care. Stroke. 2004;35:1005–9.
19. Bernhardt J, Langhorne P, Lindley RI, Thrift AG, Ellery F, Collier J, et al. Efficacy and safety of very early mobilisation within 24 h of stroke onset (AVERT): a randomised controlled trial. Lancet (London, England). 2015;386:46–55. https://doi.org/10.1016/S0140-6736(15)60690-0.
20. Lynch E, Hillier S, Cadilhac D. When should physical rehabilitation commence after stroke: a systematic review. Int J Stroke. 2014;9:468–78. https://doi.org/10.1111/ijs.12262.
21. Bernhardt J, Churilov L, Ellery F, Collier J, Chamberlain J, Langhorne P, et al. Prespecified dose-response analysis for a very early rehabilitation trial (AVERT). Neurology. 2016;86:2138–45. https://doi.org/10.1212/WNL.0000000000002459.
22. Davis MG, Fox KR. Physical activity patterns assessed by accelerometry in older people. Eur J Appl Physiol. 2007;100:581–9.
23. Mattlage AE, Redlin SA, Rippee MA, Abraham MG, Rymer MM, Billinger SA. Use of accelerometers to examine sedentary time on an acute stroke unit. J Neurol Phys Ther. 2015;39:166–71. https://doi.org/10.1097/NPT.0000000000000092.
24. Baldwin C, van Kessel G, Phillips A, Johnston K. Accelerometry shows inpatients with acute medical or surgical conditions spend little time upright and are highly sedentary: systematic review. Phys Ther. 2017;97:1044–65. https://doi.org/10.1093/ptj/pzx076.
25. Strømmen AM, Christensen T, Jensen K. Quantitative measurement of physical activity in acute ischemic stroke and transient ischemic attack. Stroke. 2014;45:3649–55. https://doi.org/10.1161/STROKEAHA.114.006496.
26. Taraldsen K, Askim T, Sletvold O, Einarsen EK, Bjastad KG, Indredavik B, et al. Evaluation of a body-worn sensor system to measure physical activity in older people with impaired function. Phys Ther. 2011;91:277–85. https://doi.org/10.2522/ptj.20100159.
27. Helsedirektoratet. Nasjonal faglig retningslinje for behandling og rehabilitering ved hjerneslag. 2010.
28. Kramer SF, Cumming T, Churilov L, Bernhardt J. Measuring activity levels at an acute stroke ward: comparing observations to a device. Biomed Res Int. 2013;2013:460482. https://doi.org/10.1155/2013/460482.
29. Gebruers N, Vanroy C, Truijen S, Engelborghs S, De Deyn PP. Monitoring of physical activity after stroke: a systematic review of accelerometry-based measures. Arch Phys Med Rehabil. 2010;91:288–97. https://doi.org/10.1016/j.apmr.2009.10.025.
30. Mijnarends DM, Meijers JM, Halfens RJ, ter Borg S, Luiking YC, Verlaan S, et al. Validity and reliability of tools to measure muscle mass, strength, and physical performance in community-dwelling older people: a systematic review. J Am Med Dir Assoc. 2013;14:170–8. https://doi.org/10.1016/j.jamda.2012.10.009.
31. van Swieten JC, Koudstaal PJ, Visser MC, Schouten HJ, van Gijn J. Interobserver agreement for the assessment of handicap in stroke patients. Stroke. 1988;19:604–7.
32. Kasner SE, Chalela JA, Luciano JM, Cucchiara BL, Raps EC, McGarvey ML, et al. Reliability and validity of estimating the NIH stroke scale score from medical records. Stroke. 1999;30:1534–7.
33. Taraldsen K, Sletvold O, Thingstad P, Saltvedt I, Granat MH, Lydersen S, et al. Physical behavior and function early after hip fracture surgery in patients receiving comprehensive geriatric care or orthopedic care--a randomized controlled trial. J Gerontol A Biol Sci Med Sci. 2014;69:338–45. https://doi.org/10.1093/gerona/glt097.
34. Lord S, Galna B, Verghese J, Coleman S, Burn D, Rochester L. Independent domains of gait in older adults and associated motor and nonmotor attributes: validation of a factor analysis approach. J Gerontol A Biol Sci Med Sci. 2013;68:820–7. https://doi.org/10.1093/gerona/gls255.

22

Rationale and Design of a Statewide Cohort to examine efficient resource utilization for patients with Intracerebral hemorrhage (EnRICH)

Farhaan S. Vahidy[1*], Ellie G. Meyer[1], Arvind B. Bambhroliya[1], Jennifer R. Meeks[1], Charles E. Begley[2], Tzu-Ching Wu[1], Jon E. Tyson[3], Charles C. Miller[3], Ritvij Bowry[4], Wamda O. Ahmed[4], Gretchel A. Gealogo[5], Louise D. McCullough[1], Steven Warach[5] and Sean I. Savitz[1]

Abstract

Background: Intracerebral hemorrhage is a devastating disease with no specific treatment modalities. A significant proportion of patients with intracerebral hemorrhage are transferred to large stroke treatment centers, such as Comprehensive Stroke Centers, because of perceived need for higher level of care. However, evidence of improvement in patient-centered outcomes for these patients treated at larger stroke treatment centers as compared to community hospitals is lacking.

Methods / design: *"Efficient Resource Utilization for Patients with Intracerebral Hemorrhage (EnRICH)"* is a prospective, multisite, state-wide, cohort study designed to assess the impact of level of care on long-term patient-centered outcomes for patients with primary / non-traumatic intracerebral hemorrhage. The study is funded by the Texas state legislature via the Lone Star Stroke Research Consortium. It is being implemented via major hub hospitals in large metropolitan cities across the state of Texas. Each hub has an extensive network of "spoke" hospitals, which are connected to the hub via traditional clinical and administrative arrangements, or by telemedicine technologies. This infrastructure provides a unique opportunity to track outcomes for intracerebral hemorrhage patients managed across a health system at various levels of care. Eligible patients are enrolled during hospitalization and are followed for functional, quality of life, cognitive, resource utilization, and dependency outcomes at 30 and 90 days post discharge. As a secondary aim, an economic analysis of the incremental cost-effectiveness of treating intracerebral hemorrhage patients at higher levels of care will be conducted.

Discussion: Findings from EnRICH will provide much needed evidence of the effectiveness and efficiency of regionalized care for intracerebral hemorrhage patients. Such evidence is required to inform policy and streamline clinical decision-making.

Keywords: Stroke, Intracerebral hemorrhage, Patient-centered outcomes, Quality of life, Readmission rate, Mortality, Cost effectiveness, Resource utilization

* Correspondence: Farhaan.Vahidy@uth.tmc.edu
[1]Department of Neurology and the Institute for Stroke and Cerebrovascular Disease, McGovern Medical School, University of Texas - Health, Houston, TX, USA
Full list of author information is available at the end of the article

Background

Introduction

Intracerebral Hemorrhage (ICH) is a devastating disease. Although ICH accounts for about 10–15% of all stroke subtypes in the United States (US), this proportion is reported to be as high as 50% in certain regions of the world [1]. The burden of disease imposed by ICH is tremendous. Approximately 50% of ICH patients do not survive beyond 30 days, and up to 80% fail to achieve functional independence [2, 3]. Furthermore, approximately 90% of ICH patients report their quality of life (QOL) to be below average, including 20% stating their QOL to be worse than death [4]. There are no class I evidence-based modalities that improve ICH outcomes. The mainstay of management revolves around hemodynamic stabilization, neurological monitoring, blood pressure titration, reversal of coagulopathy (if indicated), surgical interventions (in selected patients), secondary stroke prevention, and rehabilitation [5]. It has also been reported that the majority of hospitals do not have well-developed ICH management protocols [6]. Clinical trials for early blood pressure management and surgical interventions in ICH patients have demonstrated safety with limited and equivocal efficacy [7, 8].

There are national and regional data showing that a large number of ICH patients are transferred from smaller community hospitals to bigger stroke treatment centers, probably for a perceived need of higher level of care (HLOC) [9, 10]. Data also suggest that the proportion of transferred patients to large hospitals has been increasing periodically [10]. However, the impact of management of ICH patients at a certain level of care on long term functional, cognitive, and quality of life outcomes within the current paradigm of stroke care delivery in the US is not understood. Furthermore, a subset of ICH patients that would optimally benefit from transfer to or management at centers with HLOC, such as Comprehensive Stroke Centers (CSCs), has not been identified. Finally, the comparative effectiveness of treating ICH patients at higher-resourced centers has not been provided. The study *"Efficient Resource Utilization for Patients with Intracerebral Hemorrhage (EnRICH)"* has been designed and is being implemented to provide evidence to address these important issues.

Rationale

The American Heart Association / American Stroke Association guidelines for management of ICH were updated in 2015. These guidelines added a new Class I, level B evidence stating, *"Initial monitoring and management of ICH patients should take place in an intensive care unit or dedicated stroke unit with physician and nursing neuroscience acute care expertise"* [11]. The guidelines provide reference to three non-randomized studies as the basis for this evidence.

The first reference is made to a retrospective comparative analysis of 1038 ICH patients admitted to a general (non-neurological) intensive care unit (ICU) and those admitted to a neurological ICU (NICU) [12]. The data were collected under Project Impact that began in 1996. The duration of data collection for patients included in this study is not clear; however, since the study was published in 2001 it is assumed that the 3 years of included data are between 1996 and 2001. The study reported an odds ratio (95% Confidence Interval [CI]) of 3.43 (1.65–7.60) for inpatient mortality among ICH patients admitted to a general ICU as compared to NICUs. The authors did acknowledge that limited data from NICUs (only two were included), and voluntary participation of hospitals in the project can lead to selection bias and lack of generalizability. However, it is also pertinent to note that analyses were done at the patient level, and clustering of patients within ICUs and NICUs was not accounted for.

The second reference is made to a cross-sectional analysis of data from 49 acute care hospitals in Alberta, Canada, including 18,142 patients with diagnoses of acute myocardial infarction, congestive heart failure, chronic obstructive pulmonary disease or stroke between April 1, 1998 and March 31, 1999 [13]. The analyses were conducted with the aim of evaluating the association between nurse education and skill, continuity of care, quality of the work environment, and 30-day all-cause mortality. The authors correctly identified certain limitations pertaining to the nature of administrative data. However, it is apparent that the patient population included in this study does not allow generalizability of the results to ICH patients. Diagnosis-based stratified analyses have not been presented, and the only reported metric for stroke patients (presumably including ischemic stroke patients) is a 1% difference in 30-day mortality (15% vs. 16%) between patients discharged from low vs. high volume hospitals.

The third observational study is an analysis of the data from the Swedish Stroke Register between 2001 and 2005 [14]. It compares the risk of death, institutionalization, and dependency between 105,043 stroke patients managed at stroke units and those managed at other types of units. The authors report a benefit for ICH patients managed in stroke units in terms of mortality and dependence. However, the study does not describe the differences between stroke and other units (primary exposure in this case) in care parameters for stroke patients. More importantly, the wider generalizability of such findings from a homogenous health care system remain questionable.

It is clear that the evidence cited in the guidelines falls short in multiple domains. These studies were not conducted during the last decade and they include data from non-stroke and non-ICH patients. Furthermore, their generalizability is highly questionable – particularly to the current paradigm of stroke care delivery and stroke care certification of hospitals in the US. Finally, they largely address broad and short-term outcomes such as inpatient and 30-day mortality. These outcomes, though important administratively, may not be patient-centered.

More recent and contextually relevant evidence, evaluating the association between level of care and outcomes in ICH patients, does not clearly highlight the benefit of managing all ICH patients at a HLOC. Two analyses independently conducted at large CSCs showed that transferred patients had milder disease severity and did not significantly utilize more CSC specific treatment modalities [9, 15]. However, these data are limited by lack of outcomes for patients who are not transferred to CSCs. A direct comparison between ICH Medicare beneficiaries treated at Primary Stroke Centers (PSC) and those treated at non-certified centers did reveal a reduction in 30-day mortality for PSC patients; however, there were no differences in 30-day readmission [16]. This analysis did not consider differences between CSCs and PSCs, lacked patient-centered outcomes, and excluded patients < 65 years of age, which may constitute a considerable proportion of ICH patients. A relatively recent comparison of brain hemorrhage patients treated at CSCs vs. PSCs did not reveal any differences in 90-day mortality for ICH patients [17].

Furthermore, there are limited and conflicting data on the comparative effectiveness of ICH patient transfer for HLOC. A recent simulation-based study provided comparative effectiveness in terms of incremental cost effectiveness ratios of $47,431 per Quality Adjusted Life Years (QALY) for transferring ICH patients to a NICU under a most favorable scenario. However, these estimates are about 93% to 700% higher for less favorable scenarios [18]. Reliance on probabilistic assumptions behind simulation models, and interpretation of willingness-to-pay thresholds remain significant limitations of such analyses. Other studies based on primary data have reported that cost effectiveness of transfer of ICH patients is not clearly demonstrable, and that an evidence-based triage algorithm for optimal selection of patients is warranted [19].

Based on the above discussion, there is enough equipoise for EnRICH, which has the following aims:

1. To examine the association between level of care (as defined by certification status of the hospital) and outcomes in ICH patients
2. To estimate the health economic impact of management of ICH patients at CSCs, as compared to PSCs and / or non-certified hospitals
3. To characterize a subset of ICH patients that optimally benefits from care provision and management at HLOC (such as CSCs)

Methods / design

Study design and setting

EnRICH is designed to be an observational, prospective, multisite cohort study. It will be simultaneously operationalized at five major hubs in the state of Texas under the auspices of the Lone Star Stroke (LSS) Research Consortium of Texas. The LSS Research Consortium is a collaborative stroke research effort supported by the Texas legislature. Its mission is to conduct patient-centered stroke research across the state of Texas, with a specific focus on involving communities that generally do not have access to research, by utilizing the hub and spoke infrastructure of participating sites. One of the specific goals of the LSS charter is to *"Develop and disseminate evidence-based guidelines for safe, high-quality, and cost-effective stroke care in Texas"*. The LSS network provides an ideal infrastructure to fulfill the aims of the EnRICH study, and the EnRICH study directly supports the stipulated goal of the LSS consortium's charter. Each LSS hub is a large, academic stroke treatment center designated as a CSC in most cases. A hub has a network of multiple other spoke hospitals, which are connected to the hub in their functionality via traditional arrangements or telemedicine technology. The spokes have varying patterns of transferring ICH patients to the hub. Some spokes transfer most or all ICH patients, whereas others tend to manage ICH patients in-house. Other spokes have varying proportions of transfer / non-transfer ICH patients. The details of the network and participating sites are publically available [20]. This framework provides an opportunity to enroll ICH patients who directly present either to CSC or non-CSC hospitals, and are either transferred or not transferred for HLOC.

Study population

All male and female adult patients (≥ 18 years), of all races and ethnicities are eligible to be enrolled in EnRICH if they have a radiologically confirmed ICH (usually requiring only a non-contrast head computed tomography (CT) scan) with an etiology such as hypertension, coagulopathy or cerebral amyloidosis. We initially excluded ICH patients presenting to an index hospital 24-h after symptom onset or last seen normal, however this exclusion criteria has been removed. In our experience, decisions made at non-CSC centers to transfer radiologically confirmed ICH patients to a higher level of care are not influenced by time lapse between onset of symptoms and presentation. Among the population of transferred patients, only those patients who transfer within 24 h of their initial presentation are enrolled. Although patients with intraventricular extension of an intracerebral hemorrhage are eligible, patients with a pure or primary intraventricular hemorrhage are excluded. These patients may benefit from ventricular drainage procedures along with neurological monitoring in CSCs or other larger centers. Similarly, patients with other forms of intracranial hemorrhages, such as subdural and subarachnoid, are excluded. Patients with secondary causes of intracerebral hemorrhage - such as neoplasm, arteriovenous malformation, cerebral aneurysm, or hemorrhagic transformation of ischemic stroke - are also excluded. Secondary causes of hemorrhage are determined based on diagnostic work-up during the course of hospitalization. Potentially eligible patients are screened daily upon admission. Patients with non-primary ICH are excluded. Patients with unclear etiology are not approached, but are monitored for their diagnostic work-up and are only approached if secondary causes of ICH are excluded. If diagnostic work-up determines a secondary etiology after enrollment, patients are removed from the study. In such cases patients / their care-givers and the institutional review board (IRB) is duly notified. Detailed screening and enrollment are being maintained that track every potential ICH patient presented at an enrolling site. An IRB approved protocol amendment allows us to also enroll eligible ICH patients who die in-hospital prior to being approached for consent.

Study procedures

Eligible ICH patients with radiological confirmation of a parenchymal hemorrhage are approached to consent during their hospitalization. EnRICH is currently approved by the University of Texas Health Science Center at Houston (UTHealth) Institutional Review Board (IRB) to obtain a verbal consent from either the patient or their legally authorized representative. Upon consent, several baseline assessments are completed with the patient or by proxy, and certain preliminary information about patients – including demographic, risk factors, and initial presentation variables - is captured in the study-specific, online, secure database. Information describing inpatient management, such as treatment intensity, length of stay, procedures, laboratory investigations, and diagnostic modalities, are also captured. After discharge from acute care, consented patients are followed at 30 and 90 days via phone calls to obtain information on functional, QOL, cognitive, resource utilization, and level of dependency outcomes. A schematic representation of patient flow and information collected for EnRICH at various study phases is presented in Fig. 1.

IRB approvals and multisite implementation

The University of Texas Health Science Center at Houston IRB is the IRB of Record. The project has been approved at various study sites via IRB reciprocity, and we aim to maintain single IRB review in compliance with the current regulatory trend. An electronic study master file has been designed and implemented to facilitate inter-site communication and centralized storage of essential study documents.

Outcomes

The 90-day functional status as assessed by modified Rankin Scale (mRS) is the primary outcome. Secondary outcomes include 30-day readmission and 30-day mortality. The outcome for economic analysis is the relative cost effectiveness of ICH patient management at varying levels of care (i.e. CSCs vs. non-CSC hospitals). Cost effectiveness ratios are comprised of Cost (as determined by total costs of inpatient treatment intensity, transfer status, and post-discharge resource utilization weighted by Medicare reimbursement amounts) and effectiveness (as obtained by QALYs determined by EQ-5D QOL information). The exploratory outcomes include assessment of patients' health utility as captured by Standard Gamble, cognitive outcome determined using mini Montreal Cognitive Assessment (MoCA), and change in patient dependency status.

Statistical analysis

The primary analytical aim of EnRICH is to compare 90-day functional outcomes between ICH patients treated at CSCs and those treated and non-CSC hospitals. We propose to conduct a shift analysis of the seven point mRS (0–6) utilizing proportional odds models. Baseline variables will be assessed for imbalance between the two groups, and statistically significant ($p < 0.1$) potential confounders will be included in the multivariable models. Clinically important variables that are known to predict outcome in ICH patients (such as age, presentation National Institutes of Health Stroke Scale (NIHSS), presentation Glasgow Coma Scale (GCS), systolic blood pressure, hematoma volume, hemorrhage location, and hematoma expansion) will be included in the multivariable model regardless of their statistical significance. Model building, variable selection, and assessment of the fit of the model will be conducted utilizing methodologies described in standard texts [21]. Further analyses will also be conducted using propensity score based methods [22]. This will allow for quantification of bias and sensitivity analyses to explore robustness of the estimates to un-measured confounding. Secondary analyses based on utility weighted mRS (UW – mRS) will also be performed to provide estimates of effect size for future trials [23]. We propose to conduct multivariable modified Poisson regression and survival analyses for assessing relative risk of 30-day readmission, and hazard ratio for 30-day mortality respectively. Differences in the median scores for quality of life will be analyzed using quantile regression methods. Day-90 cost effectiveness analysis will be performed from payer's perspective using Medicare weight reimbursement rates. Long-term (1 Year) costs and outcomes will be modeled using Markov modeling. Sensitivity analyses will be conducted to determine the robustness of the incremental cost effectiveness ratio. Finally, receiver operating curve

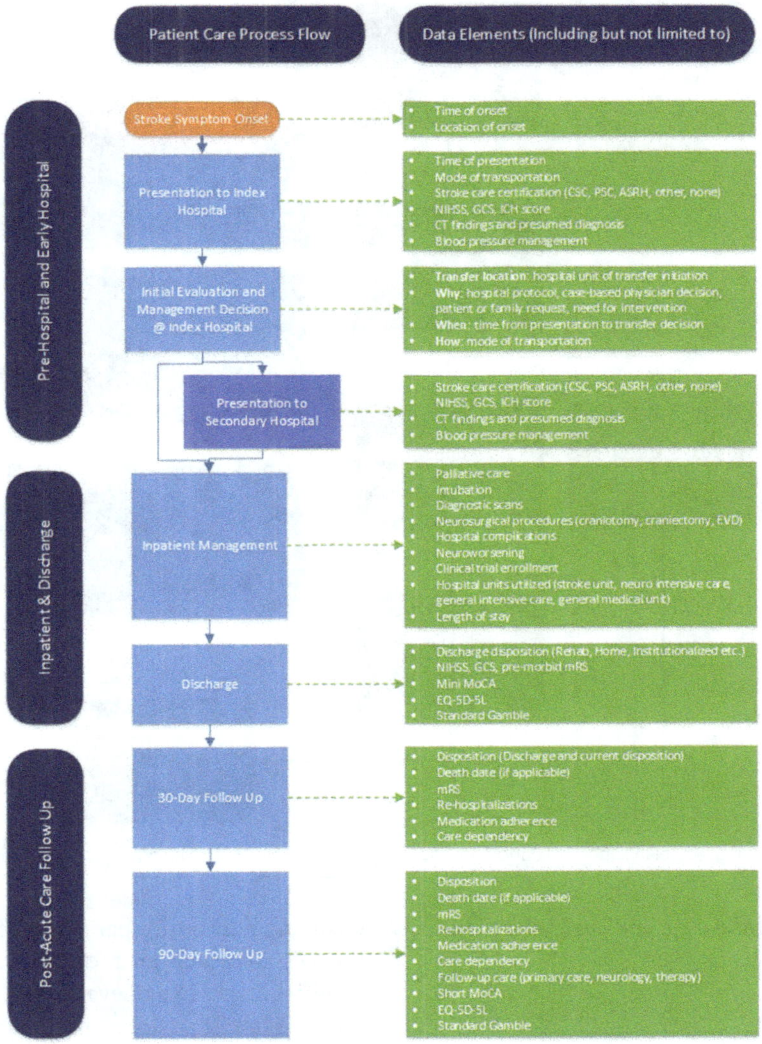

Fig. 1 Schematic representation of patient flow through various network hospitals and data elements captured at each stage. Various study phases are indicated vertically

based predictive scores will be developed for ICH patients who are likely to benefit from care at CSCs. This will help identify a subset of ICH patients optimally benefiting from HLOC.

Sample size and power

The power and sample size calculations of the study have been conducted to satisfy the primary endpoint of 90-day mRS. We determined the 90-day distribution of mRS for ICH patients using published literature [24]. In addition, based on our prior work we estimate that approximately 60% ICH patients are managed at CSCs [9]. Therefore using a ratio of 1.5 for CSC vs. Non-CSC patients, a total of 1110 patients are needed to achieve 80% power to detect a change in log odds ratio of 0.3 with the significance level of 0.05 for a two-sided test [25]. Factoring in an attrition rate of 20% we plan to enroll 1375 patients (825 CSC patients and 550 non-CSC patients) over the period of 2.5 years, such that all follow up is completed within 3 years of study duration.

Progress

Since initiation in September 2016, EnRICH has been operationalized at a total of nine hospitals in larger metropolitan areas of Houston, Austin, San Antonio, and Dallas.. Study start-up procedures are currently ongoing at two other LSS hubs. To-date, over 870 patients have been screened and 480 patients have been enrolled. The current loss to follow up rate for both the 30 and 90-day time points is less than 5%. Fig. 2 shows a flow diagram of the number and proportion of screened, approached, consented, and enrolled patients. Reasons for non-enrollment are also indicated. Since the approval and implementation of a verbal consent process in late

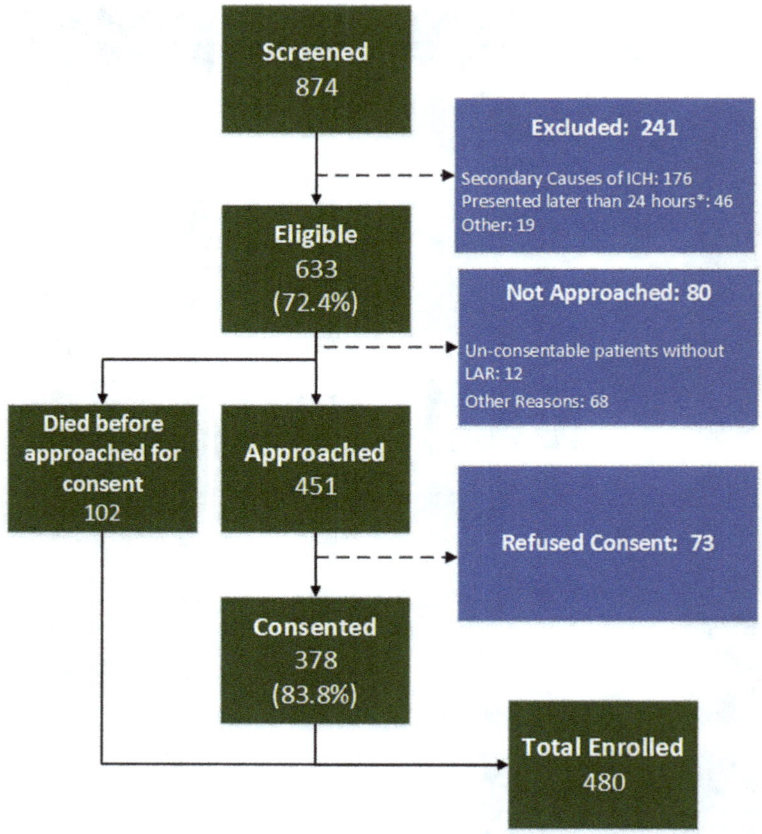

Fig. 2 Flow diagram for screening, eligibility, approach, and consent for current status of EnRICH (combined for all participating sites)

September 2016, the refusal rate for study participation has declined from 41.0% to 16.2%.

Discussion

EnRICH is a statewide cohort of ICH patients that will answer important questions regarding regionalization of care. The rationale of EnRICH stems from the gravity of the disease, lack of definitive treatment modalities for ICH patients, and current practice patterns in the absence of class I evidence. Though it remains critically important to explore novel management strategies for ICH treatment, it is perhaps even more crucial to ensure that the resources within current stroke care delivery systems are optimized to provide maximal benefit for ICH patients. On one hand, the implementation of evidence-based management practices are important, but at the same time, non-evidence based practices are necessary to be evaluated and eventually de-implemented. Parameters for management of ICH patients at a given level of care lack clarity and specificity, resulting in undue strain on systems of care, with probably little to no impact on patient-centered outcomes. Synthesized evidence supporting national guidelines and certifications should provide generalizable content and need to be contextually relevant. EnRICH will provide much needed data relevant to the changing and future paradigm of stroke care delivery in the US, in which an increasing number of stroke care facilities strive to achieve a certification status [26].

It is likely that decisions to transfer ICH patients for HLOC is an interplay of multiple patient, clinical, caregiver, physician, policy, and resource factors; with significant facilities-wide and regional variation. Recognizing the array of stakeholders in the transfer process, we conducted multiple brainstorming and focused group discussions with clinical trial design experts, analysts, stroke neurologists, neuro-intensivists, emergency care physicians, hospital administrators, members of committee for protection of human subjects, and patients and their care givers. All agreed that a trial in which patients were randomized to either stay at a certain hospital, or be transferred to a different one, was not feasible. Furthermore, there is a dearth of evidence that would establish criteria for transfer of brain hemorrhage patients to a higher level of care. The current guidelines provide extremely broad and non-precise parameters. We do hypothesize that transfer is beneficial for a certain subset of ICH patients, and believe that our work will help establish these parameters more precisely. Given this information, we continue to assess the feasibility of a step-wedge randomization design for the next phase of the study. The data from EnRICH will help us to design such a randomized trial. Therefore, despite the limitation of observational data, EnRICH is best suited to provide evidence leading to a better understanding of the impact of the level of care on outcomes for ICH patients. The design is also conducive to implementation at multiple sites, particularly those with limited resources for stroke research.

The results of the EnRICH study will have important implications for public policy and care provision, and may support evidence-based adaptation by healthcare systems. The current practice of indiscriminate patient transfer is not sustainable and is unlikely to translate into optimal societal benefit, particularly in non-urban populations with limited access to care. Economic analyses of EnRICH data will further inform rational decisions regarding the allocation of limited resources, and analyses of ICH patient outcomes - including patient quality of life - will provide direction to agencies responsible for hospital accreditation as they formulate standards and guidelines for care of ICH patients.

Abbreviations

CI: Confidence interval; CSC: Comprehensive stroke center; EQ-5D: EuroQol – 5 Dimensions; GCS: Glasgow coma scale; HLOC: Higher level of care; ICH: Intracerebral Hemorrhage; IRB: Institutional review board; LSS: Lone star stroke; MoCA: Montreal cognitive assessment; mRS: Modified rankin scale; NICU: Neurological intensive care unit; NIHSS: National institutes of health stroke scale; PSC: Primary stroke center; QALY: Quality-adjusted life years; QOL: Quality of life; US: United States; UW-mRS: Utility weighted modified rankin scale

Acknowledgments

We acknowledge contributions of Audrey 'Sarah' Cohen toward operationalization and initial acquisition of data. We acknowledge the roles of the Memorial Hermann Hospital System and Seton Healthcare Family in acquisition of data and study oversight. We acknowledge the support provided by the Biostatistics/ Epidemiology/ Research Design (BERD) component of the Center for Clinical and Translational Sciences (CCTS) for this project. CCTS is mainly funded by a grant (UL1 TR000371) from the National Center for Advancing Translational Sciences (NCATS), awarded to University of Texas Health Science Center at Houston. The content is solely the responsibility of the authors and does not necessarily represent the official views of the NCATS.

Funding

EnRICH is funded by the Texas State Legislature via the Lone Star Stroke Research Consortium. Neither the Texas State Legislature nor the Lone Star Stroke Research Consortium influenced study design, data collection and analysis, data interpretation or writing of this manuscript. The contents of this manuscript are solely the responsibility of the authors and do not necessarily represent the official views of the State of Texas.

Authors' contributions

FV conceived the study design and methods, is responsible for analysis and interpretation of study data, drafted this manuscript, gave final approval for publication, and is accountable for all aspects of the work. EM, AB, JM made contributions to the acquisition of data and study design. CB, TCW, JT, CM, LM, SW and SS substantially contributed to the conception and design. RB, WA and GG made substantial contributions to the acquisition of data. All authors read and approved the final manuscript.

Competing interests

The authors declare that they have no competing interests.

Author details

[1]Department of Neurology and the Institute for Stroke and Cerebrovascular Disease, McGovern Medical School, University of Texas - Health, Houston, TX, USA. [2]Department of Management, Policy, and Community Health, School of Public Health, University of Texas Health Science Center at Houston, Houston, TX, USA. [3]Center for Clinical Research and Evidence Based Medicine at McGovern Medical School, University of Texas Health Science Center at Houston, Houston, TX, USA. [4]Department of Neurosurgery, McGovern Medical School, University of Texas Health Science Center at Houston, Houston, TX, USA. [5]Department of Neurology, Dell Medical School, The University of Texas at Austin, Austin, TX, USA.

References

1. Krishnamurthi RV, Moran AE, Forouzanfar MH, Bennett DA, Mensah GA, Lawes CM, et al. The global burden of hemorrhagic stroke: a summary of findings from the GBD 2010 study. Glob Heart. 2014;9(1):101–6. https://doi.org/10.1016/j.gheart.2014.01.003. Epub 2014/11/30 PubMed PMID: 25432119
2. Hansen BM, Nilsson OG, Anderson H, Norrving B, Saveland H, Lindgren A. Long term (13 years) prognosis after primary intracerebral haemorrhage: a prospective population based study of long term mortality, prognostic factors and causes of death. J Neurol Neurosurg Psychiatry. 2013;84(10): 1150–5. https://doi.org/10.1136/jnnp-2013-305200. PubMed PMID: 23715913
3. van Asch CJ, Luitse MJ, Rinkel GJ, van der Tweel I, Algra A, Klijn CJ. Incidence, case fatality, and functional outcome of intracerebral haemorrhage over time, according to age, sex, and ethnic origin: a systematic review and meta-analysis. Lancet Neurol 2010;9(2):167-176. . doi: https://doi.org/10.1016/s1474-4422(09)70340-0. Epub 2010/01/09 PubMed PMID: 20056489.
4. Christensen MC, Mayer S, Ferran JM. Quality of life after intracerebral hemorrhage: results of the factor seven for acute hemorrhagic stroke (FAST) trial. Stroke. 2009;40(5):1677–82. https://doi.org/10.1161/strokeaha.108.538967. Epub 2009/03/07 PubMed PMID: 19265046
5. Thabet AM, Kottapally M, Hemphill JC 3rd. Management of intracerebral hemorrhage. Handb Clin Neurol. 2017;140:177–94. https://doi.org/10.1016/b978-0-444-63600-3.00011-8. Epub 2017/02/12 PubMed PMID: 28187799
6. Cooper D, Jauch E, Flaherty ML. Critical pathways for the management of stroke and intracerebral hemorrhage: a survey of US hospitals. Crit Pathw Cardiol. 2007;6(1):18–23. https://doi.org/10.1097/01.hpc.0000256146.81644.59. PubMed PMID: 17667882
7. Boulouis G, Morotti A, Goldstein JN, Charidimou A. Intensive blood pressure lowering in patients with acute intracerebral haemorrhage: clinical outcomes and haemorrhage expansion. Systematic review and meta-analysis of randomised trials. J Neurol Neurosurg Psychiatry. 2017;88(4):339–45. https://doi.org/10.1136/jnnp-2016-315346. Epub 2017/02/20 PubMed PMID: 28214798
8. Yang C-D, Chen Y-W, Wu H-C. Meta-analysis of randomized studies of surgery for supratentorial intracerebral hemorrhage. Formosan J Surg. 2014; 47(3):90–8.
9. Nguyen C, Mir O, Vahidy F, Wu TC, Albright K, Boehme A, et al. Resource utilization for patients with Intracerebral hemorrhage transferred to a comprehensive stroke center. J Stroke Cerebrovasc Dis. 2015;24(12):2866–74. https://doi.org/10.1016/j.jstrokecerebrovasdis.2015.08.023. PubMed PMID: 26460244; PubMed Central PMCID: PMCPMC4688147
10. Vahidy F, Albright K, Donnelly JP, Shapshak AH, Savitz SI. Abstract WMP31: National Trends in Transfer of Patients With Intracerebral Hemorrhage to Teaching Hospitals. Am Heart Assoc; 2016.
11. Hemphill JC 3rd, Greenberg SM, Anderson CS, Becker K, Bendok BR, Cushman M, et al. Guidelines for the Management of Spontaneous Intracerebral Hemorrhage: a guideline for healthcare professionals from the American Heart Association/American Stroke Association. Stroke. 2015;46(7):2032–60. https://doi.org/10.1161/STR.0000000000000069. PubMed PMID: 26022637
12. Diringer MN, Edwards DF. Admission to a neurologic/neurosurgical intensive care unit is associated with reduced mortality rate after intracerebral hemorrhage. Crit Care Med. 2001;29(3):635–40. Epub 2001/05/25. PubMed PMID: 11373434

13. Estabrooks CA, Midodzi WK, Cummings GG, Ricker KL, Giovannetti P. The impact of hospital nursing characteristics on 30-day mortality. Nurs Res. 2005;54(2):74–84. Epub 2005/03/22. PubMed PMID: 15778649
14. Terent A, Asplund K, Farahmand B, Henriksson KM, Norrving B, Stegmayr B, et al. Stroke unit care revisited: who benefits the most? A cohort study of 105,043 patients in Riks-stroke, the Swedish stroke register. J Neurol Neurosurg Psychiatry. 2009;80(8):881–7. https://doi.org/10.1136/jnnp.2008.169102. Epub 2009/04/01.PubMed PMID: 19332423
15. Kilbourn KJ, Killory BD, Fortunato G, Staff I, Sinisgalli S, Czap A, et al. Clinical characteristics and outcomes of patients with Intracerebral hemorrhage after Interhospital transfer to a designated stroke center. Conn Med. 2015; 79(6):335–41. Epub 2015/08/13. PubMed PMID: 26263713
16. Lichtman JH, Jones SB, Leifheit-Limson EC, Wang Y, Goldstein LB. 30-day mortality and readmission after hemorrhagic stroke among Medicare beneficiaries in joint commission primary stroke center-certified and noncertified hospitals. Stroke. 2011;42(12):3387–91.
17. McKinney JS, Cheng JQ, Rybinnik I, Kostis JB. Comprehensive stroke centers may be associated with improved survival in hemorrhagic stroke. J Am Heart Assoc. 2015;4(5):e001448.
18. Fletcher JJ, Kotagal V, Mammoser A, Peterson M, Morgenstern LB, Burke JF. Cost-effectiveness of transfers to centers with neurological intensive care units after intracerebral hemorrhage. Stroke. 2015;46(1):58–64. https://doi.org/10.1161/STROKEAHA.114.006653. PubMed PMID: 25477220; PubMed Central PMCID: PMC4276522
19. Nakagawa K, Galati A, Juarez DT. The excess cost of interisland transfer of intracerebral hemorrhage patients. Am J Emerg Med. 2015;33(4):512–5. https://doi.org/10.1016/j.ajem.2015.01.001. PubMed PMID: 25624077; PubMed Central PMCID: PMC4409479
20. Lone Star Stroke Consortium 2017. Available from: http://lonestarstroke.com/.
21. Hosmer Jr DW, Lemeshow S, Sturdivant RX. Applied logistic regression. New York: Wiley; 2013.
22. Guo S, Fraser MW. Propensity score analysis. Los Angeles: Sage; 2014.
23. Broderick JP, Adeoye O, Elm J. Evolution of the modified Rankin scale and its use in future stroke trials. Stroke. 2017;48(7):2007–12.
24. Palm F, Henschke N, Wolf J, Zimmer K, Safer A, Schroder RJ, et al. Intracerebral haemorrhage in a population-based stroke registry (LuSSt): incidence, aetiology, functional outcome and mortality. J Neurol. 2013; 260(10):2541–50. https://doi.org/10.1007/s00415-013-7013-0. PubMed PMID: 23812642
25. Whitehead J. Sample size calculations for ordered categorical data. Stat Med. 1993;12(24):2257–71. PubMed PMID: 8134732
26. Song S, Saver J. Growth of regional acute stroke systems of care in the United States in the first decade of the 21st century. Stroke. 2012;43(7): 1975–8. https://doi.org/10.1161/STROKEAHA.112.657809. PubMed PMID: 22669404; PubMed Central PMCID: PMCPMC3413285

23

Reliability, validity, and responsiveness of three scales for measuring balance in patients with chronic stroke

Ahmad H. Alghadir[1], Einas S. Al-Eisa[1], Shahnawaz Anwer[1*] and Bibhuti Sarkar[2]

Abstract

Background: Various outcome measures are used for the assessment of balance and mobility in patients with stroke. The purpose of the present study was to examine test-retest reliability, construct validity, and responsiveness of the Timed Up and Go Test (TUG), Berg Balance Scale (BBS), and Dynamic Gait Index (DGI) for measuring balance in patients with chronic stroke.

Methods: Fifty-six patients (39 male and 17 female) with chronic stroke participated in this study. A senior physical therapist assessed the test-retest reliability and validity of three scales, including the DGI, TUG, and BBS over two testing sessions. In addition, the third assessment of each scale was taken at the time of discharge to determine the responsiveness of the three outcome measures.

Results: The reliability of the TUG (intraclass correlation coefficient [$ICC_{2,1}$] = 0.98), DGI ($ICC_{2,1}$ = 0.98) and BBS ($ICC_{2,1}$ = 0.99) were excellent. The standard error of measurement (SEM) of the TUG, DGI, and BBS were 1.16, 0.71, and 0.98, respectively. The minimal detectable change (MDC) of the TUG, DGI, and BBS were 3.2, 1.9, and 2.7, respectively. There was a significant correlation found between the DGI and BBS (first reading [r] = 0.75; second reading [r] = 0.77), TUG and BBS (first reading [r] = −.52; second reading [r] = −.53), and the TUG and DGI (first reading [r] = 0.45; second reading [r] = 0.48), respectively.

Conclusions: The test-retest reliability of the TUG, BBS, and DGI was excellent. The DGI demonstrated slightly better responsiveness than TUG and BBS. However, the small sample size of this study limits the validity of the results.

Keywords: Dynamic gait index, Stroke, Balance, Berg balance scale, Rehabilitation, Timed up and go test

Background

Stroke is the common cerebrovascular disease with a high mortality rate and persistent disability in adults worldwide [1]. The prevalence of stroke in Saudi Arabia is relatively low compared to the Western and Asian countries [2]. A balance disorder is the commonest cause of disability in patients with stroke [3]. Previous studies have reported an increased postural sway, asymmetrical weight distribution, reduced stance capability, and impaired weight shifting ability in individuals with stroke [4–6]. These problems can impair function and activities of daily livings [7]. Therefore, interventions for enhancing balance and functional mobility is the focus of rehabilitation for the people with chronic stroke [7]. In addition, maintaining balance has been found to be a strong predictor of independent living [8] and was highly correlated with the perceived disability at the time of discharge from the rehabilitation [9]. Assessment of the balance can assist the therapists in the diagnosis, selection of appropriate interventions, and outcome measurements [10].

Various outcome measures are used for the assessment of balance and mobility in patients with stroke [7, 11–17]. The Timed Up and Go Test (TUG), Berg Balance Scale (BBS), and Dynamic Gait Index (DGI) are reliable and valid scales that clinicians commonly used to evaluate the functional abilities of lower limbs in patients with stroke. Flansbjer et al. [18] reported that the TUG test is a single-task measure involves a single 180-degree turn and straight pathway walking. In a systematic review study,

* Correspondence: anwer_shahnawazphysio@rediffmail.com; anwerphysio@gmail.com
[1]Rehabilitation Research Chair, College of Applied Medical Sciences, King Saud University, P.O.Box-10219, Riyadh 11433, Saudi Arabia
Full list of author information is available at the end of the article

Pollock et al. [19] reported that the multiple-task measure was better than a single-task measure in evaluating balance. However, multiple-task outcome measures often take a long time and could not detect specific balance deficits [20].

Previous studies suggested that impairments in the multiple tasks balance function indicates negative outcomes for instance, increased risk of fall [21–23] and reduced physical and cognitive function [24–26]. Similarly, other studies reported reduced postural stability while performing simultaneous activities of two or more balance tasks [27, 28]. Thus, assessment of balance function while performing two or more balance tasks concurrently is critical for rehabilitation of patients with stroke.

Therefore, the present study aimed to compare the single-task outcome measure such as TUG test with the multiple-task outcome measures, including the BBS and DGI for measuring balance and mobility in patients with chronic stroke.

Methods

Participants

Fifty-six patients with chronic stroke from the outpatient physiotherapy department were participated in the study. The inclusion criteria were as follows: first episode of stroke (more than 3 months of duration since onset), able to follow simple instructions, absence of comorbidities (e.g. fracture, brain tumor, severe rheumatoid arthritis, or amputation), and able to walk at least 10 m (assessed by the examiner to confirm the eligibility), with or without an assistive gait device. The institutional ethics committee, Rehabilitation Research Chair, King Saud University, Riyadh, Saudi Arabia, approved this study. An informed consent form was signed by each participant.

Procedures

A senior physical therapist administered the BBS, DGI, and TUG tests. The BBS was developed to evaluate the balance performance and determine the fall risk in the elderly [29]. The BBS measures multi-tasking ability and includes 14 items that require participants to maintain their balance in different tasks and positions with various levels of difficulty. Each item is scored from 0 to 4 points (best possible score, 56). The inter-rater and intra-rater reliability of BBS for the patients with stroke was 0.97 and 0.98, respectively [30]. There is a high risk of falling if the score is 44 or less [30].

Table 1 Participant's characteristics

	$N = 56$
Sex, male/female	39/17
Age (mean ± SD), years	58.6 ± 9.8
Height (mean ± SD), cm	165.1 ± 5.8
Weight (mean ± SD), Kg.	63.7 ± 6.5
Affected side, right/left	33/23
Duration since onset (mean ± SD), Months	22.2 ± 18.3
Stroke type, infarction/hemorrhage, n	32/24

The DGI was designed to evaluate the dynamic balance during walking [31]. It has eight items that require participants to maintain balance during normal walking and walking with different situations (e.g., changing speed, head turn, over and around the obstacles, pivot turn, and stairs climbing). Each item is scored from 0 to 3 points (best possible score, 24). A higher total DGI score signifies a higher level of independent functional mobility. The DGI was correlated with the BBS and Activities-specific Balance Confidence Scale (ABC) [29, 32].

The TUG test is designed to measure functional mobility [33]. The test-retest reliability of the TUG was excellent for individuals with stroke (ICC = 0.95) [34]. Duration of ≥13.5 s on the TUG was associated with an increased fall risk in the elderly and persons with vestibular dysfunction [35].

The BBS, DGI, and TUG tests were administered by a single rater in two testing sessions over a period of 1 week, to assess the test-retest reliability. In addition, the third assessment of each scale was taken at the time of discharge to determine the responsiveness of the three outcome measures. The duration of the entire testing procedure was 45–60 min.

Statistics

Descriptive data, including mean and standard deviation (SD) values for each score distribution, were presented for each scale. Test-retest reliability of the TUG, total DGI scores, and BBS scores were analyzed using the $ICC_{2,1}$. The agreement between two readings of each scale was assessed using the Bland-Altman plot method [36]. The mean of the scores on the x-axis was plotted with the difference of scores on the y-axis [36]. The standard error of measurement (SEM) was determined by the following formula: SD

Table 2 Test Scores of the timed up and go test (TUG), the dynamic gait index (DGI), and the berg balance scale (BBS)

	TUG_1	TUG_2	DGI_1	DGI_2	BBS_1	BBS_2
Mean ± SD	20.1 ± 8.3	19.8 ± 8.1	14.9 ± 5.3	15.3 ± 5.3	41.4 ± 10.9	41.8 ± 10.9
Range (minimum - maximum)	8.0–44.5	8.0–43.8	4–24	4–26	5–56	9–56
*p-value	0.2139		0.0618		0.0874	

*Paired t-test

Table 3 ICCs, Confidence Intervals, Standard error of measurement (SEM), and minimal detectable change (MDC) of the timed up and go test (TUG), the dynamic gait index (DGI), and the berg balance scale (BBS) (test-retest)

	TUG	DGI	BBS
ICC (95% CI)	0.98 (0.97–0.99)	0.98 (0.97–0.99)	0.99 (0.98–0.99)
SEM	1.16	0.71	0.98
MDC	3.2	1.9	2.7

√(1– ICC) [37]. The minimum detectable change (MDC) was determined by the following formula: 1.96*√2*(SEM) [38]. In addition, the construct validity of the three outcome measures was assessed using the Pearson's correlation coefficient test. Furthermore, the responsiveness of the three outcome measures to change from baseline to discharge was determined using the standardized response mean (SRM). The magnitude of responsiveness was considered as follows: an SRM > 0.8 is large, 0.5 to 0.8 is moderate, and 0.2 to 0.5 is small [39]. A p-value of ≤0.05 was set for the statistical level of significance. All statistical analyses were done using the statistical package for the social sciences for Windows version 22 (IBM Inc., Chicago, Illinois, USA).

Results

Table 1 details the demographic data and stroke-related characteristics. The majority of the participants were male (70%). Right-sided hemiplegia was present in 59% of the participants. There were no significant differences in the mean TUG score, total DGI score, and BBS scores between measurements (Table 2). There was no history of other episodes of stroke during rehabilitation period in any patients.

Table 3 details the test-retest data. Test-retest reliability of the TUG, DGI, and BBS scores were found to be excellent. The Bland-Altman limit of agreement of each scale is presented in Figs. 1, 2 and 3 showing a reasonable agreement between test – retest score of each scale. The SEM of the TUG, DGI, and BBS were 1.16, 0.71, and 0.98, respectively. The MDC of the TUG, DGI, and BBS were 3.2, 1.9, and 2.7, respectively (as shown in Table 3). There was a significant correlation found between the DGI and BBS (first reading [r] = 0.75; second reading [r] = 0.77), TUG and BBS (first reading [r] = –.52; second reading [r] = –.53), and the TUG and DGI (first reading [r] = 0.45; second reading [r] = 0.48), respectively (Table 4). Table 5 details the correlations between demographic variables with the three scales. The participant's age was significantly correlated with DGI and BBS scores. Duration since stroke was significantly correlated with DGI scores. Type of stroke was significantly correlated with BBS scores. The responsiveness data of the three scales are given in Table 6. The change in responsiveness of the TUG, DGI, and BBS was moderate from baseline to discharge.

Discussion

Balance and mobility are the most important functional limitations in patients with chronic stroke [40]. A variety

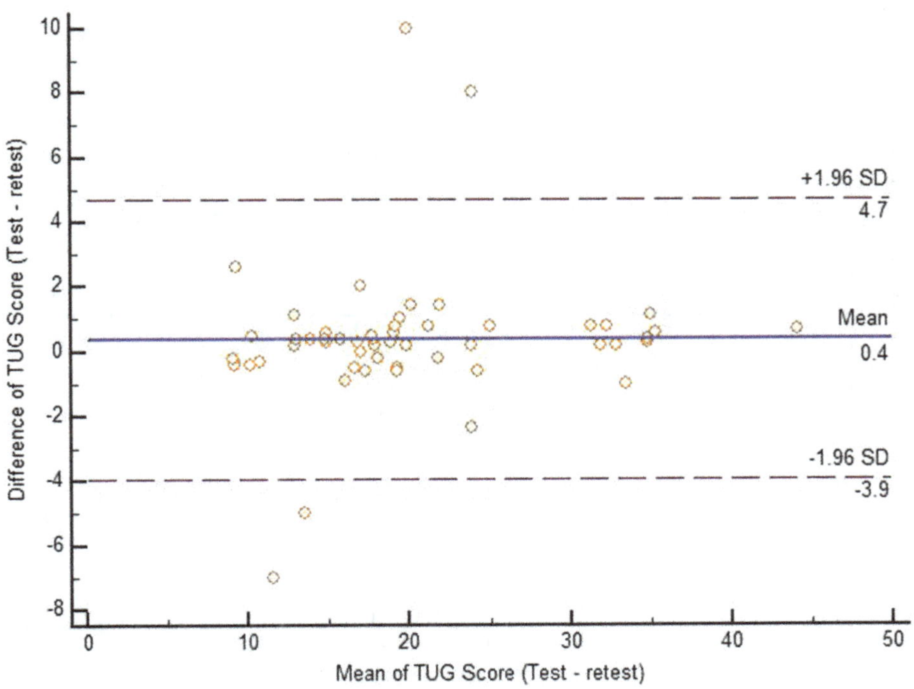

Fig. 1 Bland-Altman plot showing reliability of the Timed up and go test (TUG)

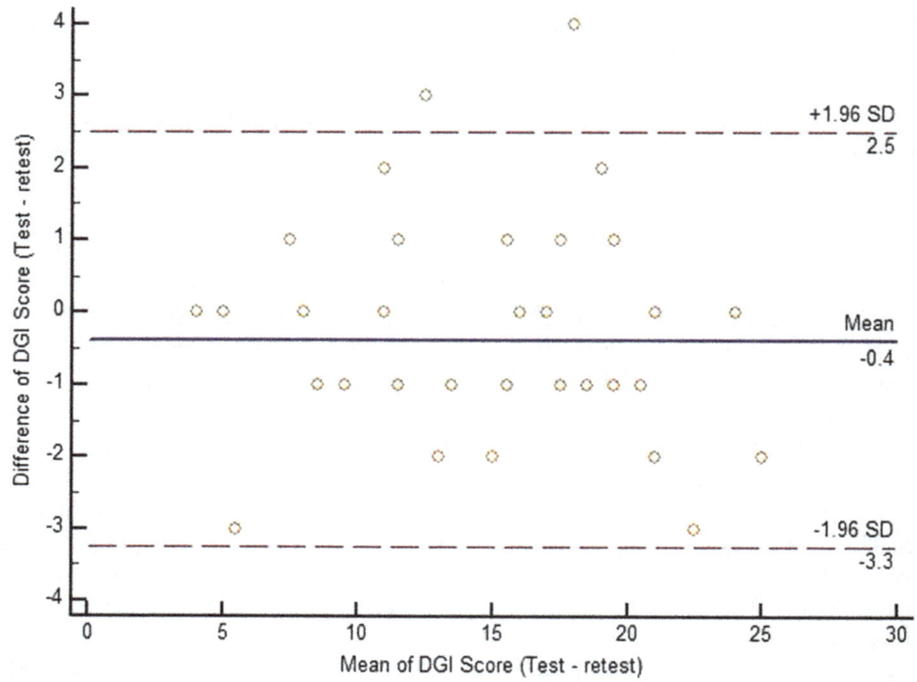

Fig. 2 Bland-Altman plot showing reliability of the Dynamic gait index (DGI)

of balance and mobility related outcomes tools available, some of them designed to measure the multiple-task outcome, while others measure a single task. For a measure to be useful, it should be easy to administer, valid, reliable, and responsive [41, 42]. In the present study, the reliability, validity, and responsiveness of the TUG test, BBS, and DGI for measuring balance and mobility was assessed in patients with chronic stroke. The test-retest reliability of the three scales including, TUG test, DGI, and BBS were excellent. Similarly, a previous

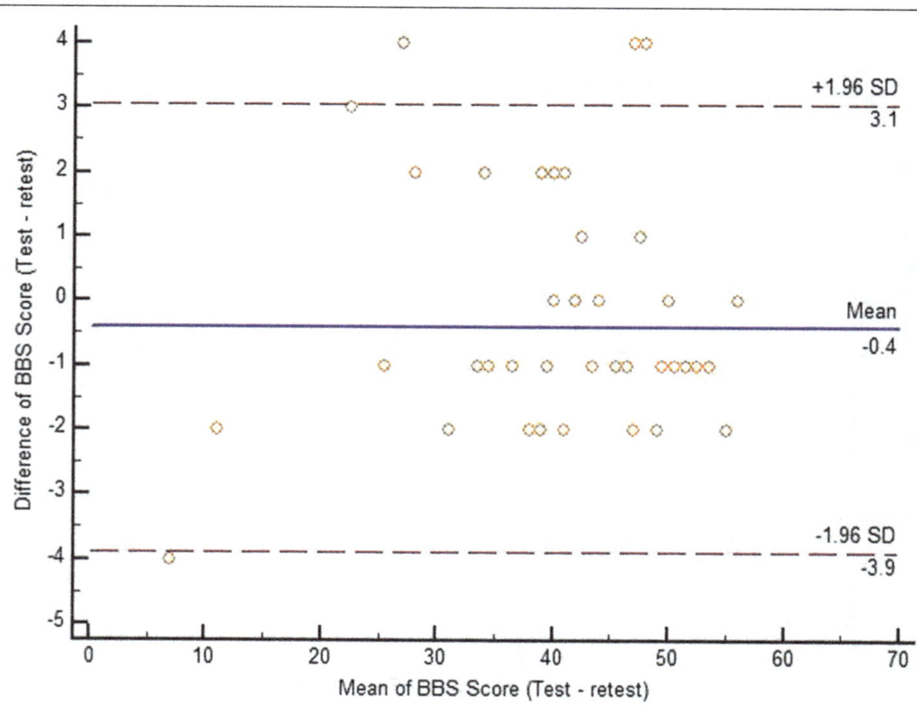

Fig. 3 Bland-Altman plot showing reliability of the Berg balance scale (BBS)

Table 4 Correlation among the timed up and go test (TUG), dynamic gait index (DGI), and the berg balance scale (BBS) at different reading

	TUG vs DGI	DGI vs BBS	TUG vs BBS
First Reading	−0.45**	0.75**	−.52**
Second Reading	− 0.48**	0.77**	−.53**

**Correlation is significant at the 0.01 level;

study reported an excellent reliability of the TUG test and the total BBS score in patients with chronic stroke [16]. The reliability of the TUG test, total DGI scores, and total BBS score in the current study were similar or near to those reported in previously published studies [7, 16, 43]. Jonsdottir and Cattaneo [7] reported an ICC value of 0.96 for total DGI scores. Hiengkaew et al. [16] reported an ICC value of 0.95 for the total BBS scores. In addition, Lin et al. [42] reported a similar test-retest reliability of the total DGI scores of individuals with chronic stroke. Blum and Korner-Bitensky [44] reported a slightly higher test-retest reliability (ICC = 0.98) of the BBS in patients with stroke. In contrast, another study reported a lower reliability of the total BBS score (ICC = 0.88) in patients with chronic stroke [45]. Similarly, Flansbjer et al. [18] reported lower test-retest reliability (ICC = 0.95) of TUG test in patients with chronic stroke. However, these studies had a higher sample size than the current study. In addition, the former study had a high proportion of left-sided hemiplegia in their participants compared to the current study in which right-sided hemiplegia was dominant. Furthermore, Ng and Hui-Chan [34] reported slightly lower test-retest reliability (ICC = 0.95) of the TUG test in patients with chronic stroke. However, Ng and Hui-Chan [34] study had a smaller sample size including only 11 subjects with chronic stroke.

In the present study, the SEM value of TUG test was slightly higher than the total DGI scores (1.16 vs. 0.71) and the total BBS scores (1.16 vs. .98). Similarly, a previous study reported lower SEM (0.97) for the total DGI scores in patients with chronic stroke [7]. Flansbjer et al. [45] reported a lower SEM score for the total BBS scores than those reported in the present study (1.49 vs. 1.93). However, Hiengkaew et al. [16] reported a higher SEM score for the TUG test than that in the present study (3.22 vs. 1.16). In the present study, the MDC value of the TUG test was lower than that in a previously published study (3.2 vs. 7.8) [16]. Similarly, the MDC value of the total BBS scores was lower than that in a previously published study (2.7 vs 4.7) [16].

In the present study, a good positive correlation was found between the DGI and BBS, and a moderate negative correlation was found between the TUG and BBS. Jonsdottir and Cattaneo [7] reported a moderate positive correlation between the DGI and BBS, and a moderate negative correlation between the DGI and TUG test. Although, in the present study, there was a slightly lower negative correlation found between the TUG test and DGI, this confirms the concurrent validity of these scales. In addition, Vistamehr et al. [46] reported a moderate positive correlation between the DGI and BBS total scores. In a future study of large cohort might give a better correlation among these scales.

The TUG, DGI, and BBS displayed a moderate degree of responsiveness from baseline to discharge, indicating they can adequately detect patients' recovery following an intervention. However, DGI showed a better responsiveness compared to the TUG and BBS. A previous study reported an acceptable level of responsiveness of BBS at various stages of recovery in patients with stroke [47]. Another study reported a moderate level of responsiveness of DGI in detecting changes at the 5-month period of intervention in patients with chronic stroke [43]. No previous study had reported the responsiveness of the TUG test in detecting changes following an intervention in patients with chronic stroke. The current study indicates that the three scales are able to detect changes in patients with chronic stroke undergoing outpatient physiotherapy.

Generalization of the present results should be limited to the individuals with chronic stroke who could walk at least 10 m with or without a walking aid. Since it is not possible to score 4 points using a walking aid in DGI assessment, it becomes a 3-points scale for those participants who used such aids. This could results a better reliability of this scale. In addition, the degree of plantar flexor tone was not measured, which could affect the present results. Furthermore, lack of data about the pre-medical stroke history, exact stroke location and size may affect the scale interpretation. Since fewer female patients participated in this study, gender influence was not considered. However, this could have some impact on the overall responsiveness of each scale. It is recommended to examine the treatment effect on the DGI,

Table 5 Correlations among demographic variables and the three scales

	Age	Height	Weight	Affected side	Duration since stroke	Type of stroke
TUG	0.225	− 0.017	0.161	−0.001	−.020	0.202
DGI	−0.386*	0.164	−0.093	0.020	−.337*	−0.166
BBS	−0.545**	0.213	0.093	0.112	−.045	−0.312*

*Correlation is significant at the 0.05 level; **Correlation is significant at the 0.01 level
TUG Timed up and go test, *DGI* Dynamic gait index, *BBS* Berg balance scale

Tables 6 Responsiveness of timed up and go test (TUG), the dynamic gait index (DGI), and the berg balance scale (BBS)

Indices of responsiveness	TUG	DGI	BBS
Baseline	20.1 ± 8.3	14.9 ± 5.3	41.4 ± 10.9
Discharge	16.9 ± 7.9	17.4 ± 4.8	45.7 ± 8.6
Mean difference	3.11	2.52	4.34
Pooled Standard Deviation	8.18	5.02	9.85
Standard Deviation of paired differences	5.87	2.82	5.37
*Effect size (ES) using pooled SD (95% CI)	0.38 (−0.57 − − 0.08)	0.50 (0.31–0.73)	0.44 (0.23–0.67)
Standardized response mean (SRM) (95%CI)	0.53 (−1.01 − − 0.03)	0.89 (0.47–1.30)	0.81 (0.47–1.01)

*Cohen's d

TUG, BBS scores, muscle strength, the degree of spasticity, and gait parameters in prospective studies in patients with chronic stroke. Additionally, the small sample size limits the validity of the results. Therefore, future parametric studies are needed with larger sample size to confirm this finding and to compare these scales to one another.

Conclusions

The test-retest reliability of the TUG, BBS, and DGI was excellent. The DGI demonstrated better responsiveness than TUG and BBS. The results of the present study support the use of these scales for measuring balance and mobility in patients with chronic stroke.

Acknowledgments
The authors are grateful to the Deanship of Scientific Research, King Saud University for funding through Vice Deanship of Scientific Research Chairs.

Funding
This project was funded by the Deanship of Scientific Research, King Saud University through Vice Deanship of Scientific Research Chairs. The funding body played no role in the study design, manuscript writing, or decision to submit the manuscript for publication.

Authors' contributions
SA: the corresponding author, participated in the study design and data collection, drafted the manuscript, and finalized the manuscript. AA: participated in the study design, helped with the ethics application and revised the manuscript critically. EA: participated in the study design and revised the manuscript critically. BS: participated in the data collection and revised the manuscript critically. All authors read and approved the final manuscript.

Competing interests
There are no competing interests reported by any authors.

Author details
[1]Rehabilitation Research Chair, College of Applied Medical Sciences, King Saud University, P.O.Box-10219, Riyadh 11433, Saudi Arabia. [2]National Institute for Locomotor Disabilities (Divyangjan), Kolkata, India.

References

1. Blomstrand A, Blomstrand C, Ariai N, Bengtsson C, Björkelund C. Stroke incidence and association with risk factors in women: a 32-year follow-up of the prospective population study of women in Gothenburg. BMJ Open. 2014;4(10):e005173.
2. Alahmari K, Paul SS. Prevalence of stroke in kingdom of Saudi Arabia - through a physiotherapist diary. MJSS. 2016;7:228–33.
3. Rode G, Tiliket C, Boisson D. Predominance of postural imbalance in left hemiparetic patients. Scand J Rehabil Med. 1997;29(1):11–6.
4. Shumwaycook A, Anson D, Haller S. Postural sway biofeedback - its effect on reestablishing stance stability in hemiplegic patients. Arch Phys Med Rehab. 1988;69(6):395–400.
5. Goldie PA, Matyas TA, Evans OM, Galea M, Bach TM. Maximum voluntary weight-bearing by the affected and unaffected legs in standing following stroke. Clin Biomech. 1996;11(6):333–42.
6. Horak FB, Esselman P, Anderson ME, Lynch MK. The effects of movement velocity, mass displaced, and task certainty on associated postural adjustments made by normal and hemiplegic individuals. J Neurol Neurosur Ps. 1984;47(9):1020–8.
7. Jonsdottir J, Cattaneo D. Reliability and validity of the dynamic gait index in persons with chronic stroke. Arch Phys Med Rehab. 2007;88(11):1410–5.
8. Lin JH, Hsieh CL, Hsiao SF, Huang MH. Predicting long-term care institution utilization among post-rehabilitation stroke patients in Taiwan: a medical Centre-based study. Disabil Rehabil. 2001;23(16):722–30.
9. Desrosiers J, Noreau L, Rochette A, Bravo G, Boutin C. Predictors of handicap situations following post-stroke rehabilitation. Disabil Rehabil. 2002;24(15): 774–85.
10. Bohannon RW, Leary KM. Standing balance and function over the course of acute rehabilitation. Arch Phys Med Rehab. 1995;76(11):994–6.
11. Berg K, Norman KE. Functional assessment of balance and gait. Clin Geriatr Med. 1996;12(4):705–23.
12. Benaim C, Perennou DA, Villy J, Rousseaux M, Pelissier JY. Validation of a standardized assessment of postural control in stroke patients - the postural assessment scale for stroke patients (PASS). Stroke. 1999;30(9):1862–8.
13. Fuglmeyer AR, Jaasko L, Leyman I, Olsson S, Steglind S. Post-stroke hemiplegic patient .1. Method for evaluation of physical performance. Scand J Rehabil Med. 1975;7(1):13–31.
14. Poole JL, Whitney SL. Motor-assessment scale for stroke patients - concurrent validity and interrater reliability. Arch Phys Med Rehab. 1988; 69(3):195–7.
15. Huang YC, Wang WT, Liou TH, Liao CD, Lin LF, Huang SW. Postural assessment scale for stroke patients scores as a predictor of stroke patient ambulation at discharge from the rehabilitation ward. J Rehabil Med. 2016; 48(3):259–64.
16. Hiengkaew V, Jitaree K, Chaiyawat P. Minimal detectable changes of the berg balance scale, Fugl-Meyer assessment scale, timed "up & go" test, gait speeds, and 2-minute walk test in individuals with chronic stroke with different degrees of ankle plantarflexor tone. Arch Phys Med Rehab. 2012; 93(7):1201–8.
17. Faria CD, Teixeira-Salmela LF, Silva EB, Nadeau S. Expanded timed up and go test with subjects with stroke: reliability and comparisons with matched healthy controls. Arch Phys Med Rehab. 2012;93(6):1034–8.
18. Flansbjer UB, Holmback AM, Downham D, Patten C, Lexell J. Reliability of gait performance tests in men and women with hemiparesis after stroke. J Rehabil Med. 2005;37(2):75–82.

19. Pollock CL, Eng JJ, Garland SJ. Clinical measurement of walking balance in people post stroke: a systematic review. Clin Rehabil. 2011;25(8):693–708.
20. Wong SST, Yam MS, Ng SSM. The figure-of-eight walk test: reliability and associations with stroke-specific impairments. Disabil Rehabil. 2013; 35(22):1896–902.
21. Beauchet O, Annweiler C, Allali G, Berrut G, Dubost V. Dual task-related changes in gait performance in older adults: a new way of predicting recurrent falls? J Am Geriatr Soc. 2008;56:181–2.
22. Lundin-Olsson L, Nyberg L, Gustafson Y. "Stops walking when talking" as a predictor of falls in elderly people. Lancet. 1997;349:617.
23. Faulkner KA, Redfern MS, Cauley JA, Landsittel DP, Studenski SA, Rosano C, et al. Multitasking: association between poorer performance and a history of recurrent falls. J Am Geriatr Soc. 2007;55:570–6.
24. Coppin AK, Shumway-Cook A, Saczynski JS, Patel KV, Ble A, Ferrucci L, et al. Association of executive function and performance of dual-task physical tests among older adults: analyses from the InChianti study. Age Ageing. 2006;35:619–24.
25. Pettersson AF, Olsson E, Wahlund LO. Effect of divided attention on gait in subjects with and without cognitive impairment. J Geriatr Psychiatry Neurol. 2007;20:58–62.
26. Manckoundia P, Pfitzenmeyer P, d'Athis P, Dubost V, Mourey F. Impact of cognitive task on the posture of elderly subjects with Alzheimer's disease compared to healthy elderly subjects. Mov Disord. 2006;21:236–41.
27. Lord SR, Castell S. Physical activity program for older persons: effect on balance, strength, neuromuscular control, and reaction time. Arch Phys Med Rehab. 1994;75:648–52.
28. Brauser SG, Woollacott M, Shumway-Cook A. The interacting effects of cognitive demand and recovery of postural stability in balance-impaired elderly persons. J Gerontol A Biol Sci Med Sci. 2001;56:M489–96.
29. Berg K, Wood-Dauphinee S, Williams J, Gayton D. Measuring balance in the elderly: preliminary development of an instrument. Physiother Can. 1989;41:304–11.
30. Berg K, Wooddauphinee S, Williams JI. The balance scale - reliability assessment with elderly residents and patients with an acute stroke. Scand J Rehabil Med. 1995;27(1):27–36.
31. ShumwayCook A, Gruber W, Baldwin M, Liao S. The effect of multidimensional exercises on balance, mobility, and fall risk in community-dwelling older adults. Phys Ther. 1997;77(1):46–57.
32. Powell LE, Myers AM. The activities-specific balance confidence (ABC) scale. J Gerontol A Biol Sci Med Sci. 1995;50A(1):M28–34.
33. Podsiadlo D, Richardson S. The timed up and go - a test of basic functional mobility for frail elderly persons. J Am Geriatr Soc. 1991;39(2):142–8.
34. Ng SS, Hui-Chan CW. The timed up & go test: its reliability and association with lower-limb impairments and locomotor capacities in people with chronic stroke. Arch Phys Med Rehab. 2005;86(8):1641–7.
35. Whitney SL, Marchetti GF, Schade A, Wrisley DM. The sensitivity and specificity of the timed "up & go" and the dynamic gait index for self-reported falls in persons with vestibular disorders. J Vestibul Res-Equil. 2004; 14(5):397–409.
36. Francq BG, Govaerts B. How to regress and predict in a bland-Altman plot? Review and contribution based on tolerance intervals and correlated-errors-in-variables models. Stat Med. 2016;35(14):2328–58.
37. Atkinson G, Nevill AM. Statistical methods for assessing measurement error (reliability) in variables relevant to sports medicine. Sports Med. 1998;26(4):217–38.
38. Haley SM, Fragala-Pinkham MA. Interpreting change scores of tests and measures used in physical therapy. Phys Ther. 2006;86(5):735–43.
39. Cohen J. Statistical power analysis for the behavior sciences. II. Hillsdale: Lawrence Erlbaum Associates; 1988.
40. Lee KB, Lim SH, Kim YD, Yang BI, Kim KH, Lee KS, et al. The contributions of balance to gait capacity and motor function in chronic stroke. J Phys Ther Sci. 2016;28(6):1686–90.
41. Bombardier C, Tugwell P. Methodological considerations in functional assessment. J Rheumatol Suppl. 1987;14(Suppl 15):6–10.
42. Kirshner B, Guyatt G. A methodological framework for assessing health indices. J Chronic Dis. 1985;38(1):27–36.
43. Lin JH, Hsu MJ, Hsu HW, Wu HC, Hsieh CL. Psychometric comparisons of 3 functional ambulation measures for patients with stroke. Stroke. 2010;41(9):2021–5.
44. Blum L, Korner-Bitensky N. Usefulness of the berg balance scale in stroke rehabilitation: a systematic review. Phys Ther. 2008;88(5):559–66.
45. Flansbjer UB, Blom J, Brogardh C. The reproducibility of berg balance scale and the single-leg stance in chronic stroke and the relationship between the two tests. PM R. 2012;4(3):165–70.
46. Vistamehr A, Kautz SA, Bowden MG, Neptune RR. Correlations between measures of dynamic balance in individuals with post-stroke hemiparesis. J Biomech. 2016;49(3):396–400.
47. Mao HF, Hsueh IP, Tang PF, Sheu CF, Hsieh CL. Analysis and comparison of the psychometric properties of three balance measures for stroke patients. Stroke. 2002;33(4):1022–7.

Re-evaluation of the stroke prognostication using age and NIH Stroke Scale index (SPAN-100 index) in IVT patients — the-SPAN 100^{65} index

Cornelia Möbius[1], Christian Blinzler[1], Stefan Schwab[1], Martin Köhrmann[2] and Lorenz Breuer[1*]

Abstract

Background: The SPAN-100 index adds patient age and baseline NIHSS-score and was introduced to predict clinical outcome after acute ischemic stroke (AIS). Even with high NIHSS-scores younger patients cannot reach a SPAN-100-positive status (index ≥100). We aimed to evaluate the SPAN-100 index among a large, contemporary cohort of i.v.-thrombolysed AIS-patients and exclusively among older patients who can at least theoretically achieve SPAN-100-positivity.

Methods: The SPAN-100 index was applied to AIS-patients receiving i.v.-thrombolysis (IVT) in our institution between 01/2006 and 01/2013. Clinical outcome and symptomatic intracerebral hemorrhage rates were compared between SPAN-100-positive and -negative patients. Furthermore we excluded patients < 65 years, without any theoretical chance to achieve SPAN-100-positivity, and re-evaluated the index ($SPAN^{65}$–100 index).

Results: SPAN-100-positive IVT-patients (124/1002) had a 9-fold increased risk for unfavorable outcome compared to SPAN-negative patients (OR 9.39; 95% CI 5.87–15.02; $p < 0.001$). The odds ratio for mortality was 7.48 (95% CI 4.90–11.43; $p < 0.001$). No association was found between SPAN-100-positivity and sICH-incidence (OR 0.88; 95% CI 0.31–2.53; $p = 0.810$).
$SPAN^{65}$–100-positivity (124/741) was associated with an 8-fold increased risk for unfavorable outcome (OR 7.6; 95% CI 4.71–12.22; $p < 0.001$) but not associated with higher sICH-rates (OR 0.86; 95% CI 0.29–2.53; $p < 0.001$).

Conclusions: Also for patients ≥65 years the SPAN-100 index can be a fast, easy method to predict clinical outcome of IVT-patients in everyday practice. However, it should not be used to determine the risk of sICH after IVT. Based on a SPAN-positive status IVT should not be withheld from AIS-patients merely because of feared sICH-complications.

Keywords: SPAN-100 index, SPAN-100^{65} index, Acute ischemic stroke, I.V.-thrombolysis, Clinical outcome, Symptomatic intracerebral hemorrhage

Background

Age and stroke severity are known major risk factors and predictors for unfavorable outcome in acute ischemic stroke (AIS) patients [1–3]. However, impact of higher age and higher initial National Institutes of Health Stroke Scale (NIHSS)-scores on clinical outcome after AIS and the way how these two factors interact with each other still remain not entirely clear. In particular data showing which individual patient will achieve favorable or unfavorable outcome is sparse. Different scores to predict clinical outcome after AIS have been introduced [4–8]. Most of them are rather complex and may therefore not be extensively used in daily routine. In order to create a fast and practical tool to predict clinical outcome of AIS patients the Stroke Prognostication using Age and NIH Stroke Scale index (SPAN-100 index) was introduced [9]. It simply combines patient age (years) and the NIHSS-Score at stroke onset. Patients with a score ≥ 100 are classified as

* Correspondence: lorenz.breuer@uk-erlangen.de
[1]Department of Neurology, Universitätsklinikum Erlangen, Schwabachanlage 6, 91054 Erlangen, Germany
Full list of author information is available at the end of the article

SPAN-100–positive and those with a score < 100 are designated as SPAN-100-negative. The index was applied to the dataset of the National Institute of Neurological Disorders and Stroke (NINDS)-tPA trials [10] and found to be of good value to predict clinical outcome and risk of intracerebral hemorrhage [9]. Since its introduction the SPAN-100-index has been evaluated several times in different patient cohorts [11–15]. However, previous investigations have in common that they included patients who could not achieve a SPAN-100-positve status at all, e.g. the original SPAN-100-evaluation [9] with a considerable proportion of younger patients. Even with very high NIHSS-scores they were not able to reach a SPAN-Index of ≥100. Including such patients might have increased selectivity of the score potentially leading to an overestimation of its benefit.

The first aim of our study was to re-evaluate reliability of the original SPAN-100 index in an independent, more recent cohort of 1002 i.v.-thrombolysed AIS-patients. The second objective was to exclude younger patients from our patient cohort to exclusively evaluate the SPAN-index among the subgroup of patients who could at least theoretically achieve SPAN-100-positivity.

Methods

The Erlangen Stroke and Thrombolysis Database is a prospective database of all AIS-patients at the University Hospital Erlangen, Germany. It contains baseline demographic and stroke related data as well as treatment specifics, imaging information and outcome parameters for each stroke patient. Outcome at day 90 was assessed using the mRS (modified Rankin Scale) evaluated by a neurologist as part of the general database independently from the present study using a semi-structured interview either in person or by telephone. Favorable clinical outcome was defined as mRS: 0–2 and/or clinical recovery to the pre-stroke mRS. Unfavorable outcome was defined as a mRS of 4–6. The study was approved by the local ethics committee. 17/1002 patients were lost to follow-up at day 90. Symptomatic intracerebral hemorrhage (sICH) was defined according to the European Cooperative Acute Stroke Study (ECASS) III criteria (sICH-definition 1) [16]. To assure comparability to the derivation cohort we additionally applied the sICH-definition (any documented decline in the neurologic status) used in the original publication [9] (sICH-definition 2). Our institutional guidelines are less restrictive than the European Medicines Agency -licence for tPA, therefore more than half of our patients receive off-label IVT. Besides that all patients were treated and monitored on our stroke unit in accordance with European guidelines [17]. Standard CT-based treatment was performed within the 4.5-h-window. For patients within an extended or unknown time window our institution uses an MRI mismatch-based algorithm as described elsewhere [18]. Follow-up imaging was performed after 24 to 36 h to evaluate for intracerebral hemorrhage and infarct distribution. NIHSS-scores were documented by NIHSS-certified stroke neurologists.

Study population

For this study we extracted all AIS-patients from the database who consecutively received IVT between 01/2006 and 01/2013. We applied the SPAN-100 index to this cohort to create two groups by adding age (years) to the NIHSS-score on admission. Patients with a score ≥ 100 were classified as SPAN-100-positive, whereas all patients with a score < 100 were designated as SPAN-100-negative. We compared clinical outcomes and sICH-rates of SPAN-100-negative and SPAN-100-positive patients. To identify patients who were eligible for the second part of our study, we subtracted the highest NIHSS-score documented in our patient cohort from the SPAN-100 cut off score of ≥100. Referring to the NIHSS-Coma Scoring Rules (as stated in the original scoring manual developed for the NINDS Trial of tPA for Acute Stroke) this was a NIHSS-score of 35 resulting in a second patient-cohort aged ≥65 years. We again compared clinical outcomes at day 90 and sICH-rates in both groups ($SPAN^{65}$–100-positive and $SPAN^{65}$–100-negative patients).

Statistical analysis

Statistical analysis was performed using PASW Statistics 19 (SPSS Inc., Chicago, Ill., USA). All data were tested for normality. Categorical variables are presented as frequencies and percentages, whereas continuous data are expressed as mean and standard deviation or as median and interquartile range as appropriate. Intergroup differences were assessed using analysis of variance for normally distributed items, the Kruskal-Wallis test for non-normal data, and the x^2-test for dichotomous variables. Binary logistic regression was performed with SPAN-100-status as independent variable. p-values ≤0.05 were considered significant.

Results

1002 AIS-patients received IVT at our institution between 01/2006 and 01/2013. After applying the SPAN-100 index 124 (12.4%) were classified as SPAN-100-positive.

Baseline characteristics

Mean age was 87 years for SPAN-100-positive and 72 years in SPAN-100-negative patients. Median NIHSS-scores on admission were 19 for SPAN-100-positive and 8 for SPAN-100-negative patients respectively. Door-to-needle-time did not differ in both groups. Compared to SPAN-100-negative patients, those in the SPAN-100-positive group were more likely to be women and to suffer from coronary artery disease and atrial fibrillation. SPAN-100-positive patients had worse pre-stroke-mRS scores than SPAN-100-negative patients. Baseline characteristics are summarized in Table 1.

Outcome comparison of SPAN-100-positive and SPAN-100-negative patients

SPAN-100-positive patients were more likely to have unfavorable outcomes (80.1% vs. 30.1%; $p < 0.001$), and only 13 of them achieved favorable outcome at day 90 (10.7% vs. 36.9% in the SPAN-100-negative group; $p < 0.001$) (Fig. 1). Mortality during hospital stay (29.8% vs. 6.4%; $p < 0.001$) and after three months (44.6% vs. 9.7%; $p < 0.001$) was significantly higher in SPAN-100-positive patients. Unadjusted binary regression analysis showed a 9-fold increase in the odds of unfavorable outcome for SPAN-100-positive patients and a 7.5-fold increase for mortality after three months (Table 2).

Area under the curve (AUC) for the SPAN-100 concerning mRS 4–6 was 0.74; 95%; $p < 0.0001$; 95% CI (0.71–0.77). Sensitivity and specificity for the cut-off of 100 was 0.27 and 0.96 respectively.

SICH comparison between SPAN-100-positive and SPAN-100-negative patients

Of 36 sICH (sICH-definition 1) 4 (3.2%) occurred in SPAN-100-positive and 32 (3.7%) in SPAN-100-negative patients, respectively ($p = 1.000$). The binary logistic regression analysis showed that SPAN-100-positive status was not predictive for sICH-incidence regardless if sICH-definition 1 or 2 were applied (Table 2).

Table 1 Baseline characteristics of SPAN-100-positive and SPAN-100-negative patients

Variable	Total ($n = 1002$)	SPAN pos. ($n = 124$)	SPAN neg. ($n = 878$)	p-value
Age (years), median (IQR)	73 (18)	87 (8)	72 (17)	< 0.001
Sex (female), n (%)	473 (47.2%)	81 (65.3%)	392 (44.6%)	< 0.001
Risk factors, n (%)				
Hypertension	872 (87.0%)	111 (89.5%)	761 (86.7%)	0.475
Hypercholesterolemia	571 (57.3%)	47 (37.9%)	524 (60.0%)	< 0.001
Nicotine	145 (14.5%)	7 (5.6%)	138 (15.7%)	0.002
Diabetes	330 (32.9%)	40 (32.3%)	290 (33.0%)	0.919
Coronary artery disease	283 (28.2%)	46 (37.1%)	237 (27.0%)	0.025
Previous myocardial infarction	112 (11.2%)	19 (15.3%)	93 (10.6%)	0.128
Previous stroke/TIA	241 (24.1%)	33 (26.6%)	208 (23.7%)	0.501
Atrial fibrillation	412 (41.1%)	86 (69.4%)	326 (37.1%)	< 0.001
door-to-needle time [min.] Median (IQR)	32 (26)	34,5 (24)	32 (26)	0.543
NIHSS-score on admission Median (IQR)	10 (10)	19 (6)	8 (8)	< 0.001
Pre-stroke mRS: 0–1, n (%)	753 (75.1%)	57 (46.0%)	696 (79.3%	< 0.001
Vital signs/laboratory findings				
Temperature on admission [°C] median (IQR)	36.6 (1.0)	36.4 (1.0)	36.7 (0.9)	0.004
Blood glucose on admission [mg/dl] median (IQR)	117 (41)	118 (34)	116 (43)	0.509
Systolic blood pressure on admission [mmHg], median (IQR)	160 (36)	160 (37)	160 (35)	0.748
Diastolic blood pressure on admission [mmHg], median (IQR)	88.5 (23)	85 (19)	89 (23)	0.028
Leucocytes on admission [$\times 10^3/\mu l$] median (IQR)	8.40 (3.73)	8.63 (3.61)	8.31 (3.79)	0.073
CRP on admission [mg/l],median (IQR)	4.3 (8.1)	6.85 (13.2)	4.0 (7.8)	0.001
Platelet count on admission [$\times 10^3$] median (IQR)	234 (98)	243.5 (102)	232 (97))	0.205
Triglycerides [mg/dl] median (IQR)	115 (71)	106 (49)	118 (78)	0.055
Stroke subtype				0.001
Large artery disease	92 (9.3%)	8 (6.5%)	84 (9.7%)	
Cardioembolic	440 (44.3%)	88 (71%)	352 (40.5%)	
Small-vessel disease	36 (3.6%)	3 (2.4%)	33 (3.8%)	
Other	36 (3.6%)	0	36 (4.1%)	
Unknown	389 (39.2%)	25 (20.2%)	364 (41.9%)	

Abbreviations SPAN = Stroke Prognostication using Age and NIH Stroke Scale, *NIHSS* = NIH Stroke Scale, *TIA* = transient ischemic attack, *CRP* = C-reactive protein

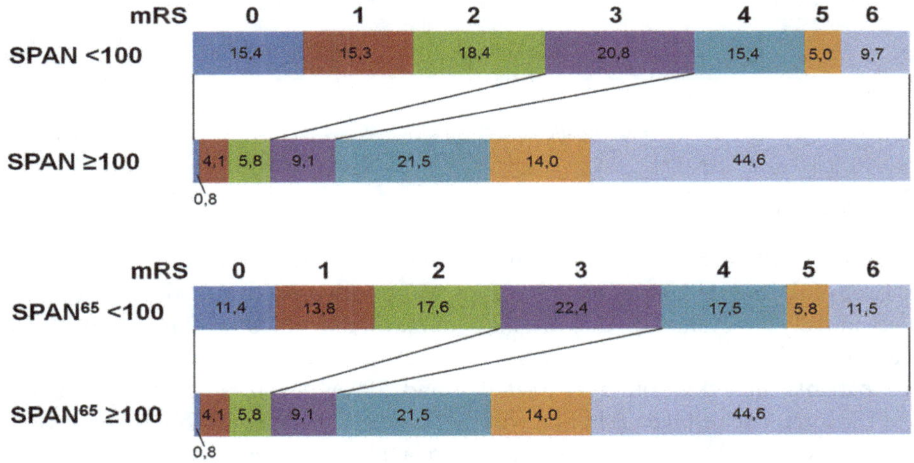

Fig. 1 Comparison of functional outcome according to the mRS between SPAN-100-positive and SPAN-100-negative patients as well as between SPAN-100^{65}-positive and SPAN-100^{65}-negative patients. Abbreviations: SPAN = Stroke Prognostication using Age and NIH Stroke Scale; mRS = modified Rankin scale

Evaluation of the SPAN-100 index in patients ≥65 years (SPAN-100^{65} index)

741/1002 (74%) patients were ≥ 65 years old. After applying the SPAN^{65}–100 index, we identified 617 (83.3%) SPAN^{65}–100-negative and 124 (16.7%) SPAN^{65}–100-positive patients. Selected baseline characteristics for both subgroups are shown in Table 3.

Outcome results of the SPAN^{65}-cohort did not substantially differ from the findings of the total cohort. Mortality during hospital stay (29.8% vs. 7.1%; $p <$ 0.001) and after three months (44.6% vs. 11.5%; $p <$ 0.001) was higher for SPAN^{65}–100-positive patients. Patients in the SPAN^{65}–100-positive group were more likely to achieve unfavorable outcomes (80.1% vs. 34.8%; $p <$ 0.001) and only 13 patients in the SPAN-100-positive group achieved a favorable outcome at 90 days (10.7% vs. 42,8% in the SPAN 100 negative group; $p <$ 0.001) (Fig. 1). SICH (sICH-definition 1) occurred in 4 (3.2%) and 23 (2.7%) of the SPAN^{65}–100-positive and SPAN^{65}–100-negative patients, respectively (p = 1.000). Binary regression analysis revealed patients with SPAN^{65}–100-positive status to have an 8-fold increased risk in the odds for unfavorable outcome. AUC for the SPAN^{65}–100 was 0.73; 95%; $p <$ 0.0001; 95% CI (0.69–0.76). Sensitivity and specificity for the cut-off of 100 was 0.32 and 0.94 respectively. No significant association was found between SPAN^{65}–100-status and sICH-incidence regardless which sICH-definition was used. (Table 4).

Table 2 Association between SPAN-100-positivity and outcome

variable	OR	95% CI	*p*-value
mRS 4–6	9.39	5.869–15.021	< 0.001
mortality at 3 months	7.48	4.901–11.427	< 0.001
sICH-Def. 1	0.88	0.305–2.527	0.810
sICH-Def. 2	1.01	0.389–2.638	0.978

Abbreviations SPAN = Stroke Prognostication using Age and NIH Stroke Scale, *mRS* = modified Rankin scale, *sICH* = symptomatic intracranial hemorrhage, *OR* = odds ratio, *CI* = confidence interval

Discussion

The SPAN-100 index was introduced by Saposnik et al. to facilitate treatment decisions in stroke patients [9]. With age and stroke severity it combines two main predictors for unfavorable stroke outcome. After applying the index to the patients in the NINDS-tPA trials [10] SPAN-100-positivity was found to be associated with worse outcomes. Besides that higher ICH-rates were seen in SPAN-100-positive compared to SPAN-negative patients whether they had received IVT before or not. An IVT-benefit was described for SPAN-100-negative, but not for SPAN-100-positive patients [9]. However, several conditions may have influenced these results. First, the number of SPAN-positive patients who received IVT was rather small (n = 36). Second, the population of the NINDS-trials does not reflect current treatment standards, e.g. patients were randomized to tPA or placebo within 3-h after symptom onset [10].

Several additional studies evaluated the SPAN-100 index after its first introduction [11–15, 19]. Overall they confirmed that SPAN-100-positive patients are less likely to achieve favorable outcome compared to SPAN-negative patients. Only one Chinese study found a low prediction power of the SPAN-100 index for 3- and 12-month outcome [19].

However, data concerning the predictive power of the SPAN-100 index for sICH are inconsistent. Krishnan et al. found higher intracerebral hemorrhage-rates in SPAN-100-positive patients compared to the SPAN-negative patients [9, 13] while Abilleira et al. observed similar sICH-rates [11]. In contrast two other studies

Table 3 Baseline characteristics of SPAN^{65}–100-positive and SPAN^{65}–100-negative patients

Variable	Total (n = 741)	SPAN^{65} pos. (n = 124)	SPAN^{65} neg. (n = 617)	p-value
Age (years), median (IQR)	78 (12)	87 (8)	76 (10)	< 0.001
Sex (female), n (%)	385 (52%)	81 (65.3%)	304 (49.3%)	< 0.001
NIHSS-score on admission,median (IQR)	10 (11)	19 (6)	8 (8)	< 0.001

Abbreviations SPAN = Stroke Prognostication using Age and NIH Stroke Scale, *NIHSS* = NIH Stroke Scale, *IQR* inter quartile Range

comparing performance of different sICH-scores found a poor predictive power of the SPAN-100 index [14, 20].

In our study, we initially re-evaluated the original SPAN-100 index among a larger, more contemporary cohort of 1002 IVT-patients, including off-label treated patients. In terms of outcome our results are in line with previous studies. Patients with SPAN-100-positive status had a 9-fold increased risk of unfavorable outcome at three months.

Irrespective of the used sICH-definition SPAN-100-positive status was not associated with a higher risk of sICH.

Therefore our data do not support the hypothesis by Saposnik et al. who suggested that the SPAN-100 index might help to evaluate the risk of ICH after IVT [9]. This discrepancy might possibly be explained by the fact that advances concerning diagnostic and treatment infrastructure were achieved since the NINDS trials [10]. Continued development of imaging techniques might account for lower sICH-rates despite inclusion of off-label treated patients, e.g. patients with prolonged or unknown time window.

Previous evaluations of the SPAN-100-Index did not differentiate between patients who could a priori reach a SPAN-positive status and those who could not. Even with very high NIHSS-scores, younger patients are unable to reach the SPAN-100 index cut off score of 100. In the analysis by Saposnik et al. 219/624 (35.1%) patients in the SPAN-negative group were younger than 65 years [9]. This might have biased the SPAN-negative group towards a better outcome potentially increasing selectivity of the index and leading to an overestimation of its benefit. In the second part of our study we addressed this issue by removing patients younger than 65 years from our data set and applying the SPAN-100^{65} index to the resulting new patient-cohort aged ≥65 years.

Table 4 Association between SPAN-100^{65}-positivity and outcome

variable	OR	95% CI	p-value
mRS 4–6	7.58	4.708–12.222	< 0.001
mortality at 3 months	6.18	3.996–3.996	< 0.001
sICH-Def. 1	0.86	0.291–2.526	0.781
sICH-Def. 2	1.22	0.488–3.031	0.674

Abbreviations SPAN = Stroke Prognostication using Age and NIH Stroke Scale, *mRS* = modified Rankin scale, *sICH* = symptomatic intracranial hemorrhage, *OR* = odds ratio, *CI* = confidence interval

Similar to the results of the total cohort, SPAN^{65}–100-positive patients had an 8–fold higher risk to reach unfavorable outcome. But even in IVT-patients ≥65 years sICH-rates did not differ between SPAN^{65}–100-positive and SPAN^{65}–100-negative patients. Hence, unfavorable outcome in our SPAN-100-positive patients was not related to hemorrhagic complications of thrombolytic therapy suggesting that IVT should not be withheld from older stroke patients with high NIHSS-scores merely because of safety reasons. This is in line with results from the SITS-ISTR Registry which show no excess risk of cerebral hemorrhage in patients with NIHSS-score > 25 [21]. Besides that several observational studies indicate safety and efficacy of tPA-treatment in stroke patients > 80 years [22–25] and the results of the third international stroke trial (IST-3) suggest that age should not be a barrier to IVT [26].

Our study has several limitations, primarily the single-center approach and the use of our institutional diagnostic and treatment guidelines as well as the retrospective design. However, including off-label patients might increasingly reflect common daily routine.

Conclusions

Our findings confirm the value of the SPAN-100 index. Also after excluding younger patients who a priori cannot reach a SPAN-positive status the SPAN-100 index can be an easy to use, readily available calculator in everyday clinical practice to predict clinical outcome in IVT patients. However, in our cohort SPAN-100-positive status was not predictive for the risk of sICH after IVT. Based on a positive SPAN-100 status IVT should not be withheld from patients merely because of feared sICH complications.

Abbreviations

AIS: Acute ischemic stroke; AUC: Area under the curve; CI: Confidence interval; CRP: C-reactive protein; i.v.: Intravenous; IVT: Intravenous thrombolysis; mRS: Modified Rankin Scale; NIHSS: National Institutes of Health Stroke Scale; NINDS: National Institute of Neurological Disorders and Stroke; OR: Odds ratio; sICH: Symptomatic intracerebral hemorrhage; SPAN-100 index: Stroke Prognostication using Age and NIH Stroke Scale-100 index; SPAN-10065 index: SPAN-100 index evaluated in patients ≥65 years; TIA: Transient ischemic attack; tPA: Tissue type plasminogen activator

Authors' contributions

CM Data acquisition, literature search, manuscript preparation. CB Data analysis, manuscript editing and review. SS Data analysis, manuscript editing and review. MK Study concept, manuscript editing and review. LB Study concept, data acquisition, data analysis, literature search manuscript editing and review. All authors read and approved the final manuscript.

Competing interests

CM and CB reported no conflict of interest. SS reported having received speaker honoraria from Bayer, BMS Pfizer and Boehringer Ingelheim. MK reported having received advisory board and speaker honoraria and travel grants from Boehringer Ingelheim, BMS/Pfizer, Bayer and Novartis. LB reported having received speaker honoraria and travel grants from Bayer and travel grants from Boehringer Ingelheim.

Author details

[1]Department of Neurology, Universitätsklinikum Erlangen, Schwabachanlage 6, 91054 Erlangen, Germany. [2]Department of Neurology, Universitätsklinikum Essen, Hufelandstr. 55, 45147 Essen, Germany.

References

1. Predicting outcome after acute ischemic stroke. An external validation of prognostic models. Neurology. 2004;62(4):581–5.
2. Konig IR, Ziegler A, Bluhmki E, Hacke W, Bath PM, Sacco RL, Diener HC, Weimar C. Predicting long-term outcome after acute ischemic stroke: a simple index works in patients from controlled clinical trials. Stroke. 2008;39(6):1821–6.
3. Weimar C, Konig IR, Kraywinkel K, Ziegler A, Diener HC. Age and National Institutes of Health stroke scale score within 6 hours after onset are accurate predictors of outcome after cerebral ischemia: development and external validation of prognostic models. Stroke. 2004;35(1):158–62.
4. Kent DM, Selker HP, Ruthazer R, Bluhmki E, Hacke W. The stroke-thrombolytic predictive instrument: a predictive instrument for intravenous thrombolysis in acute ischemic stroke. Stroke. 2006;37(12):2957–62.
5. Lou M, Safdar A, Mehdiratta M, Kumar S, Schlaug G, Caplan L, Searls D, Selim M. The HAT score: a simple grading scale for predicting hemorrhage after thrombolysis. Neurology. 2008;71(18):1417–23.
6. Ntaios G, Faouzi M, Ferrari J, Lang W, Vemmos K, Michel P. An integer-based score to predict functional outcome in acute ischemic stroke: the ASTRAL score. Neurology. 2012;78(24):1916–22.
7. Saposnik G, Kapral MK, Liu Y, Hall R, O'Donnell M, Raptis S, Tu JV, Mamdani M, Austin PC. IScore: a risk score to predict death early after hospitalization for an acute ischemic stroke. Circulation. 2011;123(7):739–49.
8. Strbian D, Meretoja A, Ahlhelm FJ, Pitkaniemi J, Lyrer P, Kaste M, Engelter S, Tatlisumak T. Predicting outcome of IV thrombolysis-treated ischemic stroke patients: the DRAGON score. Neurology. 2012;78(6):427–32.
9. Saposnik G, Guzik AK, Reeves M, Ovbiagele B, Johnston SC. Stroke prognostication using age and NIH stroke scale: SPAN-100. Neurology. 2013;80(1):21–8.
10. Tissue plasminogen activator for acute ischemic stroke. The National Institute of Neurological Disorders and Stroke rt-PA stroke study group. N Engl J Med. 1995;333(24):1581–7.
11. Abilleira S, Ribera A, Quesada H, Rubiera M, Castellanos M, Vargas M, Gomis M, Krupinski J, Delgado-Mederos R, Gomez-Choco M, et al. Applicability of the SPAN-100 index in a prospective and contemporary cohort of patients treated with intravenous rtPA in Catalonia. Neurologia. 2016;31(9):592–8.
12. Almekhlafi MA, Davalos A, Bonafe A, Chapot R, Gralla J, Pereira VM, Goyal M. Impact of age and baseline NIHSS scores on clinical outcomes in the mechanical thrombectomy using solitaire FR in acute ischemic stroke study. AJNR Am J Neuroradiol. 2014;35(7):1337–40.
13. Krishnan P, Saposnik G, Ovbiagele B, Zhang L, Symons S, Aviv R. Contribution and additional impact of imaging to the SPAN-100 score. AJNR Am J Neuroradiol. 2015;36(4):646–52.
14. Li M, Wang-Qin RQ, Wang YL, Liu LB, Pan YS, Liao XL, Wang YJ, Xu AD. Symptomatic intracerebral hemorrhage after intravenous thrombolysis in chinese patients: comparison of prediction models. J Stroke Cerebrovasc Dis. 2015;24(6):1235–43.
15. Ovbiagele B, Reeves MJ, Nasiri M, Johnston SC, Bath PM, Saposnik G. A simple risk index and thrombolytic treatment response in acute ischemic stroke. JAMA Neurol. 2014;71(7):848–54.
16. Hacke W, Kaste M, Bluhmki E, Brozman M, Davalos A, Guidetti D, Larrue V, Lees KR, Medeghri Z, Machnig T, et al. Thrombolysis with alteplase 3 to 4.5 hours after acute ischemic stroke. N Engl J Med. 2008;359(13):1317–29.
17. European Stroke Organisation (ESO) Executive Committee and ESO Writing Committee. Guidelines for management of ischaemic stroke and transient ischaemic attack. Cerebrovasc Dis. 2008;25(5):457–507.
18. Breuer L, Schellinger PD, Huttner HB, Halwachs R, Engelhorn T, Doerfler A, Kohrmann M. Feasibility and safety of magnetic resonance imaging-based thrombolysis in patients with stroke on awakening: initial single-Centre experience. Int J Stroke. 2010;5(2):68–73.
19. Pan Y, Jing J, Zhang R, Zhao X, Liu L, Wang H, Liu G, Wang C, Wang Y. Poor performance of stroke prognostication using age and National Institutes of Health stroke Scale-100 to predict 3- and 12-month outcomes of ischemic stroke in China National Stroke Registry. J Stroke Cerebrovasc Dis. 2014; 23(9):2335–40.
20. Strbian D, Michel P, Seiffge DJ, Saver JL, Numminen H, Meretoja A, Murao K, Weder B, Forss N, Parkkila AK, et al. Symptomatic intracranial hemorrhage after stroke thrombolysis: comparison of prediction scores. Stroke. 2014; 45(3):752–8.
21. Mazya MV, Lees KR, Collas D, Rand VM, Mikulik R, Toni D, Wahlgren N, Ahmed N. IV thrombolysis in very severe and severe ischemic stroke: results from the SITS-ISTR registry. Neurology. 2015;85(24):2098–106.
22. Mishra NK, Ahmed N, Andersen G, Egido JA, Lindsberg PJ, Ringleb PA, Wahlgren NG, Lees KR. Thrombolysis in very elderly people: controlled comparison of SITS international stroke thrombolysis registry and virtual international stroke trials archive. BMJ. 2010;341:c6046.
23. Ringleb PA, Schwark C, Kohrmann M, Kulkens S, Juttler E, Hacke W, Schellinger PD. Thrombolytic therapy for acute ischaemic stroke in octogenarians: selection by magnetic resonance imaging improves safety but does not improve outcome. J Neurol Neurosurg Psychiatry. 2007;78(7):690–3.
24. Toni D, Lorenzano S, Agnelli G, Guidetti D, Orlandi G, Semplicini A, Toso V, Caso V, Malferrari G, Fanucchi S, et al. Intravenous thrombolysis with rt-PA in acute ischemic stroke patients aged older than 80 years in Italy. Cerebrovasc Dis. 2008;25(1–2):129–35.
25. Vatankhah B, Dittmar MS, Fehm NP, Erban P, Ickenstein GW, Jakob W, Bogdahn U, Horn M. Thrombolysis for stroke in the elderly. J Thromb Thrombolysis. 2005;20(1):5–10.
26. Sandercock P, Wardlaw JM, Lindley RI, Dennis M, Cohen G, Murray G, Innes K, Venables G, Czlonkowska A, Kobayashi A, et al. The benefits and harms of intravenous thrombolysis with recombinant tissue plasminogen activator within 6 h of acute ischaemic stroke (the third international stroke trial [IST-3]): a randomised controlled trial. Lancet. 2012;379(9834):2352–63.

25

Decompressive craniectomy for herpes simplex encephalitis complicated by frank intracerebral hemorrhage

Yoon Hwan Byun[1], Eun Jin Ha[1], Sang-Bae Ko[2] and Kyung Hyun Kim[1*]

Abstract

Background: Herpes simplex encephalitis is the most common type of sporadic encephalitis worldwide. Frank intracerebral hemorrhage complicating the disease course in herpes simplex encephalitis patients is rare, especially cases where surgical decompression is necessary. Here, we report a previously healthy female with herpes simplex encephalitis who underwent surgical decompression due to temporal lobe hemorrhage.

Case presentation: A previously healthy 34-year-old Korean female presented with fever, myalgia and severe headache. Brain MRI showed a high T2 signal intensity change and diffuse swelling of the right temporal lobe. Polymerase chain reaction testing of the cerebrospinal fluid confirmed the presence of herpes simplex virus 1. The patient was admitted for close observation and intravenous acyclovir. On hospital day 3, she had a sudden onset of vomiting and severe headache. Brain CT showed frank temporal lobe hemorrhage. Despite aggressive medical treatment, she became increasingly drowsy. Ultimately, she underwent emergency right decompressive craniectomy, expansile duraplasty and intracranial pressure monitor insertion. The patient recovered fully without any neurological deficits or neuropsychological problems. She was discharged after completion of 2 weeks of acyclovir and returned 2 months later for cranioplasty.

Conclusions: Patients with severe herpes simplex encephalitis complicated by intracerebral hemorrhage or malignant cerebral edema should undergo aggressive medical treatment. Surgical decompression should also be actively considered in these severe cases to prevent further neurological deterioration.

Keywords: Herpes simplex encephalitis, Intracerebral hemorrhage, Surgical decompression

Background

Herpes simplex encephalitis (HSE) is a severe viral infection of the human central nervous system caused by either herpes simplex virus (HSV) 1 or 2. This infection is known to be the most frequent form of sporadic encephalitis worldwide, accounting for 10–20% of all cases [1]. Patients with HSE frequently present with fever, headache, seizure or focal neurological deficits [2]. Encephalitis characterized by cerebral edema and hemorrhagic necrosis typically involves the temporal lobe, which is best visualized by magnetic resonance imaging (MRI) of the brain [3, 4]. The diagnosis of HSE is confirmed by positive polymerase chain reaction (PCR) results for HSV DNA in the cerebrospinal fluid (CSF) [5]. The fatality rate of HSE has been reduced to 5–15% from 70% with the development of viral therapy [6]. However, even after initiation of acyclovir treatment, cerebral edema may progress and cause mass effects, increased intracranial pressure (ICP) and uncal herniation [7]. Frank intracerebral hematoma formation complicating the disease course of HSE is reported to be rare. We report a case of delayed temporal lobe hemorrhage in an immunocompetent patient with HSE who ultimately underwent surgical decompression.

* Correspondence: ds4ckd@daum.net
[1]Department of Neurosurgery, Seoul National University Hospital, 101 Daehak-ro, Jongno-gu, Seoul 03080, Republic of Korea
Full list of author information is available at the end of the article

Case presentation

A previously healthy 34-year-old Korean female was admitted to a regional hospital for fever, myalgia and severe headache that had started 2 weeks ago. Brain MRI showed a high T2 signal intensity change and diffuse swelling of the right temporal lobe, insula and hippocampus (Fig. 1). Lumbar puncture showed lympho-dominant pleocytosis. The patient was started on intravenous (iv) dexamethasone and acyclovir under a high suspicion of viral encephalitis.

She was transferred to our institution 4 days later due to persistent headache despite treatment. A noncontrast computed tomography (CT) brain scan taken at our institution showed a hemorrhagic transformation of the right temporal lobe, which was not observed on the initial MRI (Fig. 2a, b). Follow-up lumbar puncture showed 510 white cells per mm^3 (82% lymphocytes), 144 mg/dL protein and 61 mg/dL glucose. CSF culture studies were negative for bacteria, fungi and tuberculosis. PCR of the CSF confirmed the presence of HSV1. The patient was free of neurological symptoms, with a Glasgow Coma Scale of E4M6V5, and was admitted for close observation and continuation of iv acyclovir. Corticosteroid treatment was discontinued upon her admission. On day 3 of hospitalization, the patient presented with a sudden onset of vomiting and severe headache. Brain CT showed an increased amount of temporal lobe hemorrhage and a leftward shift in the midline (Fig. 2c, d). Mannitol was administered but did not seem to have a significant effect. The patient became increasingly drowsy, and her right pupil became dilated. She underwent emergency right decompressive craniectomy, expansile duraplasty and ICP monitor insertion. Postoperative brain CT showed alleviation of midline shifting (Fig. 2d, e). The patient recovered fully 5 days after the surgery. Apart from mild intermittent headache and dizziness, she did not show any other significant clinical symptoms, including neuropsychological problems. There were no significant neurologic deficits upon neurological examinations performed by the attending neurosurgeon and neurologist. The patient was discharged after completion of 2 weeks of acyclovir and returned 2 months later for cranioplasty. She was followed up 3 more times after cranioplasty. She was stable, without any neuropsychological problems or neurologic deficits, and was able to successfully return to work as a public official.

Discussion and conclusions

Petechial cortical hemorrhages in HSE are common. However, frank hematoma formation in HSE is rare, especially in cases requiring surgical decompression. To the best of our knowledge, only 8 similar adult cases [8–14] have been reported in the English literature; these cases are summarized in Table 1. Acyclovir was started promptly upon admission in all cases, and the mean interval from admission to hematoma formation was 8 days. The exact mechanism of hemorrhage has not been found, but a few hypotheses have been proposed. These hypotheses include the rupture of small vessels due to either vasculitis or transient hypertension caused by increased ICP [15].

In HSE patients, administration of acyclovir should be initiated immediately to prevent further viral replication in the brain [16]. Acyclovir significantly improves the outcomes achieved by HSE patients, and late initiation of viral

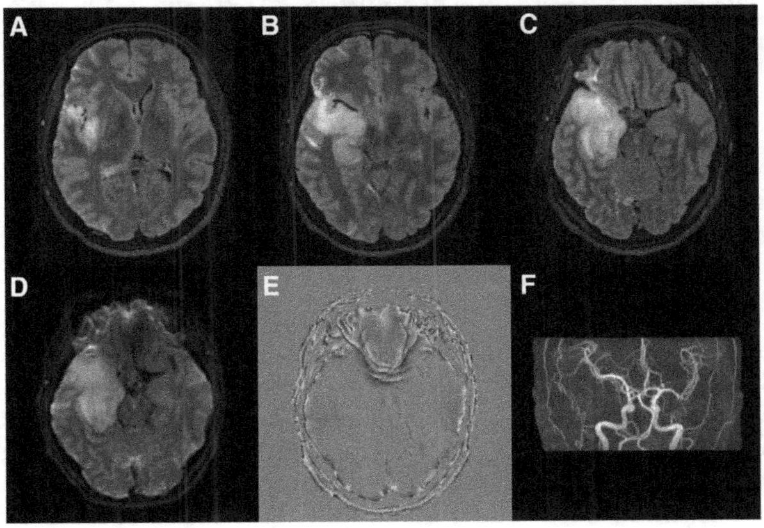

Fig. 1 Initial brain MRI (2017.12.15). T2 weighted image shows diffuse swelling and high signal intensity changes of the right (**a**) insula (**b**) hippocampus (**c**) temporal lobe. **d** Diffusion weighted image (DWI) shows diffusion restriction of the right temporal lobe lesion (**e**) Susceptibility weighted angiography (SWAN) shows no evidence of hemorrhage (**f**) Brain MR Angiography shows no steno-occlusive lesion or aneurysm in intracranial vessels

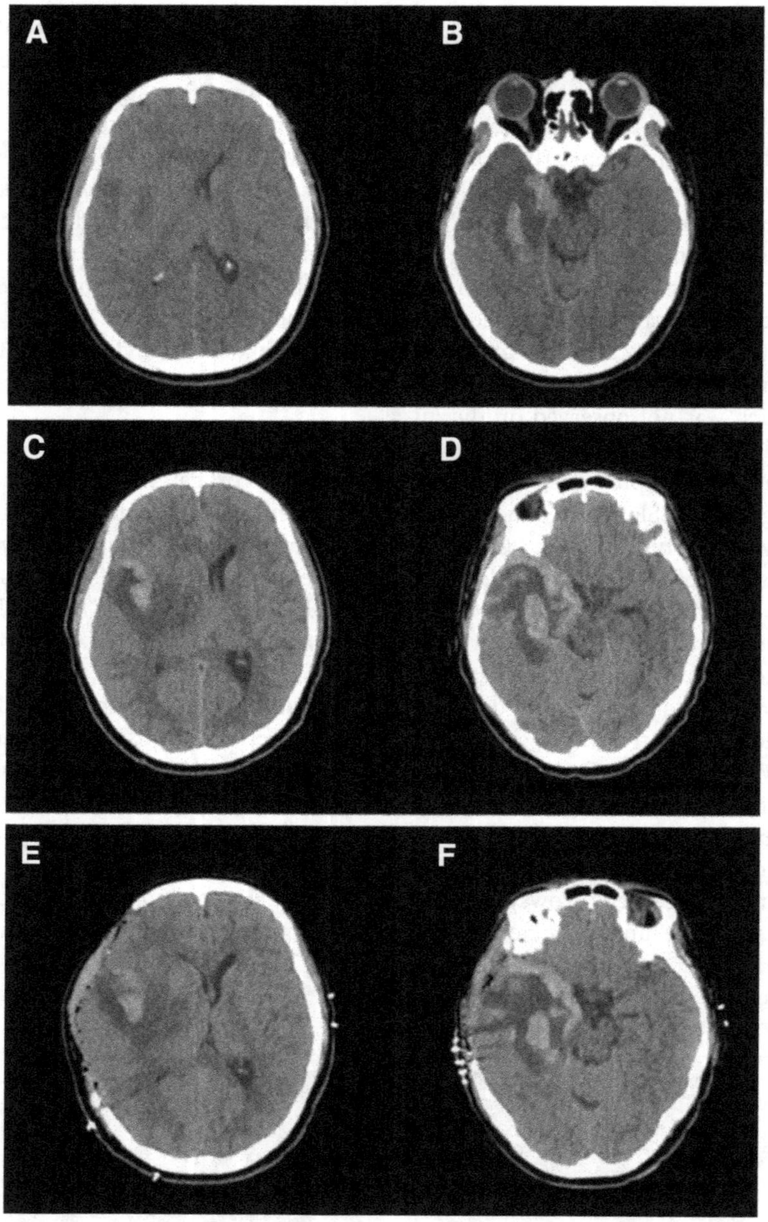

Fig. 2 Serial follow up noncontrast brain CT. **a**, **b**: Brain CT taken on the day of admission to our institution (2017.12.19) shows a hemorrhagic transformation of the right temporal lobe lesion. **c**, **d**: Brain CT taken on day 3 of hospitalization (2017.12.22) shows an increased amount of temporal lobe hemorrhage and a leftward shift in the midline. **e**, **f**: Postoperative brain CT (2017.12.23) shows an improvement in midline shift with no significant increase of temporal lobe hemorrhage

treatment can lead to significant morbidity and mortality. The Infectious Disease Society of America (IDSA) recommends 2–3 weeks of intravenous acyclovir at 10 mg/kg/8 h depending on the clinical course [17]. Some HSE patients present with atypical symptoms and/or normal initial CSF analysis, which may hinder physicians from reaching the correct diagnosis. Repeated clinical and laboratory tests are recommended when encephalitic syndromes are suspected, and acyclovir should be considered in these patients even before proven diagnosis [18].

Any worsening of initial symptoms or manifestation of new neurologic deficits despite adequate viral treatment, especially during the second week of admission, warrants the need for neuroimaging study [8]. Aggravation of cerebral edema and formation of new intracerebral hemorrhage should be ruled out. In addition, acyclovir resistance and acyclovir side effects should be considered in the differential diagnosis.

Medical treatment to control increased ICP due to cerebral edema or hematoma includes hyperventilation,

Table 1 Patients who underwent surgical decompression for HSE complicated by intracerebral hemorrhage

Reference	Age/ Sex	Initial clinical presentation	Admission to hemorrhage lapse (days)	New symptoms associated with hemorrhage	Location	Treatment				Outcome	Other medical condition
						Medical			Surgical		
						Acyclovir	Mannitol	Steroid			
Rodriguez-Sainz et al. [8]	45/F	fever, headache, incoherent speech	9	lt third nerve palsy, rt. hemiparesis, severe aphasia	lt temporal	ACV 10 mg/kg 8 h x 21d	o	x	DC + HE	rt hemiparesis, motor aphasia	hepatitis C
Yan [9]	37/M	fever, headache, bizarre behavior, hallucination, memory problem	8	altered mental status, anisocoric pupil	lt temporal	ACV 10 mg/kg/8 h x 18d	x	x	TL	full recovery	
	48/F	headache, altered mental status, hemianopsia	10	rt hemiparesis, anisocoric pupil	lt temporal	ACV 10 mg/kg/8 h x 12d	x	x	DC + TL	mild stuttering	
Counsell et al. [10]	32/M	fever, headache, seizure	10	altered mental status, partial rt. third nerve palsy	rt fronto-temporal	ACV 10 mg/kg/d x 3d +10d (post-operative)	x	o	TL	full recovery	
Jabbour et al. [11]	27/M	fever, headache, seizure	9	altered mental status, partial rt. third nerve palsy	rt temporal	ACV 10 mg/kg/12 h (duration not specified)	x	x	HE	full recovery	iv heparinization for pulmonary embolism
Li et al. [12]	56/M	seizure, impairment in memory	6	altered mental status	lt temporal	ACV x 28d	x	x	DC + HE	impairment in word finding, memory impairment	HIV (+)
Lo et al. [13]	46/M	fever, headache, vomiting, confusion	6	rt hemiparesis, anisocoric pupil	lt temporal	ACV 10hg/kg/d x 36d	x	o	TL + HE + delayed DC	full recovery	
Mueller et al. [14]	40/F	fever, headache, nausea, photophobia	7	altered mental status, lt hemiparesis	rt temporal	ACV x 21d	x	x	DC + TL	not specified	
Current case	34/F	fever, headache, myalgia	7	altered mental status, anisocoric pupil	rt temporal	ACV x 14d	o	o	DC	full recovery	

ACV acyclovir, *Lt* Left, *Rt* Right, *DC* decompressive craniectomy, *HE* hematoma evacuation, *TL* temporal lobectomy, *HIV* human immunodeficiency virus

corticosteroids and hyperosmolar therapy. The use of corticosteroids in HSE is controversial due to its potential to increase viral replication, resulting in further cell damage [19]. However, previously reported studies generally support the use of corticosteroids in severe cases of HSE after the initiation of antiviral therapy [20]. Corticosteroids may benefit these patients by inhibiting the inflammatory cascades that lead to vasogenic edema in the latter part of the disease course. There is no concrete evidence regarding the use of mannitol or hypertonic saline in HSE, and the use of hyperosmolar therapy to reduce ICP in these situations is extrapolated from traumatic brain injury guidelines [21]. However, we postulate that hyperosmolar therapy may help alleviate cytotoxic edema caused by viral replication early in the course of HSE.

There is a lack of literature concerning the utilization of surgical decompression, such as decompressive craniectomy or temporal lobectomy, in patients with severe HSE. Nonetheless, presently available data generally support the use of surgical decompression in viral encephalitis with severe life-threatening neurological symptoms [22]. Our patient underwent surgical decompression due to neurological deterioration despite aggressive medical treatment and was able to recover fully without neurological deficits. We support the use of surgical decompression in severe HSE cases complicated by malignant cerebral edema or intracerebral hemorrhage.

In conclusion, frank intracerebral hemorrhage in HSE is a rare complication. This occurrence can cause neurological deterioration due to a mass effect or increased ICP. Neuroimaging studies should be conducted in HSE patients who show unchanged or worsened symptoms even after the initiation of acyclovir. Patients with severe HSE complicated by intracerebral hemorrhage or malignant cerebral edema should undergo aggressive medical treatment. Surgical decompression should also be actively considered in such severe cases to prevent further neurological deterioration.

Abbreviations

CSF: Cerebrospinal fluid; CT: Computed tomography; HSE: Herpes simplex encephalitis; HSV: Herpes simplex virus; ICP: Intracranial pressure; MRI: Magnetic resonance imaging; PCR: Polymerase chain reaction

Acknowledgements

None

Funding

This work did not receive any specific grant from funding agencies in the public, commercial, or non-profit sectors.

Authors' contributions

YHB: analysis and interpretation of patient's data, drafting the manuscript. EJH, SBK, KHK: interpretation of patient's data, revising the manuscript. All authors read and approved the final manuscript.

Competing interests

The authors declare that they have no competing interests.

Author details

[1]Department of Neurosurgery, Seoul National University Hospital, 101 Daehak-ro, Jongno-gu, Seoul 03080, Republic of Korea. [2]Department of Neurology, Seoul National University Hospital, 101 Daehak-ro, Jongno-gu, Seoul 03080, Republic of Korea.

References

1. Whitley RJ, Gnann JW. Viral encephalitis: familiar infections and emerging pathogens. Lancet. 2002;359(9305):507–13. https://doi.org/10.1016/S0140-6736(02)07681-X.
2. Whitley RJ. Herpes simplex encephalitis: adolescents and adults. Antivir Res. 2006;71(2–3):141–8. https://doi.org/10.1016/j.antiviral.2006.04.002.
3. Solbrig MV, Hasso AN, Jay CA. CNS viruses—diagnostic approach. Neuroimaging Clin N Am 2008;18 1:1–18; vii; doi: https://doi.org/10.1016/j.nic.2007.12.008.
4. Adamo MA, Deshaies EM. Emergency decompressive craniectomy for fulminating infectious encephalitis. J Neurosurg. 2008;108(1):174–6. https://doi.org/10.3171/JNS/2008/108/01/0174.
5. Tyler KL. Acute viral encephalitis. N Engl J Med. 2018;379(6):557–66. https://doi.org/10.1056/NEJMra1708714.
6. Sili U, Kaya A, Mert A, Group HSVES. Herpes simplex virus encephalitis: clinical manifestations, diagnosis and outcome in 106 adult patients. J Clin Virol. 2014;60(2):112–8. https://doi.org/10.1016/j.jcv.2014.03.010.
7. Singhi P, Saini AG, Sahu JK, Kumar N, Vyas S, Vasishta RK, et al. Unusual clinical presentation and role of decompressive Craniectomy in herpes simplex encephalitis. J Child Neurol. 2015;30(9):1204–7. https://doi.org/10.1177/0883073814546688.
8. Rodriguez-Sainz A, Escalza-Cortina I, Guio-Carrion L, Matute-Nieves A, Gomez-Beldarrain M, Carbayo-Lozano G, et al. Intracerebral hematoma complicating herpes simplex encephalitis. Clin Neurol Neurosurg. 2013; 115(10):2041–5. https://doi.org/10.1016/j.clineuro.2013.06.016.
9. Yan HJ. Herpes simplex encephalitis: the role of surgical decompression. Surg Neurol. 2002;57(1):20–4.
10. Counsell CE, Taylor R, Whittle IR. Focal necrotising herpes simplex encephalitis: a report of two cases with good clinical and neuropsychological outcomes. J Neurol Neurosurg Psychiatry. 1994;57(9):1115–7.
11. Jabbour PM, Ojemann SG. Herpes simplex encephalitis. Is anticoagulation safe? Neurologist. 2005;11(3):187–9. https://doi.org/10.1097/01.nrl.0000159761.57148.70.
12. Li JZ, Sax PE. HSV-1 encephalitis complicated by cerebral hemorrhage in an HIV-positive person. AIDS Read. 2009;19(4):153–5.
13. Lo WB, Wilcock DJ, Carey M, Albanese E. Neurological picture. Herpes encephalitis complicated by cerebral haemorrhage. J Neurol Neurosurg Psychiatry. 2013;84(12):1404–6. https://doi.org/10.1136/jnnp-2013-305552.
14. Mueller K, Ryan JE, Tai A, Armonda RA. Delayed temporal lobe hemorrhage after initiation of acyclovir in an immunocompetent patient with herpes simplex Virus-2 encephalitis: a case report. Cureus. 2017;9(1):e980. https://doi.org/10.7759/cureus.980.
15. ElShimy G, Mariyam Joy C, Berlin F, Lashin W. Intracranial hemorrhage complicating herpes simplex encephalitis on antiviral therapy: a case report and review of the literature. Case Rep Infect Dis. 2017;2017:6038146. https://doi.org/10.1155/2017/6038146.
16. Baringer JR. Herpes simplex infections of the nervous system. Neurol Clin 2008;26 3:657–674, viii; doi: https://doi.org/10.1016/j.ncl.2008.03.005.
17. Skelly MJ, Burger AA, Adekola O. Herpes simplex virus-1 encephalitis: a review of current disease management with three case reports. Antivir Chem Chemother. 2012;23(1):13–8. https://doi.org/10.3851/IMP2129.
18. Vachalova I, Kyavar L, Heckmann JG. Pitfalls associated with the diagnosis of herpes simplex encephalitis. J Neurosci Rural Pract. 2013;4(2):176–9. https://doi.org/10.4103/0976-3147.112756.
19. Ramos-Estebanez C, Lizarraga KJ. Merenda a. a systematic review on the role of adjunctive corticosteroids in herpes simplex virus encephalitis: is timing critical for safety and efficacy? Antivir Ther. 2014;19(2):133–9. https://doi.org/10.3851/imp2683.
20. Safain MG, Roguski M, Kryzanski JT, Weller SJ. A review of the combined medical and surgical management in patients with herpes simplex encephalitis. Clin Neurol Neurosurg. 2015;128:10–6. https://doi.org/10.1016/j.clineuro.2014.10.015.

26

Autoantibodies against neuronal surface proteins in spontaneous subarachnoid and intracerebral haemorrhage

Harald Hegen[1], Raimund Helbok[1], Mario Kofler[1], Bettina Pfausler[1], Alois Schiefecker[1], Erich Schmutzhard[1] and Ronny Beer[1,2*]

Abstract

Background: Brain autoimmunity has been reported in patients with preceding infection of the central nervous system by *herpesviridae*. It has been hypothesized that neuronal damage releasing antigens might trigger secondary immune response. The objective of the study was to investigate whether brain damage due to spontaneous subarachnoid haemorrhage (SAH) or intracerebral haemorrhage (ICH) induces reactivity against neuronal surface proteins.

Methods: Patients with spontaneous SAH and ICH, who had cerebrospinal fluid (CSF) and serum sampling within 2 weeks after disease onset (baseline) and afterwards at least 10 days later (follow-up), were included. Antibodies against NMDA, GABA-B, AMPA-1/– 2 receptor, LGI1 and CASPR2 were determined by indirect immunofluorescence.

Results: A total of 43 SAH and 11 ICH patients aged 62 (±12) years (65% females) had simultaneous CSF/ serum sampling median 5 and 26.5 days after disease onset. At baseline, all CSF samples were collected via ventricular drainage, at follow-up 20 (37.0%) patients had CSF collection by lumbar puncture because ventricular drain had been already removed. All CSF and serum samples at baseline and follow-up tested negative for antibodies against NMDA, GABA-B, AMPA-1/– 2 receptor, LGI1 and CASPR2.

Conclusions: Immunoreactivity against common neuronal surface proteins was not observed within the early disease course of spontaneous SAH and ICH.

Keywords: Subarachnoid haemorrhage, Intracerebral haemorrhage, Immunoreactivity, Neuronal surface proteins, NMDA receptor, $GABA_B$ receptor, AMPA receptor, LGI-1, CASPR-2

Background

Spontaneous subarachnoid haemorrhage (SAH) and spontaneous intracerebral haemorrhage (ICH) are both severe neurological disorders that result in brain injury due to several mechanisms including primary mechanical tissue damage caused by the bleeding and secondary effects such as inflammatory processes, oxidative stress responses, brain edema and in case of SAH delayed cerebral ischemia [1, 2].

With cell injury and blood brain barrier disruption antigens are released into the intrathecal space and, therefore, abundantly presented to the immune system. This may result in breaking tolerance and in the formation of an immune response. Brain autoimmunity has been observed in patients with preceding infections of the central nervous system (CNS) by *herpesviridae* [3–8]. In these patients, antibodies against N-methyl-D-aspartate (NMDA) receptor and other, so far unknown neuronal surface antigens, appeared between one to several weeks after disease onset [3]. It has been hypothesized that antigens being released through neuronal damage trigger secondary immune reactivity [9].

In the present study, we aimed to investigate whether acute brain damage due to spontaneous SAH or ICH induces the formation of antibodies against neuronal surface proteins in the early and post-acute phase.

* Correspondence: ronny.beer@i-med.ac.at
[1]Department of Neurology, Medical University of Innsbruck, Innsbruck, Austria
[2]Neurological Intensive Care Unit, Department of Neurology, Medical University of Innsbruck, Anichstrasse 35, A-6020 Innsbruck, Austria

Methods

Patients and samples

Patients with spontaneous SAH and ICH admitted within 24 h of disease onset to the neuro-intensive care unit of Medical University of Innsbruck have been recorded in a computerized database since April 2010 and July 2011, respectively. Diagnoses were confirmed by computed tomography of the head and traumatic causes were excluded. Only patients who had ventricular cerebrospinal fluid (CSF) and serum sampling within 2 weeks after disease onset (baseline) and afterwards at least 10 days later (follow-up), were included into this retrospective analysis. At follow-up, also lumbar CSF analysis was eligible in case of lacking ventricular CSF sampling (Fig. 1). All CSF and serum samples were withdrawn simultaneously and stored at – 20 °C until analysis.

Immunofluorescence assay

Antibodies against NMDA, γ-aminobutyric acid type B ($GABA_B$), α-amino-3-hydroxy-5-methyl-4-isoxazolepropionic acid (AMPA)-1, AMPA-2 receptor and against the voltage-gated potassium channel (VGKC)-associated proteins leucine-rich glioma inactivated 1 (LGI1) and contactin-associated protein 2 (CASPR2) were determined in CSF and serum at baseline and follow-up by commercially available cell-based indirect immunofluorescence assays (Cat.No. FA112d-1010-51, FA112l-1005-50, FA112k-1005-1 and FA1439–1005-1; Euroimmun, Lübeck, Germany).

Briefly, CSF and serum samples were added to an object plate containing human embryonic kidney cells, which express the respective antigen on their surface. After incubation, detection of patients' autoantibodies was achieved by fluorescein isothiocyanate-conjugated anti-human immunoglobulin G antibodies that were finally visualized by fluorescence microscopy.

Statistical analysis

We performed statistical analysis using SPSS 23.0 (SPSS Inc., Chicago, IL). Distribution of data was assessed by Kolmogorov-Smirnov test and, accordingly, data were displayed as mean ± standard deviation (SD) or as median and interquartile range (IQR).

Results

A total of 43 SAH and 11 ICH patients aged 62 (±12) years comprising 65% females had simultaneous CSF and serum sampling at baseline, median 5 (IQR 3–8) days after disease onset, and at follow-up after 26.5 (19–35.5) days. At baseline, all CSF samples were collected via ventricular drainage. At follow-up, 15 (34.9%) SAH and 5 (45.5%) ICH patients had CSF collection by lumbar puncture because ventricular drain had been already removed. Demographic and main sample characteristics for each disease group are displayed in Table 1.

Negative antibodies against neuronal surface proteins

All CSF and serum samples at baseline and follow-up were tested negative for antibodies against NMDA, $GABA_B$, AMPA-1, AMPA-2 receptor and against the VGKC-associated proteins LGI1 and CASPR2.

Discussion

According to recent reports on patients with CNS infection by *herpesviridae* who developed secondary brain autoimmunity as shown by the detection of anti-NMDA receptor antibodies and other so far unknown neuronal surface antibodies within weeks after disease onset [3–8], one might hypothesize that neuronal damage in other CNS disorders might also result in the formation of a secondary immune response. In the present study, we screened for antibodies against NMDA, $GABA_B$, AMPA-1, AMPA-2 receptors and against the VGKC-associated proteins LGI1

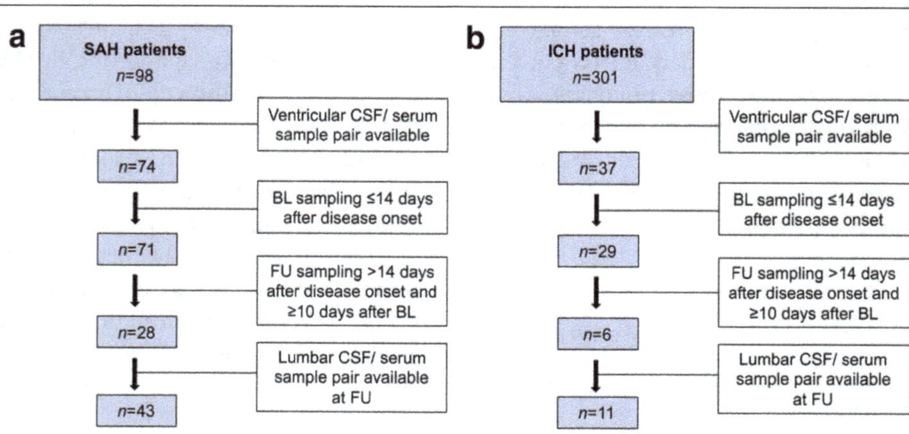

Fig. 1 Sample Flow Chart. **a** Subarachnoid haemorrhage patient cohort; **b** Intracerebral haemorrhage patient cohort. A total of 43 SAH and 11 ICH patients had simultaneous CSF and serum sampling at baseline and at follow-up

Table 1 Demographic data and cerebrospinal fluid characteristics at baseline and follow-up

	SAH	ICH
n	43	11
Age, years; mean ± SD (range)	60.7 ± 12.2 (28–86)	67.6 ± 9.3 (55–85)
Sex, female; n (%)	29 (67.4)	6 (54.5)
Hunt & Hess, n (%)		
Grad I-II	6 (14.0)	
Grad III	12 (27.9)	
Grad IV-V	25 (58.1)	
Time between disease onset and BL sampling, days	5 (3–8)	6 (4–9)
Time between disease onset and FU sampling, days	27 (19–39)	26 (19–33)
Baseline CSF findings		
RBC, /µl	32,000 (10667–96,000)	30,000 (3093–130,000)
WBC, /µl	91 (28–371)	73 (35–363)
Total protein, mg/l	1910 (880–2870)	2520 (1040–4280)
FU CSF findings		
RBC count, /µl	106 (13–419)	72 (3–3072)
WBC count, /µl	9 (2–18)	18 (10–36)
Total protein, mg/l	410 (320–690)	840 (445–1625)

Data are given as median (interquartile range) unless otherwise specified
BL baseline, *CSF* cerebrospinal fluid, *FU* follow-up, *ICH* intracerebral haemorrhage, *RBC* red blood cell, *SAH* subarachnoid haemorrhage, *WBC* white blood cell

and CASPR2 in the CSF and serum of patients with spontaneous SAH and ICH. Within a median time period of approximately 4 weeks after disease onset, we did not obtain any positive result.

There might be several reasons for the absence of a secondary immune response in our cohort of SAH and ICH patients. First, the aetiology of the evolution of anti-NMDA receptor antibodies in patients with preceding *herpesviridae* encephalitis is still unknown [9]. Although it has been hypothesized that a release of antigens by viral neuronal cell lysis triggers an immune response that is misdirected against a structurally similar epitope present in the NMDA receptor [9], there might be other or additional, so far unknown factors required for the initiation of CNS autoimmunity that are lacking or altered in patients with intrathecal bleeding. Secondly, immune reactivity with detectable levels of autoantibodies could start after the observation period of our patients (in our cohort only 10 out of 54 patients had follow-up sample later than 6 weeks).

There are some limitations of the study, e.g. the small number of patients. One could argue that autoantibodies against neuronal surface proteins might occur at a low frequency, and, therefore, were not detected. Although a higher patient number would strengthen the (negative) results, one has still to consider a false positive rate of the immunofluorescence test of up to 1% (as determined in healthy individuals) [10, 11]. Furthermore, as only a small proportion of the entire SAH and ICH cohort was eligible for determination of neuronal surface antibodies depending on availability of CSF and serum samples, it cannot be excluded that a selection bias has been introduced. Even though patients requiring ventricular drainage usually present with a more severe disease course, i.e. show more extensive brain damage, that possibly predisposes to secondary immune response formation, these patients typically show more intrathecal blood. It is unclear whether the presence of intrathecal blood might hamper the local establishment of a specific immune reactivity due to its potential ability of blocking epitopes.

Finally, antibodies against neuronal surface proteins cover only a small part of possible antigens against an immune response can be directed. Therefore, screening for antibodies against neuropil as well as determination of antibodies against intracellular epitopes has to be done in a further study.

Conclusions

Immunoreactivity against common neuronal surface proteins was not observed within the early disease course of spontaneous SAH and ICH.

Abbreviations

AMPA: α-amino-3-hydroxy-5-methyl-4-isoxazolepropionic acid; CASPR2: contactin-associated protein 2; CNS: central nervous system; CSF: cerebrospinal fluid; $GABA_B$: γ-aminobutyric acid type B; ICH: intracerebral haemorrhage; LGI1: leucine-rich glioma inactivated 1; NMDA: N-methyl-D-aspartate; SAH: subarachnoid haemorrhage; VGKC: voltage-gated potassium channel

Funding
This study has received funding from the Austrian Science Fund (FWF) under project number KLI 375.

Authors' contributions

HH has participated in the conception and design of the study, acquisition and statistical analysis of the data, and in drafting the manuscript. RH has participated in reviewing the manuscript for intellectual content. MK has participated in reviewing the manuscript for intellectual content. BP has participated in reviewing the manuscript for intellectual content. AS has participated in reviewing the manuscript for intellectual content. ES has participated in the conception and design of the study, and in reviewing the manuscript for intellectual content. RB has participated in the conception and design of the study, and in reviewing the manuscript for intellectual content. All authors read and approved the final manuscript.

Competing interests

H. Hegen declares to have no competing interests.
R. Helbok declares to have no competing interests.
M. Kofler declares to have no competing interests.
B. Pfausler declares to have no competing interests.
A. Schiefecker declares to have no competing interests.
E. Schmutzhard declares to have no competing interests.
R. Beer declares to have no competing interests.

References

1. Mracsko E, Veltkamp R. Neuroinflammation after intracerebral hemorrhage. Front Cell Neurosci. 2014;8:388.
2. Macdonald RL. Delayed neurological deterioration after subarachnoid haemorrhage. Nat Publ Group. 2014;10(1):44–58.
3. Armangue T, Leypoldt F, Málaga I, Raspall-Chaure M, Marti I, Nichter C, et al. Herpes simplex virus encephalitis is a trigger of brain autoimmunity. Ann Neurol. 2014;75(2):317–23.
4. Leypoldt F, Titulaer MJ, Aguilar E, Walther J, Bönstrup M, Havemeister S, et al. Herpes simplex virus-1 encephalitis can trigger anti-NMDA receptor encephalitis: case report. Neurology. 2013;81(18):1637–9.
5. Hacohen Y, Deiva K, Pettingill P, Waters P, Siddiqui A, Chretien P, et al. N-methyl-D-aspartate receptor antibodies in post-herpes simplex virus encephalitis neurological relapse. Mov Disord. 2014;29(1):90–6.
6. Mohammad SS, Sinclair K, Pillai S, Merheb V, Aumann TD, Gill D, et al. Herpes simplex encephalitis relapse with chorea is associated with autoantibodies to N-methyl-D-aspartate receptor or dopamine-2 receptor. Mov Disord. 2014;29(1):117–22.
7. Armangue T, Titulaer MJ, Málaga I, Bataller L, Gabilondo I, Graus F, et al. Pediatric anti-N-methyl-D-aspartate receptor encephalitis-clinical analysis and novel findings in a series of 20 patients. J Pediatr. 2013;162(4):850–2.
8. Linnoila JJ, Binnicker MJ, Majed M, Klein CJ, McKeon A. CSF herpes virus and autoantibody profiles in the evaluation of encephalitis. Neurol Neuroimmunol Neuroinflamm. 2016;3(4):e245.
9. Höftberger R, Armangue T, Leypoldt F, Graus F, Dalmau J. Clinical neuropathology practice guide 4-2013: post-herpes simplex encephalitis: N-methyl-Daspartate receptor antibodies are part of the problem. Clin Neuropathol. 2013;32(4):251–4.
10. Dahm L, Ott C, Steiner J, Stepniak B, Teegen B, Saschenbrecker S, et al. Seroprevalence of autoantibodies against brain antigens in health and disease. Ann Neurol. 2014;76(1):82–94.
11. Lang K, Prüss H. Frequencies of neuronal autoantibodies in healthy controls: estimation of disease specificity. Neurol Neuroimmunol Neuroinflamm. 2017;4(5):e386.

27

Cerebral microbleeds shouldn't dictate treatment of acute stroke: a retrospective cohort study evaluating risk of intracerebral hemorrhage

Martin A. Chacon-Portillo[1], Rafael H. Llinas[2] and Elisabeth B. Marsh[2*]

Abstract

Background: Intravenous tissue plasminogen activator (IV tPA) after acute ischemic stroke carries the risk of symptomatic intracerebral hemorrhage (sICH). Cerebral microbleeds (CMBs) may indicate increased risk of hemorrhage and can be seen on magnetic resonance imaging (MRI). In this study, we examined the association between CMBs and sICH, focusing on the predictive value of their presence, burden, and location.

Methods: Records from all patients presenting to two academic stroke centers with acute ischemic stroke treated with IV tPA over a 5-year period were retrospectively reviewed. Demographic, medical, and imaging variables were evaluated. The presence, number, and location (lobar vs nonlobar) of CMBs were noted on gradient echo MRI sequences obtained during the admission. Univariable and multivariable statistical models were used to determine the relationship between CMBs and hemorrhagic (symptomatic and asymptomatic) transformation.

Results: Of 292 patients (mean age 62.8 years (SD 15.3), 49% African-American, 52% women), 21% ($n = 62$) had at least one CMB, 1% ($n = 3$) had > 10 CMBs, and 1% ($n = 3$) were diagnosed with probable cerebral amyloid angiopathy. After treatment, 16% ($n = 46$) developed hemorrhagic transformation, of which 6 (2%) were sICH. There was no association between CMB presence ($p = .135$) or location ($p = .325$) with sICH; however, those with a high CMB burden (> 10 CMB) were more likely to develop sICH (OR 37.8; 95% CI: 2.7–539.3; $p = .007$).

Conclusions: Our findings support prior findings that a high CMB burden (> 10) in patients with acute stroke treated with IV tPA are associated with a higher risk of sICH. However, the overall rate of sICH in the presence of CMB is very low, indicating that the presence of CMBs by itself should not dictate the decision to treat with thrombolytics.

Keywords: Cerebral microbleed, Intracerebral hemorrhage, Intravenous thrombolysis, Stroke, Thrombolytic therapy

Background

Early treatment with intravenous tissue plasminogen activator (IV tPA) (< 4.5 h from symptom onset) increases the proportion of patients who survive with a favorable outcome after ischemic stroke [1]. Though treatment is associated with better outcomes, the most feared complication is hemorrhagic transformation (HT), or bleeding into the area of ischemia when the tissue is reperfused. When the ischemic volume is large enough, this can result in a symptomatic intracerebral hemorrhage (sICH) that worsens morbidity and mortality [2, 3].

Cerebral microbleeds (CMBs) are small areas of signal void, 2–10 mm in diameter [4–6] that can be seen on gradient echo magnetic resonance imaging (MRI) sequences, mostly representing blood products commonly associated with disorders such as hypertension or cerebral amyloid angiopathy (CAA). Along with other known risk factors for hemorrhage such as age, renal disease, and stroke volume [7], CMBs may also be associated with hemorrhage risk [8, 9] .The reported prevalence of CMBs on pre-IV tPA imaging ranges from 15 to 40% [10, 11]. This is clinically relevant, as it is becoming increasingly common to

* Correspondence: ebmarsh@jhmi.edu
[2]Department of Neurology, Johns Hopkins University School of Medicine, 600 N Wolfe St, Phipps 446, Baltimore, MD 21287, USA
Full list of author information is available at the end of the article

perform an MRI as part of the acute work-up of ischemic stroke [12]. In addition, there is increasingly rapid electronic access to patient's prior MR imaging that may show incidental CMBs. Understanding the associated risk of sICH may, therefore, be of significant clinical impact when considering the use of thrombolytics.

There is an existing literature on the association between CMBs and intracerebral hemorrhage with varying results [10, 13–16]. This discordance between studies may be due to the varied methodologies. Increased burden and patterns of location have been analyzed differently across studies, or not at all. Of note, higher CMB burdens, particularly in the lobar location, are more highly suggestive of CAA, as described by the Boston criteria [17], and may indicate a group of individuals at a higher risk of HT following thrombolysis. There may be other factors that are helpful in determining the likelihood of CAA over hypertension and related relative risk associated with each.

The use of thrombolytic therapy in the acute setting of ischemic stroke continues to grow and information regarding a patient's CMB status is more commonly known. Given the lack of consensus in the literature regarding the relationship between CMBs and sICH in this study, we examine the association of CMBs with hemorrhage, taking into account presence, burden, location, and the likelihood of CAA, to predict hemorrhage in patients treated with IV tPA.

Methods

Patients

The Johns Hopkins Institutional Review Board approved this study. Data for all stroke patients hospitalized at two large academic stroke centers are kept in separate databases approved for both clinical research and quality assurance purposes. Within these datasets, we retrospectively reviewed the records of all patients presenting with acute ischemic stroke and treated with IV tPA between January 1, 2011, and December 31, 2015. Patients were excluded if they went to intra-arterial lysis (mechanical thrombectomy), or did not have a brain MRI during their hospital stay. Image acquisition time was within 72-h of tPA administration for 98% of patients, with a maximum of 6 days post-tPA. Demographic variables (sex, race, age); medical information (history of: hypertension, diabetes mellitus, stroke, transient ischemic attack, coronary artery disease, tobacco use, alcohol use, atrial fibrillation, congestive heart failure, hyperlipidemia, chronic kidney disease, liver disease, cancer; admission systolic blood pressure, serum glucose and creatinine); stroke characteristics (admission National Institutes of Health Stroke Scale (NIHSS) score [2], etiology as defined by the Trial of ORG 10172 in Acute Stroke Treatment (TOAST) criteria [18], degree of white matter disease as defined by the Cardiovascular Health Study (CHS) score [19], imaging characteristics including CMB analysis as below; and outcomes (discharge and 90-day NIHSS and modified Rankin Score (mRS)) were collected [2, 20].

Imaging methods and variable definitions

As part of our stroke protocol, all patients underwent MRI of the brain including diffusion-, T1-, and T2-weighted sequences. All but 21 (7%) patients had susceptibility weighted gradient echo sequences (SWI) for CMB analysis (slice thickness: 5 mm, TR: 27, TE: 20, flip angle: 15). MRI examinations were performed using 3 Tesla MRI scanners (Siemens, PA). A trained investigator (MACP) reviewed all MRIs and a subset of cases was reviewed by a vascular neurologist (EBM) with an excellent inter-rater reliability (kappa = 0.87). Investigators reviewed differing values jointly and a consensus was reached.

Cerebral microbleed characterization

CMBs were identified as areas of signal void 2–10 mm in diameter on gradient echo sequences with associated blooming [5, 6]. Mimics (i.e. vessels, mineralization of the globus pallidus and dentate nuclei, air-borne interfaces, hemorrhages within the area of infarction, old deep intracerebral hemorrhages) were differentiated from "definite CMBs" using the Microbleed Anatomical Rating Scale [5, 6]. The distribution of the CMBs was described as lobar, deep, and infratentorial per the previously mentioned guideline [5]. CMBs located in deep and infratentorial structures were combined as "nonlobar" for CMB location analysis. Patients with CMBs in both locations were classified as having a mixed distribution. CMB burden was defined as mild-moderate (1–10 CMBs) and high (> 10 CMBs). Patients with no CMBs on imaging were used as a reference group for the analyses. Patients were defined as having probable CAA by the primary team due to clinical/imaging characteristics based on the Boston criteria [17].

Ischemic burden

Stroke volume was estimated on diffusion-weighted imaging using the formula: [(length) (width) (number of slices) (slice thickness)]/2 [21]. Infarct location was divided into anterior, posterior, or mixed circulations. Lesions were further classified depending on the depth of the stroke as: lobar (cortex and subcortical white matter of the frontal, parietal, temporal, occipital and insular lobes), deep (basal ganglia, thalamus, internal capsule, external capsule, corpus callosum, deep and periventricular white matter- typically due to lacunar disease) and mixed (usually large vessel occlusions involving an entire vascular territory). The degree of white matter disease was also divided into 9 categories of increasing severity using the CHS score [19].

Hemorrhagic transformation

Any HT after IV tPA was identified by the presence of a lesion on gradient echo MRI sequences or hyperdensity on non-contrast CT within the first 24 h post-thrombolysis [2, 22], and their radiologic classification was defined per the European Cooperative Acute Ischemic Stroke Study II [3]. sICH occurrence was determined by the primary team, as defined by the National Institute of Neurological Disorders and Stroke r-tPA Stroke Study Group [2, 22].

Statistical analysis

Statistical analyses were performed using Stata version 13.0. Continuous variables were described using mean ± standard deviation (SD), or median (interquartile range) and analyzed through univariable comparisons using Student's t-tests or Mann-Whitney U test for independent variables, as appropriate. Categorical variables were described as percentages and analyzed using Pearson's chi-square or Fisher's exact analyses. Logistic regression was used to determine the influence of multiple risk factors. Variables significant in the univariable analysis and those of particular clinical interest were included in the multivariable modeling, with a p-value of 0.05 considered statistically significant.

Results

Patient characteristics

Over a 5-year period, 365 patients were identified as having been treated with IV tPA for acute stroke at our two centers. Of these 365 patients, 45 did not have an MRI, 22 underwent intra-arterial therapy, and 6 had been wrongly classified, leaving 292 for further analysis. The mean age of the cohort was 63 years (SD 15), 49% (n = 142) were black, and 52% (n = 151) were women. The mean initial NIHSS score was 8 (SD 5.5). The mean stroke volume was 15cm^3 (SD 38). The mean CHS score was 3 (SD 1.7). Following administration of IV tPA, there was no evidence of diffusion restriction in 30% (n = 87) of patients. By TOAST criteria [18], 12% (n = 36) were due to small vessel disease, 23% (n = 68) large vessel disease, 29% (n = 83) cardioembolic, and 36% (n = 105) due to other or undetermined etiology. From the 205 patients with a visible stroke, a purely cortical stroke was found in 18% (n = 37), deep lacune in 38% (n = 77), and 44% (n = 91) had a larger stroke involving both cortical and deep structures. Anterior circulation infarcts occurred in 77% (n = 157), posterior circulation strokes in 19% (n = 39), and 4% (n = 9) had both distributions involved.

Some form of HT occurred in 16% (n = 46) of our cohort, though only 2% (n = 6) were defined as symptomatic. Of these 46 cases, 45 (98%) occurred within the area of ischemia including 5 sICH cases; 3 (7%) were parenchyma hematoma type 1 (PH1), 2 (4%) were parenchymal hematoma type 2 (PH2), 28 (61%) were hemorrhagic infarct type 1 (HI1), and 13 (28%) were hemorrhagic infarct type 2 (HI2). Sixty-two patients (21%) had at least one CMB on post-treatment MRI. The distribution of the CMBs was: 11% (n = 7) purely lobar, 57% (n = 35) purely nonlobar and 32% (n = 20) mixed distribution. The majority, 95% (n = 59), had 1 to 10 CMBs, while only 5% (n = 3) had > 10 CMBs. Of the CAA cases, 67% (n = 2) had a high CMB burden and 33% (n = 1) had a mild-moderate CMB burden [17]. These CAA patients did not have a prior history of lobar intracerebral hemorrhage or a diagnosis of CAA prior to receiving IV tPA.

Factors associated with hemorrhage

Factors associated with HT and sICH occurrence are shown in Table 1. Advanced age (p = .006), black race (p = .041), large vessel occlusion (p = .006), higher NIHSS scores (at admission p < .001, at discharge p = .016), elevated discharge mRS score (p = .032), larger stroke volumes (p = .001), anterior circulation stroke location (p < .001), CAA (p = .019), lower platelet counts (p = .039), and atrial fibrillation (p < .001) were associated with HT. After adjusting for covariates, higher initial NIHSS (OR 1.07; 95% CI 1.002–1.15; p = .044), lower platelet counts (OR 0.99; 95% CI 0.99–0.999; p = .038) and large vessel disease (OR 2.38; 95% CI 1.10–5.14; p = .027) remained significant predictors of HT (Table 2). After univariable analysis, the only predictor of sICH was a high CMB burden (p < .001).

Factors associated with CMBs

Advanced age (p = .011), higher CHS scores (p < .001), and elevated baseline systolic blood pressure (p = .046) were associated with the presence of CMB. Advanced age was also associated with a higher CMB burden (0 CMBs: mean age 61.57 (SD 15.93), 1–10 CMBs: mean age 67.36 (SD 12.12), > 10 CMBs: mean age 68.67 (SD 9.07); p = .028).

Role of CMB in HT and sICH

A test for independence was performed between HT and sICH with the three variables of interest: CMB presence, burden, and location, shown in Table 3. High CMB burden was most significantly associated with sICH (OR 37.83; 95% CI; 2.65–539.25; p = .007). Of note, 1 of 3 patients diagnosed with CAA experienced a sICH, and a second patient experienced an asymptomatic hemorrhage.

Long-term outcomes

A total of 219/292 (75%) patients had a follow-up mRS at a median of 90 days (45–160 days) from symptom onset. From these, 156/219 (71%) had a mRS < 2 at follow-up and 63/219 (29%) had a mRS > 2. CMB presence, was comparable between both groups of patients, 35/156 (24%) versus 16/58 (28%) (p = .739).

Table 1 Factors associated with hemorrhagic transformation and symptomatic intracerebral hemorrhage

	All *n* = 292	No HT *n* = 246	HT *n* = 46	*P* value	No sICH *n* = 286	sICH *n* = 6	*P* value
Demographics							
Age, years	63 ± 15	62 ± 15	68 ± 15	**.006**	63 (51–75)	61 (59–65)	.944
Female, % (n)	52 (151)	50 (124)	59 (27)	.302	52 (148)	50 (3)	.932
Black, % (n)	49 (142)	51 (126)	35 (16)	**.041**	48 (138)	67 (4)	.437
LVD, % (n)	23 (68)	20 (50)	39 (18)	**.006**	23 (66)	33 (2)	.891
Clinical Scales							
Initial NIHSS	7.9 ± 5.5	7.4 ± 5.3	11 ± 5.7	**< .001**	2 (4–10)	11 (6–12)	.373
Discharge NIHSS	3.7 ± 5.1	3.2 ± 4.6	5.7 ± 6.7	**.016**	2 (0–4)	2.5 (1–9)	.373
Follow-up NIHSS	1.3 ± 2.6	1.2 ± 2.4	1.9 ± 3.7	.331	0 (0–2)	0 (0–2)	.994
Discharge mRS	2.6 ± 1.6	2.5 ± 1.6	3.1 ± 1.6	**.032**	2 (1–4)	3 (2–5)	.363
Follow-up mRS	1.5 ± 1.6	1.5 ± 1.5	1.8 ± 1.7	.338	1 (0–3)	2 (0–4)	.755
Imaging Parameters							
Stroke Size, mililiters	15 ± 38	11 ± 35	33 ± 46	**< .001**	1 (0–9)	19 (3–42)	.050
CHS Score	2 (2–3)	2 (2–3)	3 (2–3)	.143	2 (2–3)	2.5 (2–3)	.911
Anterior Circulation, % (n)	54 (157)	48 (117)	87 (40)	**< .001**	53 (151)	100 (6)	.218
Clinical Parameters							
SBP, mmHg	157 ± 30	157 ± 31	155 ± 24	.731	153 (136–172)	153 (145–189)	.437
Glucose, mg/dL	135 ± 71	133 ± 70	150 ± 76	.136	113 (97–148)	111 (103–116)	.924
Cr, mg/dL	1.2 ± 0.7	1.2 ± 0.7	1.1 ± 0.4	.834	1 (0.8–1.3)	1.1 (0.8–1.3)	.893
Platelets, K/cu mm	241 ± 74	244 ± 74	220 ± 66	**.039**	237 (191–276)	232 (217–253)	.957
Risk Factors							
CAA, % (n)	1 (3)	1 (1)	4 (2)	.073	1 (2)	17 (1)	.064
HTN, % (n)	79 (230)	80 (194)	78 (36)	.848	79 (225)	83 (5)	.999
DM, % (n)	27 (77)	27 (65)	26 (12)	.938	26 (75)	33 (2)	.658
Tobacco, % (n)	29 (85)	29 (72)	28 (13)	.893	29 (82)	50 (3)	.473
Alcohol, % (n)	24 (70)	26 (62)	17 (8)	.498	24 (68)	33 (2)	.725
Afib, % (n)	20 (58)	16 (40)	39 (18)	**< .001**	19 (55)	50 (3)	.098
Stroke History, % (n)	22 (63)	22 (54)	20 (9)	.884	21 (61)	33 (2)	.801
HLD, % (n)	51 (149)	51 (126)	50 (23)	.859	51 (146)	50 (3)	.999

Continuous data is described as mean ± standard deviation or as median (interquartile range), as appropriate per its distribution
Afib atrial fibrillation, *CAA* cerebral amyloid angiopathy, *CHS* Cardiovascular Health Study criteria, *Cr* creatinine, *DM* diabetes mellitus, *HLD* hyperlipidemia, *HT* hemorrhagic transformation, *HTN* hypertension, *LVD* large vessel disease etiology, *mRS* modified Rankin Score, *NIHSS* National Institute of Health Stroke Scale, *sICH* symptomatic intracerebral hemorrhage, *SBP* systolic blood pressure, *SD* standard deviation
Bold data indicates statistical significant ($p<.05$)

Discussion

This study was designed to evaluate the relationship between the presence, burden, and location of CMBs and HT following treatment with IV tPA for acute ischemic stroke. Our sICH rate was low at only 2%, but comparable to what has been reported in a prior multicenter stroke thrombolysis register of 7% [7] and a national registry of 5% [23]. Consistent with prior studies, we found that older patients, with larger [24], more clinically severe strokes [11, 25], lower platelet counts [26, 27], and a history of atrial fibrillation [11] were more likely to develop any HT; while a high CMB burden (> 10 CMBs) was the only predictor of sICH.

Looking specifically at the relationship between CMB and hemorrhage, we found an association between high CMB burden and sICH that is consistent with previously published studies. The 10 CMBs threshold was chosen based on the methodology of two recent meta-analyses and a recent multicenter trial [14, 15, 28]. Rates of sICH were comparable across studies: those without CMBs 2% [15] (ours: 1%), mild-moderate burden 6% [15] (ours: 3%), and high burden 29–50% [14, 15] (ours: 33%). One possible explanation is that these individuals had CAA, putting them at higher risk for hemorrhage due to their underlying vascular pathology.

Table 2 Multivariate logistic regression for risk factors for hemorrhagic transformation

	Hemorrhagic Transformation	
	OR (95% CI)	*P*-value
Age, per 1-y increase	1.01 (0.98–1.03)	.577
Black Race	0.56 (0.27–1.17)	.121
Initial NIHSS	1.07 (1.002–1.15)	**.044**
Stroke Size	1.00 (1.00–1.01)	.509
Platelet Count	0.99 (0.99–0.999)	**.038**
Stroke Location	1.60 (0.95–2.68)	.075
CAA	5.67 (0.45–71.97)	.181
Afib	1.66 (0.66–4.16)	.277
LVD	2.38 (1.10–5.14)	**.027**

Afib atrial fibrillation, *CAA* cerebral amyloid angiopathy, *NIHSS* National Institute of Health Stroke Scale, *LVD* large vessel disease
Bold data indicates statistical significant ($p<.05$)

The advantage of our smaller study was the ability to explore the association between patterns of CMB and the diagnosis of CAA, on hemorrhage risk in a population, while determining the absolute risk within a stroke cohort of similar size and composition to many urban hospital settings. Most prior meta-analyses did not take the diagnosis of CAA into account within their analyses. In our study, only 3 patients were diagnosed with CAA, but of these, one (33%) had a hemorrhage that was symptomatic. Higher numbers of CMBs may indicate a higher propensity for the breakdown of the blood brain barrier, or "leaky vessels" that may also predispose to greater risk of HT. A recent meta-analysis including CAA in its analysis supports an association between greater numbers of CMB and increased rates of HT [29].

In our population, 21% of patients had at least one CMB present on imaging, consistent with previously published rates. While this observation might suggest that we should screen for the presence of microhemorrhages when considering treatment, it is also important to point out that CMB presence alone was not associated with either HT or sICH, and that the number of patients with > 10 CMB was very low (n = 3, 1%), consistent with prior cohorts [15]. Additionally, despite a CMB prevalence of 1 in 5, our rate of sICH rate was very low. These results suggest that the presence of CMBs by itself should not be considered a predictor for sICH and that MRI in the acute setting to evaluate for their existence is likely unnecessary given low rates of numerous CMBs.

Our findings are consistent with many prior studies; [10, 16] however, three recent large meta-analyses [13, 15, 29] do report CMB presence as an independent risk factor for HT. These meta-analyses were large, and predominantly used univariable modeling to evaluate a relationship between HT and only the presence of microbleeds. Data were described mainly in aggregate, with wide confidence intervals, as they were unable to account for population characteristics varying by center [30]. Charidimou and colleagues did evaluate CMB burden and found, similar to our study, that larger numbers were associated with increasing hemorrhage risk and poorer outcome [29]. Along with our study, these studies all emphasize that larger numbers of microbleeds, in many cases suggestive of CAA, is associated with HT, but that the rate of hemorrhage after tPA is low enough that a very large number of patients must to be treated to see the effect, calling into question the true clinical significance.

We also considered the importance of the location of CMBs with respect to the likelihood of HT. Our findings indicate that location is not independently associated with either symptomatic or any HT. Though this finding might also be secondary to our sample size, previous groups have had similar results [11, 15, 16, 28].

The importance of determining the association between CMB and HT after treatment with IV tPA is increasing. Historically, non-contrast head CT has been preferred over MRI in the work-up of acute stroke due to increased availability, lower cost, and more rapid time acquisition [31]. However, the use of MRI as part of the acute stroke work-up, as well as the number of patients who have had a previous MRI for another clinical indication and whose CMB status is known, is growing [12]. Understanding the relationship between CMB and HT is, therefore, critical. We have shown that individuals with a high CMB burden do have an increased risk of sICH after treatment with IV tPA; however, that the absolute risk is quite low and in most cases should not preclude treatment. While risk quantification provides clinicians with the data to make informed decisions regarding the risk/benefit ratio, other

Table 3 Cerebral microbleed location, burden, and presence stratified by hemorrhage type

	No CMB (n = 209)	CMB (n = 62)	*p* value	> 10 CMBs (n = 3)	1–10 (n = 59)	*p* value	Nonlobar (n = 35)	Lobar (n = 7)	Mixed (n = 20)	*p* value
No HT, n (%)	175 (84)	50 (81)	.707	2 (67)	48 (81)	.508	29 (83)	7 (100)	14 (70)	.309
HT, n (%)	34 (16)	12 (19)		1 (33)	11(19)		6 (17)	0 (0)	6 (30)	
No sI CH, n (%)	206 (99)	59 (95)	.567	2 (67)	57 (97)	.023	33 (94)	7 (100)	19 (95)	.189
sI CH n (%)	3 (1)	3 (5)		1 (33)	2 (3)		2 (6)	0 (0)	1 (5)	

HT hemorrhagic transformation, *sICH* symptomatic intracerebral hemorrhage

variables such as stroke size and severity, and age of the patient should continue to be the key factors driving treatment decisions [32, 33].

Our study is not without limitations. Our sample size was relatively small, potentially limiting the strength of our results due to a lack of statistical power rather than lack of an association; and from two academic tertiary referral centers in an urban setting, a distinct population. However, our population is similar to many stroke centers across the United States; and, despite a small number of sICH events, our cohort allows real life clinical application of the post-thrombolytic hemorrhage risk, both symptomatic and asymptomatic, associated with CMBs to centers of similar or smaller size and composition. In addition, for the majority of cases, imaging sequences were obtained post-IV tPA, which does not differentiate between CMBs present before IV tPA and those which appear afterward. Post-IV tPA MRIs may not be the ideal method to document CMBs due to the fact that new CMBs have been documented to occur during the first 7 days after acute ischemic stroke symptom onset in 5–13% of patients [34–36]. However, considering that for our study that would mean an additional 14–38 individuals did not have CMB on admission, we feel that our results nicely illustrate both the relatively low rate of CMB on presentation, *and* more importantly the low risk of sICH regardless of microbleed status, rendering screening prior to treatment an unnecessary use of both time and resources.

Conclusion

Our results indicate that the overall risk of sICH following IV tPA is low, even in the presence of CMBs, which are not uncommon. Given a relative increased risk, a CMB burden of > 10 may be taken into consideration when stratifying the risk for sICH, but that even then the relative risk increase should be carefully weighed against the risks of not treating given the low absolute risk.

Abbreviations

CAA: Cerebral amyloid angiopathy; CHSC: Ardiovascular health study; CMBs: Cerebral microbleeds; HT: Hemorrhagic transformation; IV tPA: Intravenous tissue plasminogen activator; mRS: Modified rankin score; NIHSS: National institutes of health stroke scale; SD: Standard deviation; sICH: Symptomatic intracerebral hemorrhage; TOAST: Trial of ORG 10172 in acute stroke treatment

Acknowledgements

Not applicable

Funding

Not applicable

Authors' contributions

MACP: data collection, drafted and wrote the manuscript, performed data interpretation and analysis. RHL: study concept, study design, and preparation of manuscript. EBM: help with data collection and interpretation, study concept, and preparation of the manuscript. All authors read and approved the last version of the manuscript.

Competing interests

All authors declare that they have no competing interests.

Author details

[1]Division of Congenital Heart Surgery, Texas Children's Hospital, Michael E. DeBakey Department of Surgery, Baylor College of Medicine, Houston, Texas, USA. [2]Department of Neurology, Johns Hopkins University School of Medicine, 600 N Wolfe St, Phipps 446, Baltimore, MD 21287, USA.

References

1. Wardlaw JM, Murray V, Berge E, del Zoppo G, Sandercock P, Lindley RL, et al. Recombinant tissue plasminogen activator for acute ischaemic stroke: an updated systematic review and meta-analysis. Lancet. 2012;3799834:2364–72.
2. Tissue plasminogen activator for acute ischemic stroke. The National Institute of Neurological Disorders and Stroke rt-PA stroke study group. N Engl J Med. 1995;33324:1581–7.
3. Hacke W, Kaste M, Fieschi C, von Kummer R, Davalos A, Meier D, et al. Randomised double-blind placebo-controlled trial of thrombolytic therapy with intravenous alteplase in acute ischaemic stroke (ECASS II). Second European-Australasian acute stroke study investigators. Lancet. 1998; 3529136:1245–51.
4. Greenberg SM, Vernooij MW, Cordonnier C, Viswanathan A, Al-Shahi Salman R, Warach S, et al. Cerebral microbleeds: a guide to detection and interpretation. Lancet Neurol. 2009;82:165–74.
5. Gregoire SM, Chaudhary UJ, Brown MM, Yousry TA, Kallis C, Jager HR, et al. The microbleed anatomical rating scale (MARS): reliability of a tool to map brain microbleeds. Neurology. 2009;7321:1759–66.
6. Wardlaw JM, Smith EE, Biessels GJ, Cordonnier C, Fazekas F, Frayne R, et al. Neuroimaging standards for research into small vessel disease and its contribution to ageing and neurodegeneration. Lancet Neurol. 2013;128:822–38.
7. Mazya M, Egido JA, Ford GA, Lees KR, Mikulik R, Toni D, et al. Predicting the risk of symptomatic intracerebral hemorrhage in ischemic stroke treated with intravenous alteplase: safe implementation of treatments in stroke (SITS) symptomatic intracerebral hemorrhage risk score. Stroke. 2012;436:1524–31.
8. Marsh EB, Gottesman RF, Hillis AE, Maygers J, Lawrence E, Llinas RH. Predicting symptomatic intracerebral hemorrhage versus lacunar disease in patients with longstanding hypertension. Stroke. 2014;456:1679–83.
9. Senior K. Microbleeds may predict cerebral bleeding after stroke. Lancet. 2002;3599308:769.
10. Fiehler J, Albers GW, Boulanger JM, Derex L, Gass A, Hjort N, et al. Bleeding risk analysis in stroke imaging before thromboLysis (BRASIL): pooled analysis of T2*-weighted magnetic resonance imaging data from 570 patients. Stroke. 2007;3810:2738–44.
11. Yan S, Jin X, Zhang X, Zhang S, Liebeskind DS, Lou M. Extensive cerebral microbleeds predict parenchymal haemorrhage and poor outcome after intravenous thrombolysis. J Neurol Neurosurg Psychiatry. 2015;8611:1267–72.
12. Burke JF, Kerber KA, Iwashyna TJ, Morgenstern LB. Wide variation and rising utilization of stroke magnetic resonance imaging: data from 11 states. Ann Neurol. 2012;712:179–85.
13. Charidimou A, Shoamanesh A, Wilson D, Gang Q, Fox Z, Jager HR, et al. Cerebral microbleeds and postthrombolysis intracerebral hemorrhage risk updated meta-analysis. Neurology. 2015;8511:927–4.
14. Shoamanesh A, Kwok CS, Lim PA, Benavente OR. Postthrombolysis intracranial hemorrhage risk of cerebral microbleeds in acute stroke patients: a systematic review and meta-analysis. Int J Stroke. 2013;85:348–56.
15. Tsivgoulis G, Zand R, Katsanos AH, Turc G, Nolte CH, Jung S, et al. Risk of symptomatic intracerebral hemorrhage after intravenous thrombolysis in patients with acute ischemic stroke and high cerebral microbleed burden: a meta-analysis. JAMA Neurol. 2016;736:675–83.
16. Turc G, Sallem A, Moulin S, Tisserand M, Machet A, Edjlali M, et al. Microbleed status and 3-month outcome after intravenous thrombolysis in 717 patients with acute ischemic stroke. Stroke. 2015;469:2458–63.

17. Knudsen KA, Rosand J, Karluk D, Greenberg SM. Clinical diagnosis of cerebral amyloid angiopathy: validation of the Boston criteria. Neurology. 2001;564:537–9.
18. Adams HP Jr, Bendixen BH, Kappelle LJ, Biller J, Love BB, Gordon DL, et al. Classification of subtype of acute ischemic stroke. Definitions for use in a multicenter clinical trial. TOAST. Trial of org 10172 in acute stroke treatment. Stroke. 1993;241:35–41.
19. Manolio TA, Kronmal RA, Burke GL, Poirier V, O'Leary DH, Gardin JM, et al. Magnetic resonance abnormalities and cardiovascular disease in older adults. The cardiovascular health study. Stroke. 1994;252:318–27.
20. van Swieten JC, Koudstaal PJ, Visser MC, Schouten HJ, van Gijn J. Interobserver agreement for the assessment of handicap in stroke patients. Stroke. 1988;195: 604–7.
21. Sims JR, Gharai LR, Schaefer PW, Vangel M, Rosenthal ES, Lev MH, et al. ABC/2 for rapid clinical estimate of infarct, perfusion, and mismatch volumes. Neurology. 2009;7224:2104–10.
22. A systems approach to immediate evaluation and management of hyperacute stroke. Experience at eight centers and implications for community practice and patient care. The National Institute of Neurological Disorders and Stroke (NINDS) rt-PA stroke study group. Stroke. 1997;288:1530–40.
23. Hill MD, Buchan AM. Canadian Alteplase for stroke effectiveness study I. Thrombolysis for acute ischemic stroke: results of the Canadian Alteplase for stroke effectiveness study. CMAJ. 2005;17210:1307–12.
24. Selim M, Fink JN, Kumar S, Caplan LR, Horkan C, Chen Y, et al. Predictors of hemorrhagic transformation after intravenous recombinant tissue plasminogen activator: prognostic value of the initial apparent diffusion coefficient and diffusion-weighted lesion volume. Stroke. 2002;338:2047–52.
25. Kent DM, Ruthazer R, Decker C, Jones PG, Saver JL, Bluhmki E, et al. Development and validation of a simplified stroke-thrombolytic predictive instrument. Neurology. 2015;8511:942–9.
26. Fugate JE, Rabinstein AA. Absolute and relative contraindications to IV rt-PA for acute ischemic stroke. Neurohospitalist. 2015;53:110–21.
27. Prodan CI, Stoner JA, Cowan LD, Dale GL. Lower coated-platelet levels are associated with early hemorrhagic transformation in patients with non-lacunar brain infarction. J Thromb Haemost. 2010;86:1185–90.
28. Zand R, Tsivgoulis G, Singh M, McCormack M, Goyal N, Ishfaq MF, et al. Cerebral microbleeds and risk of intracerebral hemorrhage post intravenous thrombolysis. J Stroke Cerebrovasc Dis. 2017;263:538–44.
29. Charidimou A, Turc G, Oppenheim C, Yan S, Scheitz JF, Erdur H, et al. Microbleeds, cerebral hemorrhage, and functional outcome after stroke thrombolysis: individual patient data meta-analysis. Stroke. 2017;48:2084–90.
30. Jones AP, Riley RD, Williamson PR, Whitehead A. Meta-analysis of individual patient data versus aggregate data from longitudinal clinical trials. Clin Trials. 2009;61:16–27.
31. Wintermark M, Sanelli PC, Albers GW, Bello J, Derdeyn C, Hetts SW, et al. Imaging recommendations for acute stroke and transient ischemic attack patients: a joint statement by the American society of neuroradiology, the American college of radiology, and the society of neuroInterventional surgery. AJNR. 2013;3411:E117–27.
32. Andersen KK, Andersen ZJ, Olsen TS. Predictors of early and late case-fatality in a nationwide Danish study of 26,818 patients with first-ever ischemic stroke. Stroke. 2011;4210:2806–12.
33. Vogt G, Laage R, Shuaib A, Schneider A, Collaboration V. Initial lesion volume is an independent predictor of clinical stroke outcome at day 90 an analysis of the virtual international stroke trials archive (VISTA) database. Stroke. 2012;435: 1266–72.
34. Jeon SB, Kwon SU, Cho AH, Yun SC, Kim JS, Kang DW. Rapid appearance of new cerebral microbleeds after acute ischemic stroke. Neurology. 2009;7320:1638–44.
35. Kimura K, Aoki J, Shibazaki K, Saji N, Uemura J, Sakamoto Y. New appearance of extraischemic microbleeds on T2*-weighted magnetic resonance imaging 24 hours after tissue-type plasminogen activator administration. Stroke. 2013;4410: 2776–81.
36. Yan S, Chen Y, Zhang X, Liebeskind DS, Lou M. New microbleeds after thrombolysis: contiguous thin-slice 3T MRI. Medicine. 2014;9320:e99.

28

Posterior reversible encephalopathy syndrome complicated with subarachnoid hemorrhage in an eclamptic pregnant patient

Dan Hu[1], Jing Xiong[1], Yunfei Zha[2] and Zhaohui Zhang[1*]

Abstract

Background: Posterior reversible encephalopathy syndrome (PRES) is a neurotoxic condition which comprises various neurological symptoms. This syndrome could be complicated by intracranial hemorrhage including subarachnoid hemorrhage (SAH). However, SAH is rarely seen in eclamptic patients with PRES.

Case presentation: A 34-weeks-pregnant woman at the age of 33 was admitted to the obstetrics department because of an episode of generalized tonic-clonic seizure. Before the seizure, the patient had a headache and was found to have an abnormal systolic blood pressure of 160 mmHg. On admission, systolic and diastolic blood pressures were up to 182 and 99 mmHg, respectively. Emergent cesarean section was then performed. On hospital day (HD) 2, cranial non-contrast computed tomography (CT) revealed the existence of SAH. Multiple areas of high signals on T2-weighted and fluid attenuated inversion recovery (FLAIR) sequences were shown by cranial magnetic resonance imaging (MRI) performed 2 days later. CT-angiography studies didn't reveal intracranial aneurysm. After anti-hypertensive treatment, arterial blood pressure of the patient was gradually tapered to normal values. Eventually, the patient was discharged without any residual symptoms.

Conclusions: SAH is a rare complication of PRES in eclamptic patients. In patients with PRES, occurrence of SAH is related to increased morbidity and mortality especially when the hemorrhage is diffuse or massive. Our patient had a minor hemorrhage. The good prognosis might also be due to immediate elimination of the risk factor of PRES by emergent delivery.

Keywords: Posterior reversible encephalopathy syndrome, Subarachnoid hemorrhage, Eclampsia

Background

Posterior reversible encephalopathy syndrome (PRES) is a distinct clinico-radiological disease entity typically comprising a variety of symptoms such as headache, visual loss, impaired consciousness and epileptic seizures. This syndrome mainly occurs in the setting of hypertension, sepsis, eclampsia, autoimmune diseases or immunosuppressive therapy [1–3]. Cerebral imaging often present as a unique pattern of subcortical white matter edema with typical parietal-occipital predominance [4]. Recognition of subarachnoid hemorrhage as an atypical imaging appearance has recently increased [5, 6]. There are, however, few reports of such an occurrence in eclamptic patients with PRES. Here, we report a case of 34-weeks-pregnant woman who developed eclampsia and PRES as well as subarachnoid hemorrhage.

Case presentation

A 34-weeks-pregnant woman at the age of 33 was admitted to the obstetrics department after having an episode of generalized tonic-clonic seizure accompanied by headache and transient blurred vision. 2 days before the occurrence of seizure, the patient had a headache which was relieved significantly after rest. Abnormal systolic

* Correspondence: zhzhqing1990@163.com
[1]Department of Neurology, Renmin Hospital of Wuhan University, Jiefang Road 238, Wuchang District, Wuhan 430060, China
Full list of author information is available at the end of the article

blood pressure of 160 mmHg was discovered in the latest antenatal appointment. On admission, systolic and diastolic blood pressures were 182 and 99 mmHg, respectively [mean arterial pressure (MAP) 127]. On neurologic examination the patient was conscious. The laboratory studies disclosed leukocyte 12.9×10^9/L (reference $3.5–9.5 \times 10^9$/L) and lactate dehydrogenase (LDH) 282 U/L (reference 114–240 U/L). Clotting tests showed elevated levels of plasma D-dimer 3.61 mg/L (reference 0–0.55 mg/L) and fibrinogen 4.21 g/L (reference 2–4 g/L). The platelet count, the red blood cell count and levels of serum liver enzymes were all normal. Then, the patient was transferred to the operating room for an emergent cesarean section. The baby's APGAR scores at 1 min, 5 min, and 10 min were 7, 8, and 8, respectively. On hospital day (HD) 2, the patient complained of abdominal pain without any other discomforts. Cranial non-contrast computed tomography (CT) revealed subarachnoid hemorrhage (SAH) in the right parietal-occipital sulci and hypodensities in the left frontal and parietal lobes (Fig. 1).Cranial magnetic resonance imaging (MRI) performed 2 days later showed multiple areas of high signals on T2-weighted and fluid attenuated inversion recovery (FLAIR) sequences, involving the left cerebral peduncle, the bilateral parietal and the left frontal subcortical regions (Fig. 2). There were no abnormal signals in the corresponding regions on diffusion weighted imaging (DWI) (Fig. 2). MRI susceptibility weighted imaging (SWI) confirmed the existence of SAH (Fig. 2). CT-angiography test performed thereafter was normal except for a subtle enlargement at the origin of the right posterior communicating artery (Fig. 3). During the hospitalization, the patient received oral anti-hypertensive drugs (Adalat, 30 mg per day) and arterial blood pressure was gradually tapered to normal range. When she was transferred to the department of neurology, no symptoms were observed and the neurologic examination was normal. About a few days later, a follow-up brain MRI (data not shown) showed no abnormality. Without use of any anti-hypertensive and anti-epileptic treatment, the patient was discharged eventually with normal blood pressure.

Discussion and conclusions

PRES was first described by Hinchey and colleagues in 1996 [3]. Clinically, this disease is characterized by acute or subacute onset of neurological symptoms including altered mental state, epileptic seizures, headache, visual disturbances and focal neurological deficit (eg, hemiparesis, aphasia, and even myelopathic symptoms) [7]. Our patient presented with the constellation of symptoms including headache, blurred vision, and seizure. It has been proposed that generalized seizure is related to the focal abnormality of parietal-occipital lobes [2]. For our patient, MRI showed abnormal signals in the bilateral parietal subcortical regions, which might be responsible for occurrence of seizure.

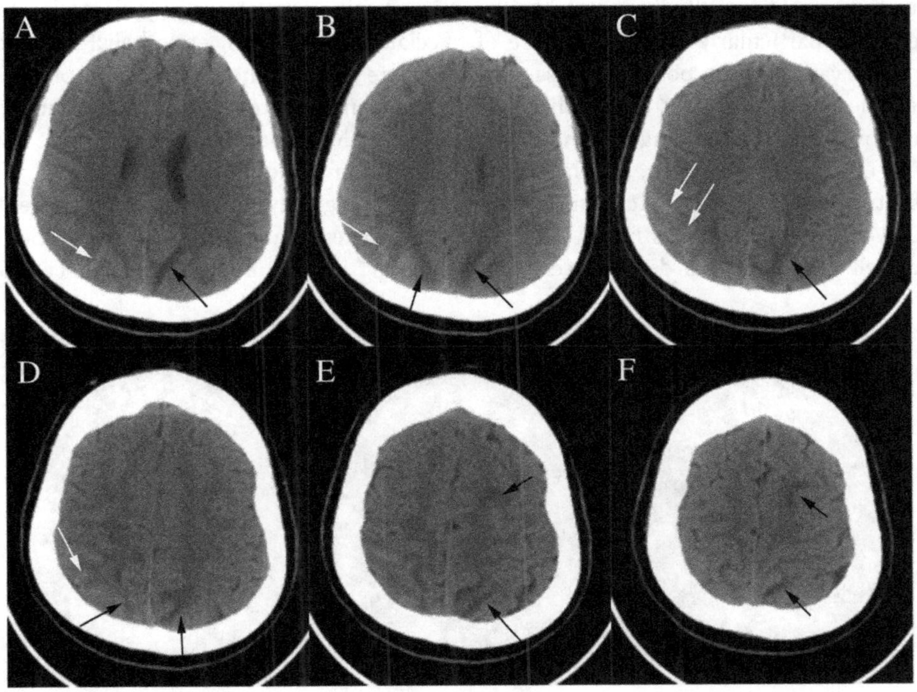

Fig. 1 CT scan (**a-f**) shows lesions with hyperdensity in the parietal-occipital sulci (white arrows) and hypodensity in the left frontal and parietal lobes (black arrows)

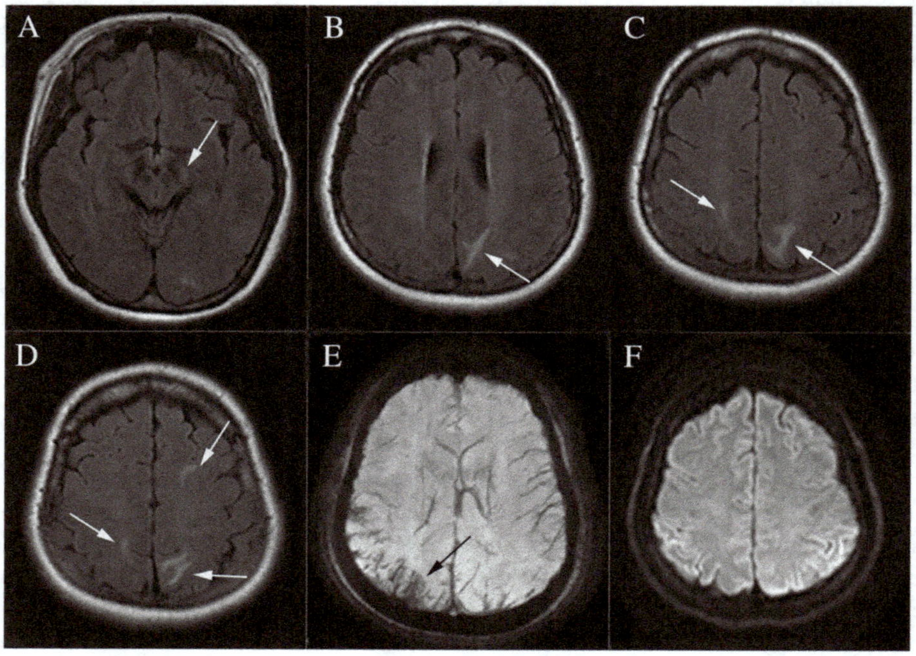

Fig. 2 Axial FLAIR (**a-d**) demonstrates PRES lesions involving multiple regions (white arrows). SWI (**e**) reveals low signals in the right parietal-occipital sulci. There are no abnormal signals in DWI (**f**)

The pathophysiology of PRES remains controversial. Rapid development of hypertension exceeds the upper limit of cerebral blood flow autoregulation, which leads to impaired cerebral autoregulation and hyperperfusion. Subsequently, the blood-brain barrier (BBB) breaks down, followed by extravasation of fluid and plasma proteins into the brain parenchyma [8]. Furthermore, the posterior head region is particularly affected because of poor sympathetic innervation in the posterior fossa. Another hypothesized mechanism involves endothelial dysfunction and vasoconstriction occurring secondary to systemic toxicity in eclampsia and sepsis, which are the common precipitants of PRES. Release of cytokines such as interleukin (IL)-1 and tumor necrosis factor (TNF-α) causes endothelial cell activation and damage, resulting in vasoconstriction and hypoperfusion [8–10]. It has been demonstrated that PRES imaging appearance commonly follows a watershed distribution [11]. Interestingly, acute hypertension without exceeding the upper limit of cerebral blood flow autoregulation (140–150 mmHg) could also lead to endothelial dysfunction in certain circumstances [12]. At least in the setting of eclampsia, however, endothelial dysfunction might contribute more to the development of PRES than hypertension, since there was no significant difference of the average MAP between the eclamptic patients with PRES and those without [13].

Radiologically, PRES typically presents as focal vasogenic edema and the posterior parietal-occipital white matter is commonly affected. Frequent frontal and

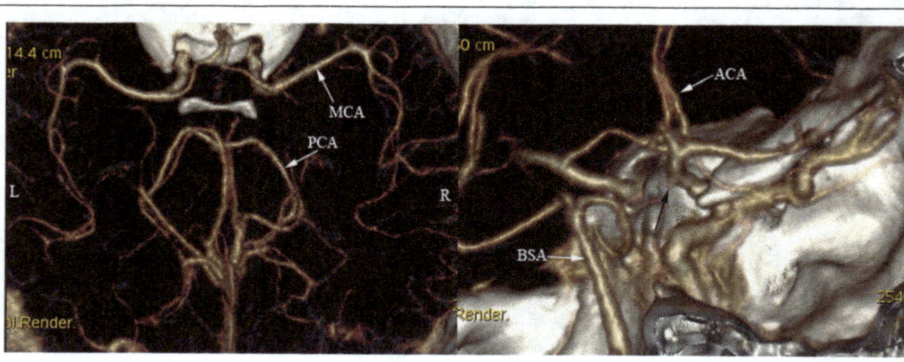

Fig. 3 CTA shows a subtle enlargement at the origin of the right posterior communicating artery (black arrow). L: Left; R: Right; ACA: Anterior cerebral artery; MCA: Middle cerebral artery; PCA: Posterior cerebral artery; BSA: Basilar artery

temporal lobe involvement has also been reported [14]. Atypical manifestations include the location of lesions in the cerebellum, basal ganglia and brainstem [15]. MRI of our patient showed abnormal T2 and FLAIR signals in the left cerebral peduncle except for the typical locations. In patients with eclampsia, the involvement of atypical brain regions might be explained by the relatively significant impact of cytokine mediated endothelial dysfunction with respect of hypertension on the development of BBB breakdown [13].

Intracranial hemorrhage is common in PRES, which has been reported with an incidence ranging from 9 to 33% [16–18]. As for the types of intracranial hemorrhage, SAH is relatively less common than intraparenchymal hemorrhage. Notably, the blood amount of SAH in PRES is mostly minimal or moderate and basal cisterns are usually spared, which is distinct from that in cases of aneurysmal rupture [5]. PRES-related hemorrhage is usually to be observed in patients with eclampsia, sepsis/recent infection, allogeneic bone marrow transplantation and those undergoing therapeutic anticoagulation [5, 12, 19]. By contrast, hypertension does not appear to be a prerequisite for the occurrence of hemorrhage [12]. The mechanism behind hemorrhage in PRES is not fully elucidated. It has been proposed that hemodynamic disturbances, endothelial dysfunction, blood brain barrier breakdown and abnormal coagulation profile might play roles in the development of hemorrhage in the setting of PRES [5]. Voetsch et al. [20] reported a case of PRES which is caused by SAH-associated vasospasm. In that case, the blood of SAH presented as a thick clot in the right Sylvian fissure and cerebral angiogram revealed a wide-necked 3 mm right middle cerebral artery (MCA) aneurysm. Aneurysmal SAH-induced PRES was also reported in another literature [21]. All of the reported patients manifested as diffuse acute SAH in basal cisterns resulting from a ruptured anterior communicating artery aneurysm. In contrast, our patient only showed a minor SAH at the cerebral convexities and subsequent CT-angiography studies did not show intracranial aneurysm. Thus, SAH was more likely to be a complication rather than a cause of PRES in our case. Reversible cerebral vasoconstriction syndrome (RCVS) is clinically characterized by thunderclap headaches. Patients with RCVS could also present with seizures and focal neurological deficits similar to that in PRES. Some of the cases are even accompanied by SAH and PRES [22]. However, diffuse segmental vasoconstrictions of the cerebral arteries, the radiological characteristic of RCVS, were not found on CT-angiography in our case.

Additionally, parenchymal edema was usually located in the ipsilateral cerebral lobe with respect to SAH in the eclamptic patients with PRES [5]. In our case, however, parenchymal edema predominantly occurred in the cerebral lobe contralateral to SAH, which is rarely seen in these cases. To our knowledge, only one reported eclamptic patient developing PRES presented with this discordant location rediologically [5].

Generally speaking, PRES has a favorable prognosis and the disorder is reversible when the predisposing factors are treated. However, it has been identified that the clinical outcome in patients with PRES is related to multiple factors including intracranial hemorrhage [23]. Hemorrhage appears to lead to increased morbidity and mortality, while it is difficult to determine the relationship in cases of minor hemorrhage [19, 23]. Our patient had a complete resolution of symptoms with a small amount of SAH, which might be associated with emergent delivery.

In the present paper, we described a case of an eclamptic patient who was diagnosed with PRES and SAH. It is rare for PRES-related SAH to occur in pregnant patients with eclampsia. This case provides us with information regarding the diagnosis, treatment, and prognosis of this kind of patients.

Abbreviations

BBB: Blood-brain barrier; CT: Computed tomography; DWI: Diffusion weighted imaging; FLAIR: Fluid attenuated inversion recovery; LDH: Lactate dehydrogenase; MAP: Mean arterial pressure; MRI: magnetic resonance imaging; PRES: Posterior reversible encephalopathy syndrome; RCVS: Reversible cerebral vasoconstriction syndrome; SAH: Subarachnoid hemorrhage; SWI: Susceptibility weighted imaging

Acknowledgements

None.

Funding

This work was supported by the National Natural Science Foundation of China (Grant No. 81401051).

Authors' contributions

DH and JX have made substantial contribution to data collection. DH and YZ were responsible for data analysis and interpretation and manuscript revision. ZZ drafted the manuscript and made substantial contribution to manuscript revision. All the authors have read and approved the manuscript for publication and agreed to be accountable for all aspects of the work.

Competing interests

The authors report no conflict of interest.

Author details

[1]Department of Neurology, Renmin Hospital of Wuhan University, Jiefang Road 238, Wuchang District, Wuhan 430060, China. [2]Department of Radiology, Renmin Hospital of Wuhan University, Jiefang Road 238, Wuchang District, Wuhan 430060, China.

References

1. Bartynski WS, Boardman JF, Zeigler ZR, Shadduck RK, Lister J. Posterior reversible encephalopathy syndrome in infection, sepsis, and shock. AJNR Am J Neuroradiol. 2006;27(10):2179–90.
2. Yoon SD, Cho BM, Oh SM, Park SH, Jang IB, Lee JY. Clinical and radiological spectrum of posterior reversible encephalopathy syndrome. J Cerebrovasc Endovasc Neurosurg. 2013;15(3):206–13.
3. Hinchey J, Chaves C, Appignani B, Breen J, Pao L, Wang A, et al. A reversible posterior leukoencephalopathy syndrome. N Engl J Med. 1996;334(8):494–500.
4. Bartynski WS. Posterior reversible encephalopathy syndrome, part 1: fundamental imaging and clinical features. AJNR Am J Neuroradiol. 2008; 29(6):1036–42.
5. Sharma A, Whitesell RT, Moran KJ. Imaging pattern of intracranial hemorrhage in the setting of posterior reversible encephalopathy syndrome. Neuroradiology. 2010;52(10):855–63.
6. Coenen F, Duprez T, Hantson P. Concomitant occurrence of posterior reversible encephalopathy syndrome and non-convexal subarachnoid haemorrhage in a renal transplant patient. Acta Neurol Belg. 2014;114(2): 159–61.
7. Fugate JE, Rabinstein AA. Posterior reversible encephalopathy syndrome: clinical and radiological manifestations, pathophysiology, and outstanding questions. Lancet Neurol. 2015;14(9):914–25.
8. Bartynski WS. Posterior reversible encephalopathy syndrome, part 2: controversies surrounding pathophysiology of vasogenic edema. AJNR Am J Neuroradiol. 2008;29(6):1043–9.
9. Benyo DF, Smarason A, Redman CW, Sims C, Conrad KP. Expression of inflammatory cytokines in placentas from women with preeclampsia. J Clin Endocrinol Metab. 2001;86(6):2505–12.
10. Aird WC. The role of the endothelium in severe sepsis and multiple organ dysfunction syndrome. Blood. 2003;101(10):3765–77.
11. Bartynski WS, Boardman JF. Distinct imaging patterns and lesion distribution in posterior reversible encephalopathy syndrome. AJNR Am J Neuroradiol. 2007;28(7):1320–7.
12. Hefzy HM, Bartynski WS, Boardman JF, Lacomis D. Hemorrhage in posterior reversible encephalopathy syndrome: imaging and clinical features. AJNR Am J Neuroradiol. 2009;30(7):1371–9.
13. Mayama M, Uno K, Tano S, Yoshihara M, Ukai M, Kishigami Y, et al. Incidence of posterior reversible encephalopathy syndrome in eclamptic and patients with preeclampsia with neurologic symptoms. Am J Obstet Gynecol. 2016;215(2):239 e1–5.
14. McKinney AM, Short J, Truwit CL, McKinney ZJ, Kozak OS, SantaCruz KS, et al. Posterior reversible encephalopathy syndrome: incidence of atypical regions of involvement and imaging findings. AJR Am J Roentgenol. 2007; 189(4):904–12.
15. Li R, Mitchell P, Dowling R, Yan B. Is hypertension predictive of clinical recurrence in posterior reversible encephalopathy syndrome? J Clin Neurosci. 2013;20(2):248–52.
16. Burnett MM, Hess CP, Roberts JP, Bass NM, Douglas VC, Josephson SA. Presentation of reversible posterior leukoencephalopathy syndrome in patients on calcineurin inhibitors. Clin Neurol Neurosurg. 2010;112(10):886–91.
17. Fugate JE, Claassen DO, Cloft HJ, Kallmes DF, Kozak OS, Rabinstein AA. Posterior reversible encephalopathy syndrome: associated clinical and radiologic findings. Mayo Clin Proc. 2010;85(5):427–32.
18. Liman TG, Bohner G, Heuschmann PU, Endres M, Siebert E. The clinical and radiological spectrum of posterior reversible encephalopathy syndrome: the retrospective Berlin PRES study. J Neurol. 2012;259(1):155–64.
19. Aranas RM, Prabhakaran S, Lee VH. Posterior reversible encephalopathy syndrome associated with hemorrhage. Neurocrit Care. 2009;10(3):306–12.
20. Voetsch B, Tarlov N, Nguyen TN, DeFusco C, Barest GD, Norbash A, et al. Asymmetric posterior reversible encephalopathy syndrome complicating hemodynamic augmentation for subarachnoid hemorrhage-associated cerebral vasospasm. Neurocrit Care. 2011;15(3):542–6.
21. Giraldo EA, Fugate JE, Rabinstein AA, Lanzino G, Wijdicks EF. Posterior reversible encephalopathy syndrome associated with hemodynamic augmentation in aneurysmal subarachnoid hemorrhage. Neurocrit Care. 2011;14(3):427–32.
22. Cappelen-Smith C, Calic Z, Cordato D. Reversible cerebral vasoconstriction syndrome: recognition and treatment. Curr Treat Options Neurol. 2017;19(6):21.
23. Alhilali LM, Reynolds AR, Fakhran S. A multi-disciplinary model of risk factors for fatal outcome in posterior reversible encephalopathy syndrome. J Neurol Sci. 2014;347(1–2):59–65.

Permissions

All chapters in this book were first published in NEUROLOGY, by BioMed Central; hereby published with permission under the Creative Commons Attribution License or equivalent. Every chapter published in this book has been scrutinized by our experts. Their significance has been extensively debated. The topics covered herein carry significant findings which will fuel the growth of the discipline. They may even be implemented as practical applications or may be referred to as a beginning point for another development.

The contributors of this book come from diverse backgrounds, making this book a truly international effort. This book will bring forth new frontiers with its revolutionizing research information and detailed analysis of the nascent developments around the world.

We would like to thank all the contributing authors for lending their expertise to make the book truly unique. They have played a crucial role in the development of this book. Without their invaluable contributions this book wouldn't have been possible. They have made vital efforts to compile up to date information on the varied aspects of this subject to make this book a valuable addition to the collection of many professionals and students.

This book was conceptualized with the vision of imparting up-to-date information and advanced data in this field. To ensure the same, a matchless editorial board was set up. Every individual on the board went through rigorous rounds of assessment to prove their worth. After which they invested a large part of their time researching and compiling the most relevant data for our readers.

The editorial board has been involved in producing this book since its inception. They have spent rigorous hours researching and exploring the diverse topics which have resulted in the successful publishing of this book. They have passed on their knowledge of decades through this book. To expedite this challenging task, the publisher supported the team at every step. A small team of assistant editors was also appointed to further simplify the editing procedure and attain best results for the readers.

Apart from the editorial board, the designing team has also invested a significant amount of their time in understanding the subject and creating the most relevant covers. They scrutinized every image to scout for the most suitable representation of the subject and create an appropriate cover for the book.

The publishing team has been an ardent support to the editorial, designing and production team. Their endless efforts to recruit the best for this project, has resulted in the accomplishment of this book. They are a veteran in the field of academics and their pool of knowledge is as vast as their experience in printing. Their expertise and guidance has proved useful at every step. Their uncompromising quality standards have made this book an exceptional effort. Their encouragement from time to time has been an inspiration for everyone.

The publisher and the editorial board hope that this book will prove to be a valuable piece of knowledge for researchers, students, practitioners and scholars across the globe.

List of Contributors

Shuolin Wu and Ning Zhang
Department of Neuropsychiatry and Behavioral Neurology and Clinical Psychology, Beijing Tiantan Hospital, Capital Medical University, Beijing, China
China National Clinical Research Center for Neurological Diseases, Beijing, China

Yuesong Pan and Wang Yong Jun
China National Clinical Research Center for Neurological Diseases, Beijing, China
Department of Neurology, Beijing Tiantan Hospital, Capital Medical University, Beijing, China
Center of Stroke, Beijing Institute for Brain Disorders, Beijing, China
Beijing Key Laboratory of Translational Medicine for cerebrovascular Disease, Beijing, China

Chunxue Wang
Department of Neuropsychiatry and Behavioral Neurology and Clinical Psychology, Beijing Tiantan Hospital, Capital Medical University, Beijing, China
China National Clinical Research Center for Neurological Diseases, Beijing, China
Department of Neurology, Beijing Tiantan Hospital, Capital Medical University, Beijing, China
Center of Stroke, Beijing Institute for Brain Disorders, Beijing, China
Beijing Key Laboratory of Translational Medicine for cerebrovascular Disease, Beijing, China

Seong-Joon Lee, Jin Soo Lee, Mun Hee Choi and Sung Eun Lee
Department of Neurology, Ajou University School of Medicine, Suwon, Republic of Korea

Dong Hoon Shin
Department of Neurology, Gachon University Gil Hospital, Incheon, Republic of Korea

Ji Man Hong
Department of Neurology, Ajou University School of Medicine, Suwon, Republic of Korea
Department of Neurology, Ajou University School of Medicine, 164, World cup-ro, Yeongtong-gu, Suwon-si, Gyeonggi-do 16499, South Korea

Gaifen Liu, Penglian Wang, Yilong Wang and Xingquan Zhao
Department of Neurology, Tiantan Comprehensive Stroke Center, Tiantan Hospital, Capital Medical University, Beijing, China
China National Clinical Research Center for Neurological Diseases, Beijing, China
Center of Stroke, Beijing Institute for Brain Disorders, Beijing, China
Beijing Key Laboratory of Translational Medicine for Cerebrovascular Disease, Beijing, China

Yuesong Pan, Hongyi Yan, Runhua Zhang and Hao Li
China National Clinical Research Center for Neurological Diseases, Beijing, China
Center of Stroke, Beijing Institute for Brain Disorders, Beijing, China

Ruijun Ji
Department of Neurology, Tiantan Comprehensive Stroke Center, Tiantan Hospital, Capital Medical University, Beijing, China
China National Clinical Research Center for Neurological Diseases, Beijing, China
Center of Stroke, Beijing Institute for Brain Disorders, Beijing, China
Beijing Key Laboratory of Translational Medicine for Cerebrovascular Disease, Beijing, China
Beijing Key Laboratory of Brain Function Reconstruction, Beijing, China

Yongjun Wang
Department of Neurology, Tiantan Comprehensive Stroke Center, Tiantan Hospital, Capital Medical University, Beijing, China
China National Clinical Research Center for Neurological Diseases, Beijing, China
Center of Stroke, Beijing Institute for Brain Disorders, Beijing, China
Beijing Key Laboratory of Translational Medicine for Cerebrovascular Disease, Beijing, China
Tiantan Comprehensive Stroke Center, Beijing Tiantan Hospital, Capital Medical University, No.6 Tiantanxili, Dongcheng District, Beijing 100050, China

Po-Chen Lin, Yung-Yang Lin and Chih-Ping Chung
Department of Neurology, Taipei Veterans General Hospital, No. 201 Sec.2, Shihpai Road, Peitou, Taipei 11217, Taiwan
National Yang Ming University, Taipei, Taiwan

Feng-Chi Chang
National Yang Ming University, Taipei, Taiwan
Department of Radiology, Taipei Veterans General Hospital, Taipei, Taiwan

Hui-Chi Huang and Jui-Yao Tsai
National Yang Ming University, Taipei, Taiwan
National Taipei University of Nursing and Health Sciences, Taipei, Taiwan

Tomoyoshi Kuribara, Takeshi Mikami, Katsuya Komatsu, Hime Suzuki and Nobuhiro Mikuni
Department of Neurosurgery, Sapporo Medical University, South1 West16, Chuo-ku, Sapporo 060-8543, Japan

Hirofumi Ohnishi
Department of Public Health, Sapporo Medical University, Sapporo, Japan

Kiyohiro Houkin
Department of Neurosurgery, Hokkaido University Graduate School of Medicine, Sapporo, Japan

Kai Shan and Wei Guo
Emergency Department, Beijing Tiantan Hospital, Capital Medical University, Beijing 100050, China

Chulho Kim, Jong-Hee Sohn and Hui-Chul Choi
Department of Neurology, Chuncheon Sacred Heart Hospital, Chuncheon-si, Gangwon-do 200-704, Republic of Korea

Adrian V. Specogna
Department of Health Professions, College of Health and Public Affairs, University of Central Florida, 12805 Pegasus Drive, Orlando, FL 32816, USA

Tanvir C. Turin
Department of Family Medicine, Cumming School of Medicine, University of Calgary, 3330 Hospital Drive NW, Calgary, AB T2N 4N1, Canada

Scott B. Patten
Department of Community Health Sciences, Cumming School of Medicine, University of Calgary, 3280 Hospital Drive NW, Calgary, AB T2N 4Z6, Canada

Michael D. Hill
Department of Clinical Neurosciences, Cumming School of Medicine, Foothills Hospital, Room 1242A, 1403 29th Street NW, Calgary, AB T2N 2T9, Canada

Guilin Meng, Xiaoye Ma, Lei Li, Yan Tan, Xiaohui Liu, Xueyuan Liu and Yanxin Zhao
Department of Neurology, Shanghai Tenth People's Hospital, Tongji University School of Medicine, Shanghai 200072, China

Laura Gioia, Ana Klahr, Mahesh Kate, Brian Buck, Thomas Jeerakathil and Kenneth Butcher
Division of Neurology, University of Alberta, 7th Floor Clinical Sciences Building, 11350-83rd Avenue, Edmonton, AB T6G 2B7, Canada

Dariush Dowlatshahi
Division of Neurology, University of Ottawa, Ottawa, ON, Canada

Derek Emery
Department of Diagnostic Imaging, University of Alberta, Edmonton, AB, Canada

Akiko Kada
Department of Clinical Trials and Research, Clinical Research Center, National Hospital Organization Nagoya Medical Center, 4-1-1 Sannomaru, Naka-ku, Nagoya, Aichi 460-0001, Japan

Kunihiro Nishimura and Fumiaki Nakamura
Center for Cardiovascular Disease Information, National Cerebral and Cardiovascular Center, Suita, Japan

Jyoji Nakagawara
Integrative Stroke Imaging Center, National Cerebral and Cardiovascular Center, Suita, Japan

Kuniaki Ogasawara
Department of Neurosurgery, Iwate Medical University, Morioka, Japan

Junichi Ono
Chiba Cardiovascular Center, Ichihara, Japan

Yoshiaki Shiokawa
Department of Neurosurgery, Kyorin University, Mitaka, Japan

Toru Aruga
Showa University, Tokyo, Japan

Shigeru Miyachi
Department of Neurosurgery, Osaka Medical College, Takatsuki, Japan

Izumi Nagata
Kokura Memorial Hospital, Fukuoka, Japan

Kazunori Toyoda
Departments of Cerebrovascular Medicine, National Cerebral and Cardiovascular Center, Suita, Japan

Shinya Matsuda
Department of Preventive Medicine and Community Health, University of Occupational and Environmental Health, Kita-Kyushu, Japan

Akifumi Suzuki
Akita Prefectural Hospital Organization Research Institute for Brain and Blood Vessels, Akita, Japan

Hiroharu Kataoka
Department of Neurosurgery, National Cerebral and Cardiovascular Center, Suita, Japan

Satoru Kamitani
Department of Public Health, Graduate School of Medicine, The University of Tokyo, Tokyo, Japan

Koji Iihara
Department of Neurosurgery, Graduate School of Medical Sciences, Kyushu University, Fukuoka, Japan

Yunchang Chen, Gancheng Li, Haiyan Fan, Shenquan Guo, Ran Li, Jian Yin, Xin Zhang, Xifeng Li and Xuying He
Department of Neurosurgery, The National Key Clinic Specialty, The Neurosurgery Institute of Guangdong Province, Guangdong Provincial Key Laboratory on Brain Function Repair and Regeneration, Zhujiang Hospital, Southern Medical University, Guangzhou 510282, China

Chuanzhi Duan
Department of Neurosurgery, The National Key Clinic Specialty, The Neurosurgery Institute of Guangdong Province, Guangdong Provincial Key Laboratory on Brain Function Repair and Regeneration, Zhujiang Hospital, Southern Medical University, Guangzhou 510282, China
Department of Neurosurgery, Southern Medical University, Zhujiang Hospital, 253# industry road, Guangzhou, Guangdong 510282, China

Hee Won Hwang, Seung Ha Lee, Chul Hyoung Lyoo and Myung Sik Lee
Department of Neurology, Gangnam Severance Hospital, Yonsei University
College of Medicine, Eonjuro 211, Gangnam-gu, Seoul, South Korea

Steffi Hillmann and Viktoria Rücker
Institute of Clinical Epidemiology and Biometry (ICE-B) Würzburg, Josef-Schneider-Str. 2/D7, 97080 Würzburg, Germany

Silke Wiedmann
Institute of Clinical Epidemiology and Biometry (ICE-B) Würzburg, Josef-Schneider-Str. 2/D7, 97080 Würzburg, Germany
Comprehensive Heart Failure Center, University of Würzburg, Straubmühlweg 2a, 97078 Würzburg, Germany

Klaus Berger
Quality Assurance Project"Stroke Register Northwest Germany", Institute of Epidemiology and Social Medicine, University of Münster, Albert-Schweitzer-Campus 1, Gebäude D3, 48149 Münster, Germany

Darius Nabavi
Department of Neurology, Vivantes Klinikum Neukölln, Berlin, Rudower Straße 48, 12351 Berlin, Germany

Ingo Bruder
Office for Quality Assurance in Hospitals (GeQiK) Stuttgart at Baden-Wuerttembergische Hospital Federation, Stuttgart, Birkenwaldstr. 151, 70191 Stuttgart, Germany

Hans-Christian Koennecke
Vivantes Klinikum im Friedrichshain, Berlin, Landsberger Allee 49, 10249 Berlin, Germany

Günter Seidel
Department of Neurology, Asklepios Klinik Nord, Hamburg,, Tangstedter Landstraße 400, 22417 Hamburg, Germany

Christine Matthis
Quality Association for Acute Stroke Treatment Schleswig-Holstein (QugSS), Institute of Social Medicine and Epidemiology, University of Lübeck, Ratzeburger Allee 160, 23538 Lübeck, Germany

Otto Busse
German Stroke Society, Berlin, Reinhardtstr. 27C, 10117 Berlin, Germany

Peter Hermanek
Bavarian Permanent Working Party for Quality Assurance, Munich, Westenriederstr.19, 80331 Munich, Germany

Peter Ulrich Heuschmann
Institute of Clinical Epidemiology and Biometry (ICE-B) Würzburg, Josef-Schneider-Str. 2/D7, 97080 Würzburg, Germany
Comprehensive Heart Failure Center, University of Würzburg, Straubmühlweg 2a, 97078 Würzburg, Germany
Clinical Trial Center Würzburg, University Hospital Würzburg, Josef-Schneider-Str. 2/D7, 97080 Würzburg, Germany

Anna Misyail Abdul Rashid
Department of Medicine, Faculty of Medicine and Health Sciences, Universiti Putra, Serdang, Malaysia

Mohamad Syafeeq Faeez Md Noh
Department of Imaging, Faculty of Medicine and Health Sciences, Universiti Putra Malaysia, Level 3, 43400 Serdang, Selangor, Malaysia

Tae Sung Lim, Jin Soo Lee, Jung Han Yoon, So Young Moon, In Soo Joo, Kyoon Huh and Ji Man Hong
Department of Neurology, School of Medicine, Ajou University, 5 San, Woncheon-dong, Yongtong-gu, Suwon-si, Kyunggi-do 442-749, Republic of Korea

Jan C. Kattenstroth
Institute for Neuroinformatik, Neural Plasticity Lab, Ruhr-University of Bochum, Bochum, Germany

Tobias Kalisch
Institute for Neuroinformatik, Neural Plasticity Lab, Ruhr-University of Bochum, Bochum, Germany
Department of Neurology, University Hospital Bergmannsheil, Ruhr-University Bochum, Bochum, Germany

Matthias Sczesny-Kaiser and Martin Tegenthoff
Department of Neurology, University Hospital Bergmannsheil, Ruhr-University Bochum, Bochum, Germany

Wolfgang Greulich
HELIOS Hospital Hagen Ambrock, Hagen, Germany

Hubert R. Dinse
Institute for Neuroinformatik, Neural Plasticity Lab, Ruhr-University of Bochum, Bochum, Germany
Department of Neurology, University Hospital Bergmannsheil, Ruhr-University Bochum, Bochum, Germany
Department of Neuroinformatik, Neural Plasticity Lab, Ruhr-University of Bochum, Building NB3, 44780 Bochum, Germany

Masashi Akamatsu, Futaba Maki, Hisanao Akiyama, Daisuke Hara, Masashi Hoshino and Yasuhiro Hasegawa
Department of Neurology, St. Marianna University School of Medicine, 2-16-1 Sugao, Miyamae, Kawasaki, Kanagawa 216-8511, Japan

Yuta Maetani, Masahiro Nakamori, Tomoaki Watanabe, Hayato Matsushima and Eiji Imamura
Department of Neurology, Suiseikai Kajikawa Hospital, 1-1-23, Higashisendamachi, Naka-ku, Hiroshima 730-0053, Hiroshima, Japan

Shinichi Wakabayashi
Department of Neurosurgery, Suiseikai Kajikawa Hospital, 1-1-23, Higashisendamachi, Naka-ku, Hiroshima 730-0053, Hiroshima, Japan

Djamel Bensmail, Didier Pradon and Nicolas Roche
Inserm Unit 1179, Team 3: Technologies and Innovative Therapies Applied to Neuromuscular diseases, UVSQ, CIC 805, Physiology–Functional Testing Ward, AP-HP, Raymond Poincaré Teaching Hospital, Garches, France

Phillippe Aegerter
Assistance Publique-Hôpitaux de Paris, Hôpital Ambroise Paré, Unité de Recherche Clinique (URC), Boulogne, France

Anthony Supiot and Maxime Geiger
Inserm Unit 1179, Team 3: Technologies and Innovative Therapies Applied to Neuromuscular diseases, UVSQ, CIC 805, Physiology–Functional Testing Ward, AP-HP, Raymond Poincaré Teaching Hospital, Garches, France
CIAMS, University Paris-Sud, Université Paris-Saclay, 91405 Orsay Cedex, France
CIAMS, Université d'Orléans, 45067 Orléans, France

Kristin Taraldsen and Xiangchun Tan
Department of Neuromedicine and Movement Science, Faculty of Medicine and health science, NTNU - Norwegian University of Science and Technology, Trondheim, Norway

Ole Petter Norvang
Department of Neuromedicine and Movement Science, Faculty of Medicine and health science, NTNU - Norwegian University of Science and Technology, Trondheim, Norway
Clinical Services, Department of Physiotherapy, St Olavs Hospital, Trondheim University Hospital, NO-7006 Trondheim, Norway

Anne Hokstad, Torunn Askim and Bent Indredavik
Department of Neuromedicine and Movement Science, Faculty of Medicine and health science, NTNU - Norwegian University of Science and Technology, Trondheim, Norway
Clinic of Medicine, Department of Stroke, St. Olavs Hospital, Trondheim University Hospital, Trondheim, Norway

Stian Lydersen
Regional Centre for Child and Youth Mental Health and Child Care, Department of Mental Health, Faculty of Medicine, NTNU - Norwegian University of Science and Technology, Trondheim, Norway

Farhaan S. Vahidy, Ellie G. Meyer, Arvind B. Bambhroliya, Jennifer R. Meeks, Tzu-Ching Wu, Louise D. McCullough and Sean I. Savitz
Department of Neurology and the Institute for Stroke and Cerebrovascular Disease, McGovern Medical School, University of Texas - Health, Houston, TX, USA

Charles E. Begley
Department of Management, Policy, and Community Health, School of Public Health, University of Texas Health Science Center at Houston, Houston, TX, USA

Jon E. Tyson and Charles C. Miller
Center for Clinical Research and Evidence Based Medicine at McGovern Medical School, University of Texas Health Science Center at Houston, Houston, TX, USA

Ritvij Bowry and Wamda O. Ahmed
Department of Neurosurgery, McGovern Medical School, University of Texas Health Science Center at Houston, Houston, TX, USA

Gretchel A. Gealogo and Steven Warach
Department of Neurology, Dell Medical School, The University of Texas at Austin, Austin, TX, USA

Ahmad H. Alghadir, Einas S. Al-Eisa and Shahnawaz Anwer
Rehabilitation Research Chair, College of Applied Medical Sciences, King Saud University, Riyadh 11433, Saudi Arabia

Bibhuti Sarkar
National Institute for Locomotor Disabilities (Divyangjan), Kolkata, India

Cornelia Möbius, Christian Blinzler, Stefan Schwab and Lorenz Breuer
Department of Neurology, Universitätsklinikum Erlangen, Schwabachanlage 6, 91054 Erlangen, German

Martin Köhrmann
Department of Neurology, Universitätsklinikum Essen, Hufelandstr. 55, 45147 Essen, Germany

Yoon Hwan Byun, Eun Jin Ha and Kyung Hyun Kim
Department of Neurosurgery, Seoul National University Hospital, 101 Daehak-ro, Jongno-gu, Seoul 03080, Republic of Korea

Sang-Bae Ko
Department of Neurology, Seoul National University Hospital, 101 Daehak-ro, Jongno-gu, Seoul 03080, Republic of Korea

Harald Hegen, Raimund Helbok, Mario Kofler, Bettina Pfausler, Alois Schiefecker and Erich Schmutzhard
Department of Neurology, Medical University of Innsbruck, Innsbruck, Austria

Ronny Beer
Department of Neurology, Medical University of Innsbruck, Innsbruck, Austria
Neurological Intensive Care Unit, Department of Neurology, Medical University of Innsbruck, Anichstrasse 35, A-6020 Innsbruck, Austria

Martin A. Chacon-Portillo
Division of Congenital Heart Surgery, Texas Children's Hospital, Michael E. DeBakey Department of Surgery, Baylor College of Medicine, Houston, Texas, USA

Rafael H. Llinas and Elisabeth B. Marsh
Department of Neurology, Johns Hopkins University School of Medicine, 600 N Wolfe St, Phipps 446, Baltimore, MD 21287, USA

Dan Hu, Jing Xiong and Zhaohui Zhang
Department of Neurology, Renmin Hospital of Wuhan University, Jiefang Road 238, Wuchang District, Wuhan 430060, China

Yunfei Zha
Department of Radiology, Renmin Hospital of Wuhan University, Jiefang Road 238, Wuchang District, Wuhan 430060, China

Index

www.ingramcontent.com/pod-product-compliance
Lightning Source LLC
LaVergne TN
LVHW080651210926
848485LV00003B/362